A Case-Based Approach to Interventional Pulmonology: A Focus on Asian Perspectives

Editors

Jamalul Azizi Abdul Rahaman

Department of Pulmonology
Serdang Hospital
Malaysia

&

Tinku Joseph

Division of Interventional Pulmonology
Amrita Institute of Medical Sciences, Kochi, Kerala
India

A Case-Based Approach to Interventional Pulmonology: A Focus on Asian Perspectives

Editors: Jamalul Azizi Abdul Rahaman and Tinku Joseph

ISBN (Online): 978-981-5124-00-2

ISBN (Print): 978-981-5124-01-9

ISBN (Paperback): 978-981-5124-02-6

First published in 2023.

Bentham Science Publishers Pte. Ltd.
80 Robinson Road #02-00
Singapore 068898
Singapore
Email: subscriptions@benthamscience.net

BENTHAM SCIENCE

CONTENTS

FOREWORD

My friend Jamalul has got a brilliant idea of writing a very original interventional pulmonology (IP) book based on clinical case scenarios. Today, evidence-based medicine and statistics are ruling our daily practice. Thus, each case is unique and each patient, somehow, follows his/her own way regardless of what the theory predicts or commands.

The Asian perspective is also of great importance given the differences in the etiologies compared to other regions of the world. Asia is the leading region in terms of population and the high incidence of certain airway and lung diseases is an amazing source for fundamental and clinical research.

Asia now possesses all the technical expertise to face this medical burden and IP experts, such as Jamalul, play a crucial role in training and spreading the knowledge. Jamalul honors me in calling me his mentor and, through me, he is part of the IP school of Marseille initiated by Jean-François Dumon, the father of interventional pulmonology. I can tell that he is a real member of this school which implies a passion for the art of bronchoscopy and IP procedures, mainly therapeutic bronchoscopy with the rigid bronchoscope.

Upon returning from Marseille, Jamalul pioneered rigid bronchoscopy amongst the pulmonologists in Malaysia. Over the past 14 years, he has dedicated himself to giving rigid bronchoscopy training to many local and overseas pulmonologists.

Tinku Joseph was one of Jamalul's former students who is now doing excellent work and regularly teaching IP fellows. He started the first exclusive IP unit in Kerala state, India which performs basic and advanced bronchoscopic procedures. He is also a recipient of many international and national awards and was the first Indian doctor to win the best overall IP procedure award from the World Association for Bronchology and Interventional Pulmonology (WABIP).

Without passion, there is no positive energy in what anyone does. Without sustained motivation, there is no transmission of knowledge to the younger generation. Jamalul and Tinku Joseph have all the necessary passion and motivation to inspire our young colleagues and this book is certainly the cornerstone of this inspiration source.

Hervé Dutau
Associate Professor of Pulmonology
Head of the Thoracic Endoscopy Unit
Thoracic Oncology, Pleural Diseases and Interventional Pulmonology Department
North University Hospital, Marseille, France

PREFACE

Our book primarily focuses on various aspects of Interventional Pulmonology (IP). To ensure an easy learning process, we have included many interesting diagnostic and therapeutic airway and pleural procedure cases. Leading experts in the field of IP from Asia, Canada and the US have contributed various cases.

Over the past 10 years, a lot of diagnostic and therapeutic innovations have taken place, paving the way for a significant boom in IP. The contents of our book have been divided into four different sections with a primary aim of case-based scenarios and solutions.

Section A consists of diagnostic IP procedures like linear and radial EBUS, navigation bronchoscopy, cryo lung biopsies and cone beam CT. We have included newer diagnostic modalities like cellvizio and robotic bronchoscopy as well.

Section B focuses on therapeutic rigid bronchoscopic procedures. Besides airway stenting and laser bronchoscopy, we have included recent interventions such as bronchial thermoplasty, bronchoscopic lung volume reduction, 3D printing and microwave ablation. Section C is dedicated to pleural procedures with the addition of the more recent ones such as indwelling pleural catheter (IPC) and fibrinolytics. Section D is dedicated to common paediatric IP procedures. The purpose of this book is not to provide the principles, theory or evidence of clinical practice of these procedures but to present actual case scenarios. We hope the book will complement the many IP books on the market that already cover the theory, principles and evidence of clinical practice.

Each case is presented with the history, including clinical, radiological, bronchoscopic/pleuroscopic findings and final outcomes. Many of these cases also have video illustrations as well. As a mark of respect to our patients, privacy identifiers have been intentionally omitted in the text and video presentations. Learning points are highlighted at the end of the case presentation.

Finally, we thank all the authors and co-authors for their hard work in making sure the work could be completed on time.

Jamalul Azizi Abdul Rahaman
Consultant Pulmonologist
Department of Pulmonology
Serdang Hospital
Malaysia

&

Tinku Joseph
Professor & Head of Interventional Pulmonology
Amrita Institute of Medical Sciences
Kochi, Kerala, India

ACKNOWLEDGEMENTS

Dr. Jamalul Azizi

I would like to thank my wife Suhani and our son Muhammad Izzat Al-Amin for allowing me to pursue my ambitions. It was not an easy job to complete the work during the COVID-19 pandemic. My gratitude to my mentor Dr. Hervé Dutau for inspiring me in the field of interventional pulmonology by imparting his skills and knowledge. A special thanks to Serdang Hospital where I work and the Malaysian Association for Bronchology and Interventional Pulmonology (MABIP) for their support building the interventional pulmonology subspecialty in Malaysia. Last but not least, my appreciation to Editor, Dr. Tinku Joseph for helping me with this project.

Dr. Tinku Joseph

Having an idea and turning it into a book is as hard as it sounds. To be honest, writing this book was harder than I thought and more rewarding than I could have ever imagined. None of this would have been possible without my supportive wife, Sania. From reading early drafts to giving me advice on the cover to keeping our little munchkin's (Nichelle and Mikhail) out of my hair so I could edit, she was as important to getting this book done as I was. Thank you so much, dear.

I am eternally grateful to my parents, in-laws and brother for being my pillar of support throughout my life. Writing and editing a book, focusing on various aspects of Interventional Pulmonology was a surreal process and I express my sincere thanks to my mentor Dr. Jamalul Azizi for giving me an opportunity to be a part of this book. Also, a special thanks to my colleagues (especially Dr. Sreeraj) at Amrita hospital where I work, and to Mr. Sam who supported us in designing this book. I must thank God and my patients most of all, because without them I wouldn't have been able to do any of this.

List of Contributors

Adnan Majid	Section of Interventional Pulmonology, Division of Thoracic Surgery, Beth Israel Deaconess Medical Center, Boston, MA 02215, USA
Aisya Natasya Musa	Respiratory Unit, Department of Internal Medicine, Faculty of Medicine, Universiti Teknologi MARA (UiTM), Malaysia
Ajit Nambiar	Department of Pathology, Amrita Institute of Medical Sciences, Kochi, Kerala, India
Alejandro Aragaki	Department of Pulmonary, Allergy and Critical Care Medicine & Transplant Center, Respiratory Institute, Cleveland Clinic, Cleveland, Ohio, USA
Alex Chee	Department of Medicine, University of Calgary, Calgary, Canada
Amanil'Ula Hassan	Paediatric Respiratory Unit, Serdang Hospital, Selangor, Selangor, Malaysia
Anantham Devanand	SingHealth Duke-NUS Lung Centre, Singapore
Andrea Ban Yu-Lin	Faculty of Medicine, National University of Malaysia, Kuala Lumpur, Malaysia
Ani Suraya Abd Ghani	Serdang Hospital, Selangor, Malaysia
Anna Marie Nathan	Division of Paediatric Respiratory & Sleep Medicine, Department of Paediatrics, University of Malaya Medical Centre, University of Malaya, Kuala Lumpur, Malaysia
Belgundi Preeti Vidyasagar	Yashoda Hospitals, Secunderabad, India
Calvin S.H. Ng	Department of Surgery, The Chinese University of Hong Kong, N.T., Hong Kong SAR
Chai Chan Sin	Division of Respiratory Medicine, Sarawak General Hospital, Kuching, Sarawak, Malaysia
Christopher Manley	Fox Chase Cancer Center, Philadelphia, PA 19111, USA
Christopher Radchenko	Department of Pulmonary, Allergy and Critical Care Medicine & Transplant Center, Cleveland Clinic, Cleveland, Ohio, USA
D. Kyle Hogarth	University of Chicago, Chicago, USA
Dayang Zuraini Sahadan	Paediatric Respiratory Unit, Serdang Hospital, Selangor, Malaysia
Eg Kah Peng	Division of Paediatric Respiratory & Sleep Medicine, Department of Paediatrics, University of Malaya Medical Centre, University of Malaya, Kuala Lumpur, Malaysia
Elaine Dumoulin	Department of Medicine, University of Calgary, Calgary, Canada
Gopan	Department of Cardiac Anaesthesia, AMRITA Institute of Medical Sciences, Kochi, Kerala, India
Hamdan Leman	Serdang Hospital, Selangor, Malaysia
Hari Kishan Gonuguntla	Yashoda Hospitals, Secunderabad, India

Hema Yamini Ramarmuty	Respiratory Department, Queen Elizabeth Hospital, Kota Kinabalu, Sabah, Malaysia
Huda Munirah Ainuddin	Paediatric Respiratory Unit, Serdang Hospital, Selangor, Malaysia
Jamalul Azizi Abdul Rahaman	Department of Pulmonology, Serdang Hospital, Selangor, Malaysia
Jayaprakash Balakrishnan	Department of Pulmonary Medicine, Trivandrum Medical College, Kerala, India
Jouke Annema	Department of Respiratory Medicine, Amsterdam UMC, Amsterdam, Netherlands
Joyce W.Y. Chan	Department of Surgery, The Chinese University of Hong Kong, N.T., Hong Kong SAR
Juan Pablo Uribe	Section of Interventional Pulmonology, Division of Thoracic Surgery, Beth Israel Deaconess Medical Center, Boston, MA 02215, USA
Kai Swenson	Section of Interventional Pulmonology, Division of Thoracic Surgery, Beth Israel Deaconess Medical Center, Boston, MA 02215, USA
Khadijah Mohd Nor	Department of Otorhinolaryngology, University Putra Malaysia, Selangor, Malaysia
Khai Lip Ng	Department of Pulmonology, Serdang Hospital, Selangor, Malaysia
Khairulamir Zainuddin	Anesthesiology Department, KPJ Selangor Specialist Hospital, Malaysia
Kho Sze Shyang	Division of Respiratory Medicine, Sarawak General Hospital, Kuching, Sarawak, Malaysia
Koh Gee Tiong	Serdang Hospital, Selangor, Malaysia
Kyle Potts	University of Chicago, Chicago, USA
Larry Ellee Nyanti	Medical Department, Faculty of Medicine and Health Sciences, Universiti Malaysia Sabah, Kota Kinabalu, Sabah, Malaysia
M.D. Varunn	Yashoda Hospitals, Secunderabad, India
Marcela Azevedo	Department of Pulmonary, Allergy and Critical Care Medicine & Transplant Center, Respiratory Institute, Cleveland Clinic, Cleveland, Ohio, USA
Mas Fazlin Mohamad Jailaini	Faculty of Medicine, National University of Malaysia, Kuala Lumpur, Malaysia
Meghana Subash	Amrita Institute of Medical Sciences, Kochi, Kerala, India
Melvin Tay Chee Kiang	SingHealth Duke-NUS Lung Centre, Singapore
Michael A. Pritchett	FirstHealth of the Carolinas and Pinehurst Medical Clinic, Pinehurst, NC, USA
Mohamed Faisal Abdul Hamid	Faculty of Medicine, National University of Malaysia, Kuala Lumpur, Malaysia
Mohammad Ashkan Moslehi	Division of Pediatric interventional pulmonology, School of Medicine, Shiraz University of Medical Sciences, Shiraz, Iran
Mohd Arif Mohd Zim	Respiratory Unit, Department of Internal Medicine, Faculty of Medicine, Universiti Teknologi MARA (UiTM), Malaysia

Mohd Faizul bin Abu Samah	Department of Pulmonology, Serdang Hospital, Selangor, Malaysia
Mona Zaria Nasaruddin	Department of Pulmonology, Serdang Hospital, Selangor, Malaysia
Muhammad Amin Ibrahim	Respiratory Unit, Department of Internal Medicine, Faculty of Medicine, Universiti Teknologi MARA (UiTM), Malaysia
Muhammad Farid Fauad	Respiratory Unit, Department of Internal Medicine, Faculty of Medicine, Universiti Teknologi MARA (UiTM), Malaysia
Muhammad Redzwan S. Rashid Ali	KPJ Johor Specialist Hospital, Johor Bahru, Malaysia
Nai-Chien Huan	Department of Pulmonology, Serdang Hospital, Selangor, Malaysia
Ng Boon Hau	Faculty of Medicine, National University of Malaysia, Kuala Lumpur, Malaysia
Nik Nuratiqah Nik Abeed	Faculty of Medicine, National University of Malaysia, Kuala Lumpur, Malaysia
Prince Ntiamoah	Department of Pulmonary, Allergy and Critical Care Medicine & Transplant Center, Respiratory Institute, Cleveland Clinic, Cleveland, Ohio, USA
Rushi Rabari	Amrita Institute of Medical Sciences, Kochi, Kerala, India
Rainbow W.H. Lau	Department of Surgery, The Chinese University of Hong Kong, N.T., Hong Kong SAR
Rosmadi Ismail	Sunway Medical Center, Selangor, Malaysia
Sadia Benzaquen	Einstein Medical Center, Jefferson University, Philadelphia, Pennsylvania, USA
Sameer Arbat	One Healthcare, Nagpur, India
Sangeta Vadivelu	Department of Pulmonology, Serdang Hospital, Selangor, Malaysia
Saraiza Abu Bakar	Department of Otorhinolaryngology, Serdang Hospital, Selangor, Malaysia
Sathish C. Reddy	AMRITA Institute of Medical Sciences, Kochi, Kerala, India
Shantini Jaganathan	Department of Otorhinolaryngology, Serdang Hospital, Selangor, Malaysia
Shuanzeng Wei	Department of Pathology, Fox Chase Cancer Center, 333 Cottman Avenue, Philadelphia, PA 19111, USA
Soo Chun Ian	University of Malaya Medical Center, Kuala Lumpur, Malaysia
Sreeraj Nair	AMRITA Institute of Medical Sciences, Kochi, Kerala, India
Suhashini Ganapaty	Department of Pathology, Serdang Hospital, Selangor, Malaysia
Syeda Samia Rasheed	Yashoda Hospitals, Secunderabad, India
Tang Jeat Thong	Department of Pulmonology, Serdang Hospital, Selangor, Malaysia
Tess Kramer	Department of Respiratory Medicine, Amsterdam University Medical Center, Netherlands
Thomas R. Gildea	Department of Pulmonary, Allergy and Critical Care Medicine & Transplant Center, Respiratory Insti tute, Cleveland Clinic, Cleveland, Ohio, USA

Tie Siew Teck	Division of Respiratory Medicine, Sarawak General Hospital, Kuching, Sarawak, Malaysia
Tinku Joseph	Professor & Head of Interventional Pulmonology, Department of Pulmonary Medicine, Amrita Institute of Medical Sciences, Kochi, Kerala, India
Tushara Madathil	Department of Cardiac Anaesthesia, Amrita Institute of Medical Sciences, Kochi, Kerala, India
Wong Soo Fen	Department of Pulmonology, Serdang Hospital, Selangor, Malaysia
Zakaria Zahari	Tunku Azizah Hospital, Kuala Lumpur, Malaysia

LIST OF ABBREVIATIONS

AFB	=	Acid Fast Bacilli
AHI	=	Apnoea Hypopnoea Index
APC	=	Argon Plasma Coagulation
BAL	=	Broncho-Alveolar Lavage
BPF	=	Bronchopleural Fistula
BT	=	Bronchial Thermoplasty
BTVA	=	Bronchoscopic Thermal Vapor Ablation
CAO	=	Central Airway Obstruction
CBCT	=	Cone Beam CT
CECT	=	Contrast-Enhanced Computed Tomography
CHP	=	Chronic Hypersensitivity Pneumonitis
CIS	=	Carcinoma *in Situ*
CLE	=	Confocal Light Endomicroscopy
COPD	=	Chronic Obstructive Pulmonary Disease
CPAP	=	Continuous Positive Airway Pressure
CRE	=	Controlled Radial Expansion
CT	=	Computed Tomography
CTA	=	Computed Tomography Angiography
CT TAP	=	Computed Tomography Thorax, Abdomen, Pelvis
CXR	=	Chest X-Ray
CTPA	=	CT Pulmonary Angiogram
DLCO	=	Diffusing Capacity for Carbon Monoxide
DLT	=	Double Lumen Tube
DNASE	=	Deoxyribonuclease
DPLD	=	Diffuse Parenchymal Lung Disease
EBUS	=	Endobronchial Ultrasound
ECMO	=	Extracorporeal Membrane Oxygenation
EDAC	=	Excessive Dynamic Airway Collapse
EGFR	=	Epidermal Growth Factor Receptor
ENB	=	Electromagnetic Navigation Bronchoscopy
ES	=	Electrosurgery
EUS-B-FNA	=	Endoscopic Ultrasound With Bronchoscope-Guided Fine Needle Aspiration
EWC	=	Extended Working Channel
EWS	=	Endobronchial Watanabe Spigot

FEV1	=	Forced Expiratory Volume in One Second
FVC	=	Forced Vital Capacity
FB	=	Foreign Body
FNA	=	Fine Needle Aspiration
FOB	=	Fibreoptic Bronchoscopy
GGO	=	Ground Glass Opacity
GS	=	Guide Sheath
HPE	=	Histopathological Examination
HRCT	=	High Resolution Computed Tomography
ICD	=	Intercostal Chest Drain
IHC	=	Immunohistochemistry
ILD	=	Interstitial Lung Disease
IPC	=	Indwelling Pleural Catheter
LB1 + 2	=	Left Upper Lobe Apicoposterior Segment
LB3	=	Left Upper Lobe Anterior Segment
LB9	=	Left Lower Lobe Lateral Basal Segment
LUL	=	Left Upper Lobe
LLL	=	Left Lower Lobe
MMRC	=	Modified Medical Research Council
MPE	=	Malignant Pleural Effusion
MRI	=	Magnetic Resonance Imaging
OR	=	Operating Room
OSA	=	Obstructive Sleep Apnoea
PA	=	Pulmonary Artery
PAP	=	Pulmonary Alveolar Proteinosis
PCR	=	Polymerase Chain Reaction
PDT	=	Photodynamic Therapy
PEEP	=	Positive End Expiratory Pressure
PET	=	Positron Emission Tomography
POCUS	=	Point of Care Ultrasound
RB1	=	Right Upper Lobe Apical Segment
RB2	=	Right Upper Lobe Posterior Segment
RB3	=	Right Upper Lobe Anterior Segment

RB7	=	Right Lower Lobe Medial Basal Segment
RB9	=	Right Lower Lobe Lateral Basal Segment
RB10	=	Right Lower Lobe Posterior Basal Segment
rEBUS	=	Radial Endobronchial Ultrasound
RLL	=	Right Lower Lobe
ROSE	=	Rapid On-Site Evaluation
RUL	=	Right Upper Lobe
SBRT	=	Stereotactic Body Radiotherapy
SPN	=	Solitary Pulmonary Nodule
SUV_{MAX}	=	Maximum Standardized Uptake Value
SVC	=	Superior Vena Cava
TB	=	Tuberculosis
TBB	=	Transbronchial Biopsy
TBLC	=	Transbronchial Lung Cryobiopsy
TBM	=	Tracheobronchomalacia
TBNA	=	Transbronchial Needle Aspiration
TKI	=	Tyrosine Kinase Inhibitor
TSTB	=	Tracheobronchial Stenosis Secondary to Endobronchial Tuberculosis
USG	=	Ultrasonography
VATS	=	Video-Assisted Thoracoscopic Surgery
V-V ECMO	=	Veno-Venous ECMO
WLL	=	Whole Lung Lavage
YAP	=	Yttrium Aluminium Perovskite

Section A

Diagnostic Interventional Pulmonology

Case 1

Linear EBUS

Not So Black and White - Principles of Staging Assessment in Non-Small Cell Lung Cancer *via* EBUS

Tay Chee Kiang Melvin[1,*], **Soo Chun Ian**[2] and **Anantham Devanand**[1]

[1] *SingHealth Duke-NUS Lung Centre, Singapore*

[2] *University of Malaya Medical Center, Kuala Lumpur, Malaysia*

Keywords: Lung cancer, Mediastinal staging, Mediastinal lymphadenopathy, EBUS, Rapid on-site cytologic examination (ROSE).

Presentation

A 76-year-old woman presents with cough and dyspnea for 2 months. No constitutional symptoms or family history of malignancy.

Comorbidities

Active smoker of 40 pack-years, hypertension.

Chest Imaging

CXR showed a rounded retrocardiac opacity (Fig. **1**). Chest computed tomography (CT) revealed enlarged left hilar, left lower paratracheal, subcarinal and right paratracheal lymph nodes (Figs. **2a-c**). There was a 7.2cm heterogeneous mass in the left lower lobe (Fig. **2d**). There were no other significant CT findings.

[*]**Corresponding author Tay Chee Kiang Melvin:** SingHealth Duke-NUS Lung Centre, Singapore; E-mail: melvin.tay.c.k@singhealth.com.sg

Jamalul Azizi Abdul Rahaman & Tinku Joseph (Eds.)

Intervention

Systematic endobronchial ultrasound (EBUS) assessment for hilar and mediastinal lymphadenopathy using convex-probe EBUS (BF-UC180F, Olympus) under topical airway anesthesia (Lignocaine 1% instilled *via* "spray-as-you-go" technique) and moderate sedation (Midazolam and Fentanyl). Linear EBUS assessment began in the right hilum (Station 10R) and continued up into the mediastinum with the right lower and upper paratracheal nodes (Stations 4R & 2R respectively).

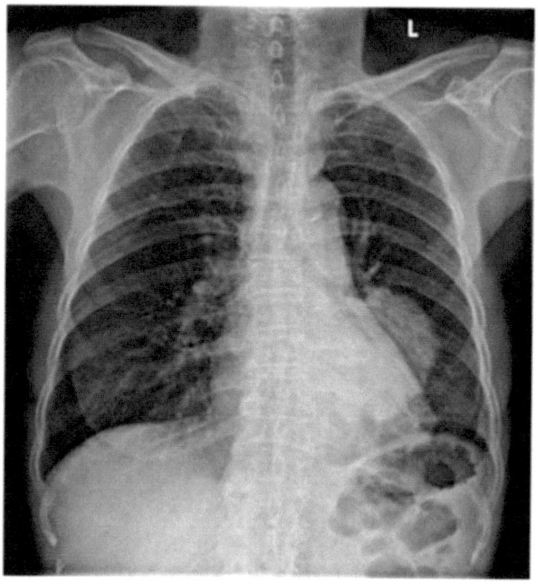

Fig. (1). Rounded retrocardiac opacity on CXR.

On EBUS, there was no lymph node ≥ 5mm in the short axis at Station 10R. However, enlarged nodes (short-axis diameter approximately 1cm) were visualized at a location cranial to the intersection between the caudal margin of the left brachiocephalic vein and the trachea. Endobronchial ultrasoundguided trans-bronchial needle aspiration (EBUS-TBNA) was performed on a Station 2R node using 22G ViziShot aspiration needle (NA-201SX-4022, Olympus). 4 passes were made, with rapid on-site cytologic examination (ROSE) confirming malignant cells and adequate cellular yield. The procedure was halted at this time.

Complications

Nil.

Post-Intervention

EBUS-TBNA Station 2R histologic results – gross description: multiple clumps of tissue measuring 0.7 x 0.6 x 0.1cm; microscopic description: clusters of epithelial cells with up to moderate nuclear atypia. On immunochemistry, the atypical cells show positivity for deltaNp63 (p40) whilst being negative for thyroid transcription factor 1 (TTF1), in keeping with squamous cell carcinoma.

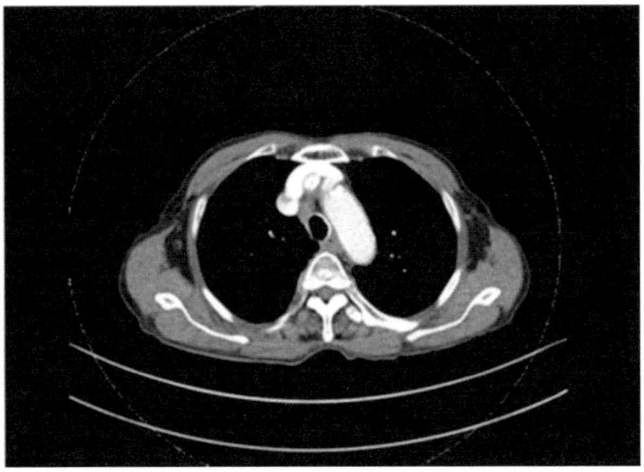

Fig. (2). (a) 2R lymph node at level of left brachiocephalic vein on CT thorax (*Note*: For most instances, the aortic arch would not be visualized at this level as it typically lies more caudal to the left brachiocephalic vein).

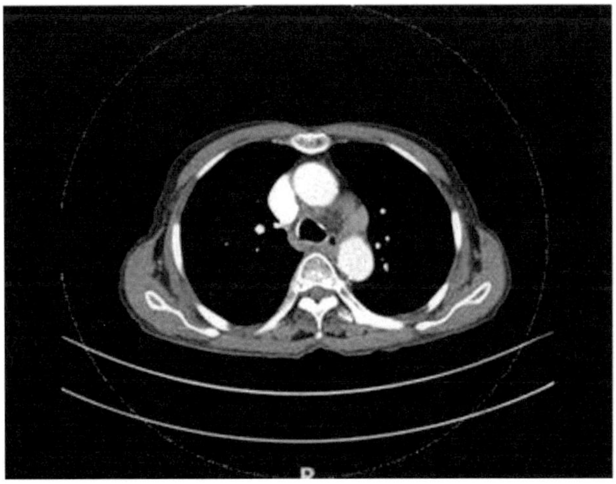

Fig. (2). (b) Small 4R lymph nodes and large 4L lymph nodes.

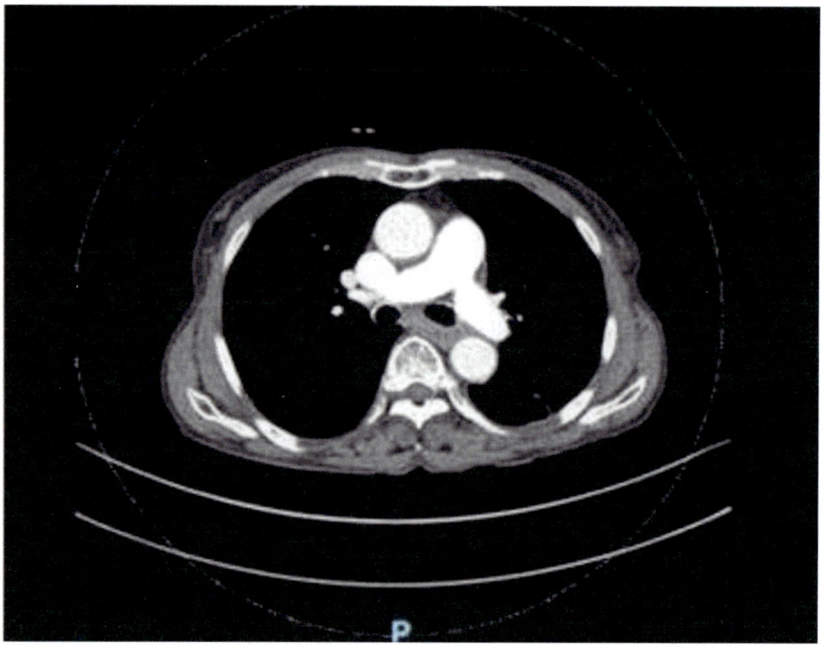

Fig. (2). (c) Subcarinal lymph node.

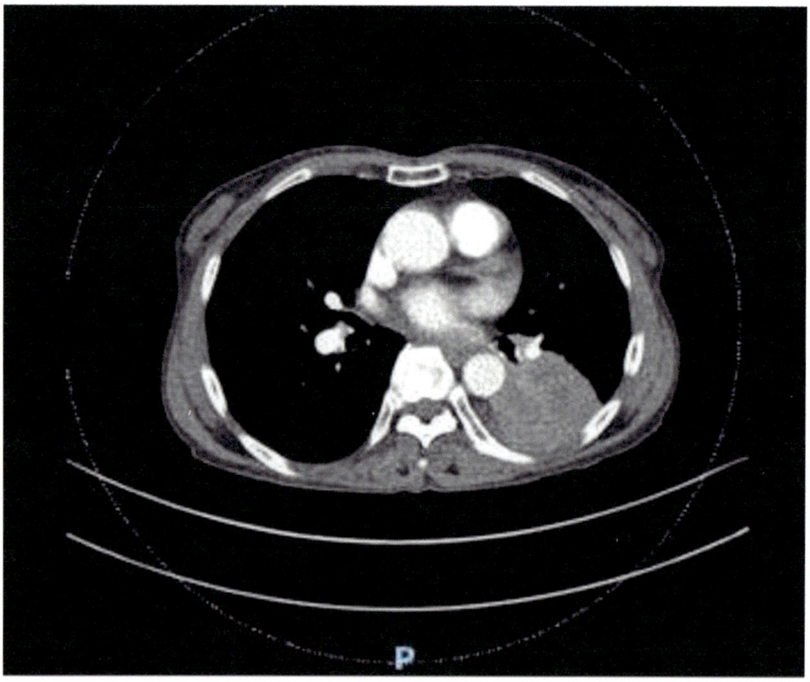

Fig. (2). (d) Left lower lobe mass in the superior segment.

Learning Points

- EBUS-TBNA is often used for both diagnosis and staging of non-small cell lung cancer during the same procedure [1]. Thorough pre-procedural planning is pivotal to the success of achieving the two aims.
- Generally, the approach to the staging examination is to sample the highest station lymph nodes first, *i.e.*, N3 level nodal stations, followed by N2 level, and lastly N1 level.
- A good understanding and appreciation of the relationship between anatomic landmarks and the various nodal stations during EBUS, and accurate classification of the latter (according to the latest edition of the International Association for the Study of Lung Cancer lymph node map) are crucial as nodal status impacts surgical candidacy.
- The choice between systematic assessment (≥ 3 passes per node or ROSE at stations 2R, 2L, 4R, 4L, and 7) *versus* selective assessment (short-axis diameter ≥ 1cm by CT/ultrasound or < 3 passes or no ROSE) in staging examination remains somewhat contentious. Nonetheless, it is our practice to sample any lymph node ≥ 5mm in the short axis, and to perform ≥ 4 passes per station to ensure adequate yield for molecular testing.

Video

EBUS TBNA of station 2R lymph node.

CONSENT FOR PUBLICATION

Not applicable.

CONFLICT OF INTEREST

The authors declare no conflict of interest, financial or otherwise.

ACKNOWLEDGEMENT

Declared none.

REFERENCE

[1] Kinsey CM, Arenberg DA. Endobronchial ultrasound-guided transbronchial needle aspiration for non- small cell lung cancer staging. Am J Respir Crit Care Med 2014; 189(6): 640-9. [http://dx.doi.org/10.1164/rccm.201311-2007CI]

Case 2

Systematic Approach to Mediastinal Node Staging with Linear EBUS

Hema Yamini Ramarmuty[1,*]

[1] *Respiratory Department, Queen Elizabeth Hospital, Kota Kinabalu, Sabah, Malaysia*

Keywords: Linear EBUS, Diagnostic, Systematic mediastinal nodal staging, Lung cancer, Invasive mediastinal staging.

Presentation

A 64-year-old lady presented with chronic cough, loss of weight and loss of appetite for 8 months duration.

Comorbidities

Hypertension for the past 4 years. She is a non-smoker.

Chest Imaging

CXR showed a large left lung mass. This was confirmed with a CECT thorax which demonstrated a left hilar mass, measuring 9.7 X 9.6cm with enlarged and necrotic mediastinal nodes (Figs. **1a** and **b**).

Intervention

Convex-probe endobronchial ultrasound (CP-EBUS) through a size 4 laryngeal mask airway (LMA) under general anaesthesia (total intravenous anaesthesia).

The mediastinal nodes were assessed using a systematic approach. The 2L node and 4L (N2) node (Fig. **2a**) were less than 1cm in size. The station 11R node (Fig. **2b**) measured 8mm while the station 7 (N2) node (Fig. **2c**) was 30mm with

*Corresponding author Hema Yamini Ramarmuty: Respiratory Department, Queen Elizabeth Hospital, Kota Kinabalu, Sabah, Malaysia; E-mail: yamini8254@hotmail.com

heterogeneous opacity. The station 4R (N3) node (Fig. **2d**) measured around 11mm with distinct margins and was heterogeneous in nature. We were unable to assess the left hilar nodes as the left main bronchus was narrowed. We proceeded to sample the station 4R node.

EBUS-TBNA Procedural Steps

1. The 22G EBUS-TBNA needle is introduced into the working channel of the CP-EBUS scope.
2. The sheath is then adjusted to the desired position (till it is visible on the endoscopic image).
3. Once the sheath is seen, the length of the needle is adjusted and the needle is advanced into the lesion. Doppler examination is performed before advancing the needle to avoid unintentional puncture of vessels. Once the needle is within the lesion, the inner stylet is used to clear the tip of the internal lumen. The stylet is removed and negative pressure is applied using a syringe.
4. Subsequently, the needle is moved back and forth within the lesion.
5. The needle is retrieved and the stylet is used to push out the aspirated material on to a glass slide. This is then smeared, air-dried and fixed with a Diff-Quik stain.
6. Rapid On-Site Evaluation (ROSE), which is performed by an on-site cytopathologist will aid in confirming the adequacy of material thus reducing the duration of the procedure and the amount of unnecessary biopsy. More samples are sent in a saline pot for cell block.

In this patient, a total of 4 passes were performed at station 4R node (Fig. **3**). ROSE showed clusters of malignant cells. We then switched to a flexible fibreoptic bronchoscope and proceeded with a thorough examination of the airways. She was found to have widening of the main carina angle and total stenosis of the right middle lobe. Mucosa over the left main bronchus (LMB) appeared oedematous and congested. Nodular deposits were seen at the entrance of the LMB. The scope could not be advanced further into the LMB to visualise the left upper lobe and left lower lobe segments as it was narrowed. A 1.1mm flexible cryoprobe was used to obtain biopsies from the nodular deposits at the LMB (Fig. **4**).

Complications

There were no procedure related adverse effects. The patient was discharged home the next day with no complications.

Post-Intervention

ROSE showed atypical cells suspicious for malignancy. Final pathology results revealed adenocarcinoma. She was diagnosed with stage IIIc (T4N3M0) adenocarcinoma and was referred to the oncologists for further management.

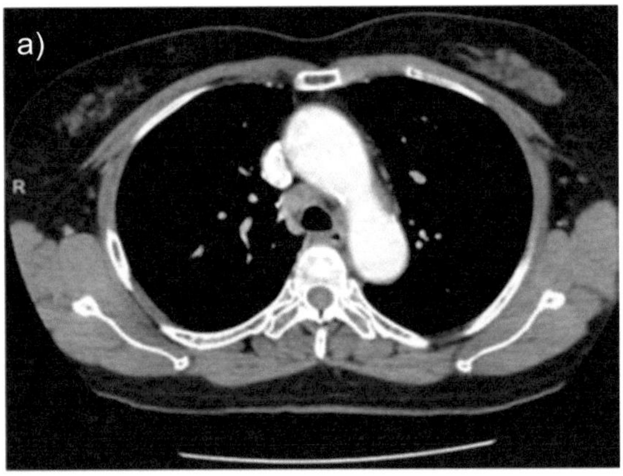

Fig. (1). (a) Axial CT thorax shows enlarged right lower paratracheal node (station 4R).

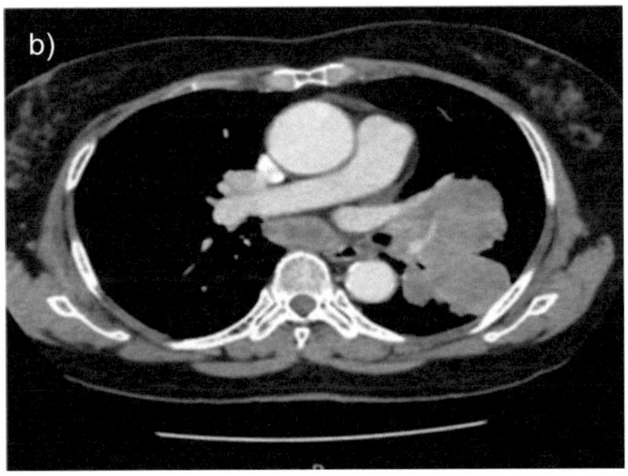

Fig. (1). (b) Axial CT thorax shows a left hilar mass and an enlarged station 7 node.

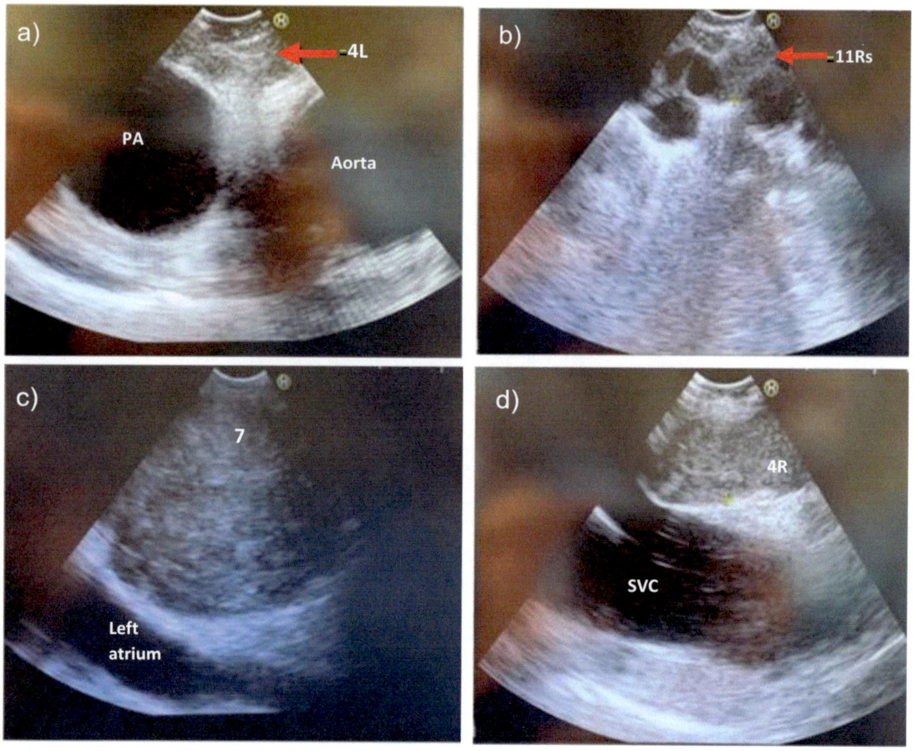

Fig. (2). **(a)** 4L node is 8mm and is seen below the aorta and above the pulmonary artery (PA). The margins are indistinct. **(b)** The 11Rs node is 8mm. The right interlobar artery is seen next to it. **(c)** Enlarged station 7 node measuring 30mm. **(d)** The 4R node is 11mm with clear margins, SVC (Superior vena cava) is seen below it.

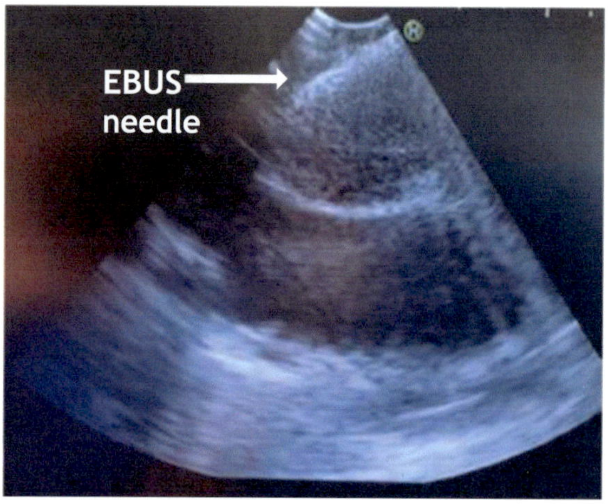

Fig. (3). EBUS needle is seen within the 4R node.

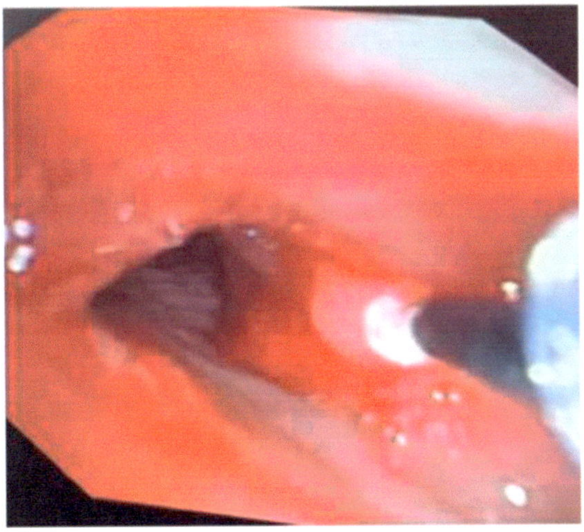

Fig. (4). Flexible cryoprobe used to obtain biopsy from the nodular mucosa at the entrance of the LMB.

Learning Points

- Accurate staging of lung cancer is important to prognosticate as well as to identify the appropriate treatment modalities that can be offered to pati-ents. In patients with lung cancer without distant metastases, assessment of mediastinal nodal involvement is critical.
- For patients with tumours measuring less than 3cm and are localized to the outer third of the lung, surgical resection is recommended along with systematic nodal dissection. The prerequisite for this is that no enlarged nodes are seen on CT and PET CT does not demonstrate any uptake within the nodes [1]. Pre-operative mediastinal staging must be done for patients with central tumours or N1 nodes [1].
- The American College of Chest Physicians (ACCP) guidelines for staging of non–small cell lung cancer recommends EBUS or endoscopic ultrasound (EUS) as the modality of choice for invasive mediastinal staging [2]. A systematic approach of sampling mediastinal nodes is considered superior to selective sampling of radiographically abnormal nodes. The order of nodal sampling should begin at the level of N3 nodes followed by N2 nodes before ending with N1 nodes [2]. This will also avoid contamination when a single needle is used for EBUS [2]. In our patient, the N3 node was sampled first. As malignant cells were seen on ROSE, further sampling of N2 and N1 nodes was not performed.

Video

EBUS-TBNA of 4R node through a laryngeal mask airway under general anaesthesia.

CONSENT FOR PUBLICATION

Not applicable.

CONFLICT OF INTEREST

The authors declare no conflict of interest, financial or otherwise.

ACKNOWLEDGEMENT

Declared none.

REFERENCES

[1] De Leyn, Christophe Dooms, Jaroslaw Kuzdzal, Didier Lardinois, Bernward Passlick, Ramon Rami-Porta, Akif Turna, Paul Van Schil, Frederico Venuta, David Waller, Walter Weder, Marcin Zielinski, Revised ESTS guidelines for preoperative mediastinal lymph node staging for non-small-cell lung cancer, European Journal of Cardio-Thoracic Surgery, Volume 45, Issue 5, May 2014, Pages 787–798.

[http://dx.doi.org/10.1093/ejcts/ezu028] [PMID: 24578407]

[2] Silvestri GA, Gonzalez AV, Jantz MA, Margolis ML, Gould MK, Tanoue LT, Harris LJ, Detterbeck FC. Methods for staging non-small cell lung cancer: diagnosis and management of lung cancer, 3rd ed: American College of Chest Physicians evidence- based clinical practice guidelines. Chest2013;143(5 Suppl):e211S–e250S.

[http://dx.doi.org/10.1378/chest.12-2355]

Case 3

Linear EBUS: Can Ultrasonographic Features of the Lymph Nodes be Used to Predict Malignancy?

Hema Yamini Ramarmuty[1,*]

[1]*Respiratory Department, Queen Elizabeth Hospital, Kota Kinabalu, Sabah, Malaysia*

Keywords: Malignancy, Ultrasound, Linear EBUS, Lymph node characteristics, Mediastinal lymphadenopathy.

Presentation

A 53 year-old mechanic presented with reduced effort tolerance and a feeling of fullness at the neck and anterior chest wall for 2 months duration. He did not report constitutional symptoms. There was no family history of malignancy. Physical examination revealed dilated veins over the neck and anterior chest wall.

Comorbidities

Hypertension and dyslipidemia. He is an active smoker of 50 pack-years.

Chest Imaging

CECT thorax demonstrated a right upper lobe mass (4 x 2.5cm) with right mediastinal and hilar nodal metastasis, superior vena cava (SVC) compression, sternal erosion and phrenic nerve palsy (Figs. **1** and **2**).

Intervention

Convex-probe endobronchial ultrasound (CP-EBUS) guided transbronchial needle aspiration (TBNA) was performed under general anaesthesia (total intravenous anaesthesia) with the airway secured using a size 4 laryngeal mask airway (LMA).

[*]**Corresponding author Hema Yamini Ramarmuty:** Respiratory Department, Queen Elizabeth Hospital, Kota Kinabalu, Sabah, Malaysia; E-mail: yamini8254@hotmail.com

Jamalul Azizi Abdul Rahaman & Tinku Joseph (Eds.)

CP-EBUS scope was inserted through the LMA and used to systematically stage the mediastinal and hilar nodes. The 11L, 10 L, 4L (Fig. **3a**) and 2L nodes were subcentimeter nodes and were not sampled. Station 11R (Fig. **3c**) and station 7 (Fig. **3b**) lymph nodes were enlarged. The margins were distinct and the nodes demonstrated heterogeneous echogenicity. The 4R node was enlarged, heterogeneous and continuous with the 2R node causing significant narrowing of the SVC. We proceeded to sample the station 4R node (Fig. **3d**).

EBUS-TBNA Procedural Steps: The 22G EchoTip ProCore EBUS needle is introduced into the working channel of the CP-EBUS scope. The sheath is then adjusted to the desired position (till it is visible on the endoscopic image). Once the sheath is seen, the desired length of the needle is adjusted and the needle is advanced into the lesion. Doppler examination is performed before advancing the needle to avoid unintentional puncture of vessels. Once the needle is within the lesion, the inner stylet is used to clear the tip of the internal lumen clogged with bronchial membrane. The stylet is removed and negative pressure is applied using a syringe.

Subsequently, the needle is moved back and forth within the lesion (multidirectional, edge to edge and without moving out completely from the node). The needle is retrieved and the stylet is used to push out the aspirated material onto a glass slide. This is then smeared, air-dried and fixed with a Diff-Quik stain.

Rapid On-Site Evaluation (ROSE), which is performed by an on-site cytopathologist will aid in confirming the adequacy of material thus reducing the duration of EBUS-TBNA and the amount of unnecessary biopsy. Histologic cores are fixed with formalin and sent to the laboratory for further analysis. A total of 4 passes were made at station 4R node.

Complications

There were no procedure-related adverse effects.

Post-Intervention

ROSE showed atypical cells suspicious of malignancy. Final pathology results revealed squamous cell carcinoma. A diagnosis of stage IVA (T3N2M1a) squamous cell carcinoma was made during the lung cancer multidisciplinary meeting. He was referred to the oncologists for further evaluation and treatment.

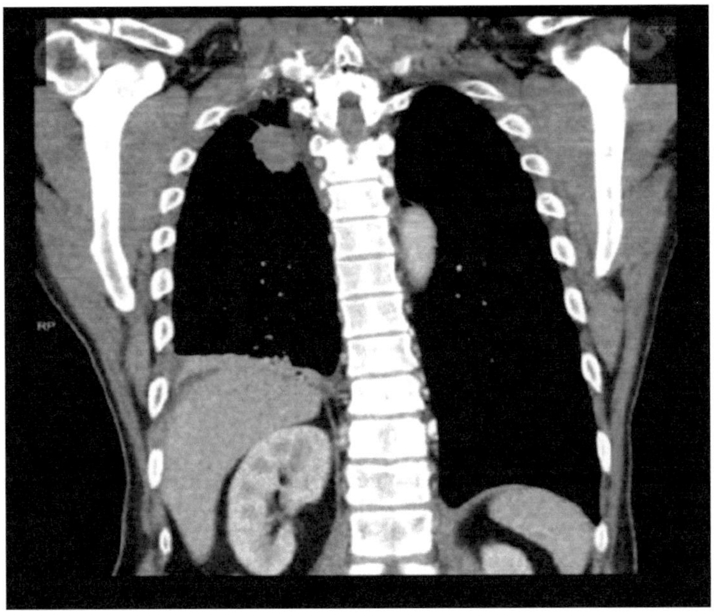

Fig. (1). Coronal CT thorax shows a 3.1cm right upper lobe mass abutting the pleura with irregular pleural thickening and elevation of right hemidiaphragm (phrenic nerve palsy).

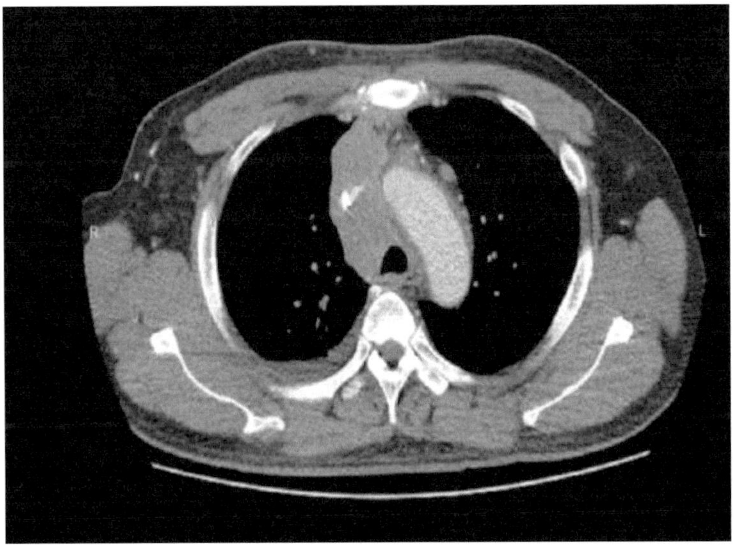

Fig. (2). Axial CT thorax shows enlarged superior mediastinal nodes (2R and 4R) causing SVC compression and erosion of the sternal manubrium.

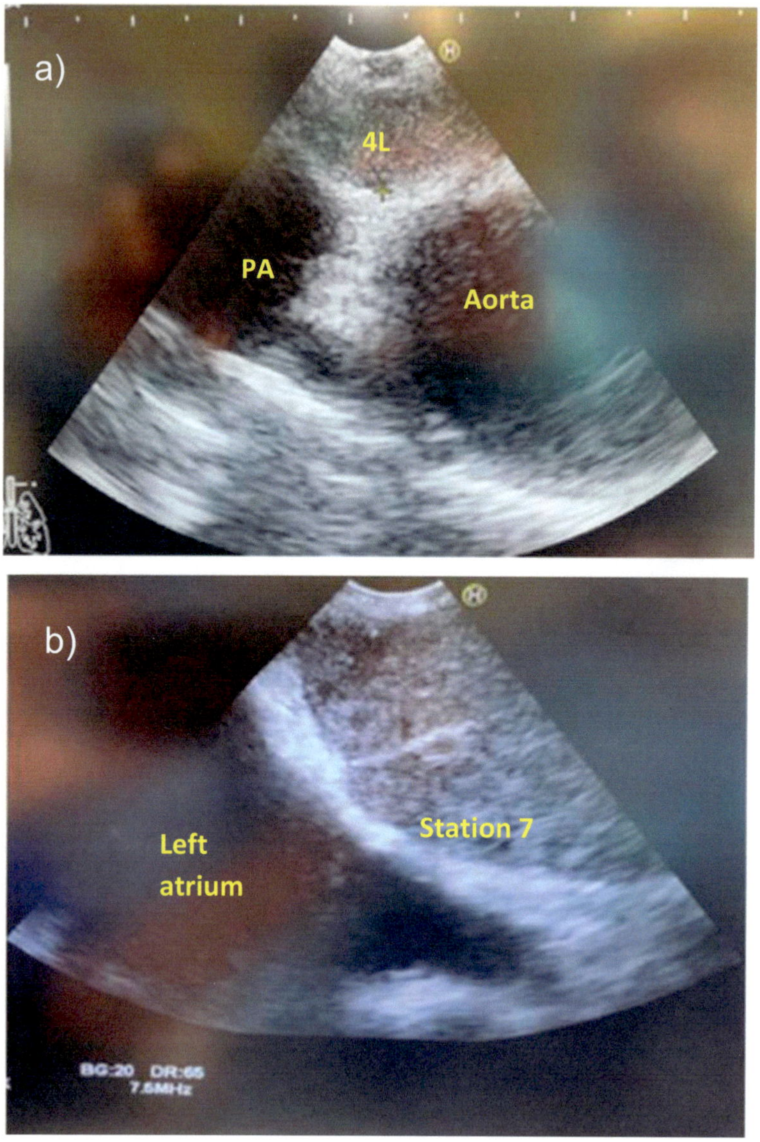

Fig. (3). (a) 4L lymph node is seen located above the pulmonary artery (PA) and below the aorta. **(b)** The station 7 node is enlarged (25mm) with a distinct margin.

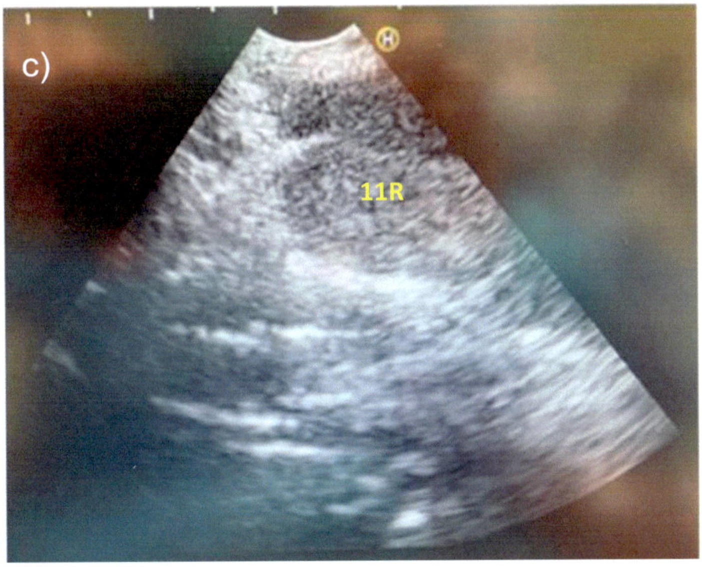

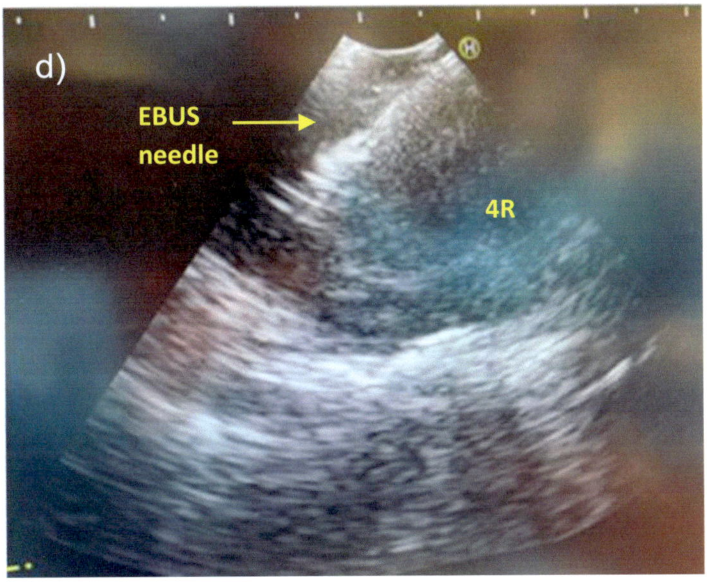

Fig. (3). **(c)** 11R node is seen measuring 17mm. **(d)** The EBUS needle is seen within the 4R node.

Learning Points

CP-EBUS is a minimally invasive, safe and well-tolerated procedure. It is particularly useful for sampling mediastinal nodes for lung cancer diagnosis and staging as well as for evaluation of mediastinal masses [1]. It is also helpful to diagnose benign diseases such as TB and sarcoidosis.

EBUS-TBNA can be performed under local anaesthesia and conscious sedation in an outpatient setting where the EBUS bronchoscope is introduced transorally with a bite block in place. It can be also performed through LMA or ETT (endotracheal tube) with the patient under general anaesthesia/deep sedation. ETT should be avoided if a higher lymph node station (1, 2R, 2L and 3p) sampling is planned as ETT will block the ultrasonographic view of the nodes [2].

Ultrasonographic features of the lymph node may be used to predict malignant and benign disease; however, it is not reliable enough to forgo a biopsy. Tissue samples are still necessary for confirmation of diagnosis [2]. Multivariate analysis showed that independent predictive factors for malignancy includes round shape, distinct margin, heterogeneous echogenicity and the presence of coagulation necrosis. In our patient, the node that proved to be malignant was noted to have distinct margins as well as heterogeneous echogenicity [2].

CONSENT FOR PUBLICATION

Not applicable.

CONFLICT OF INTEREST

The authors declare no conflict of interest, financial or otherwise.

ACKNOWLEDGEMENT

Declared none.

REFERENCES

[1] Gomez M, Silvestri GA. Endobronchial ultrasound for the diagnosis and staging of lung cancer. Proc Am Thorac Soc 2009; 6(2): 180-6.
[http://dx.doi.org/10.1513/pats.200808-081LC] [PMID: 19349486]

[2] Wahidi MM, Herth F, Yasufuku K, *et al.* Technical aspects of endobronchial ultrasound-guided transbronchial needle aspiration. Chest 2016; 149(3): 816-35.
[http://dx.doi.org/10.1378/chest.15-1216] [PMID: 26402427]

Case 4

How to Deal with Mush – Tackling the Necrotic Lymph Node During Endobronchial Ultrasound-Guided Transbronchial Needle Aspiration?

Tay Chee Kiang Melvin[1,*], **Soo Chun Ian**[2] and **Anantham Devanand**[1]

[1] *SingHealth Duke-NUS Lung Centre, Singapore*

[2] *University of Malaya Medical Center, Kuala Lumpur, Malaysia*

Keywords: Necrosis, Mediastinal lymphadenopathy, EBUS, Elastography, Rapid on-site cytologic examination (ROSE).

Presentation

A 47-year-old man was referred by colorectal surgery for bilateral lung nodules and mediastinal lymphadenopathy on chest computed tomography (CT). These findings were partly detected on CT abdomen and pelvis (CTAP) performed to evaluate the patient's recent change in bowel habit. Primary rectal malignancy was suspected as irregular concentric mural thickening of the mid to upper rectum with associated luminal stenosis was noted on CTAP (Fig. **1**). No gastrointestinal scopes had been done yet. Otherwise, he did not have respiratory symptoms or any family history of colorectal cancer.

Comorbidities

Ex-smoker 10 pack-years, quit 5 years ago.

Chest Imaging

Chest CT revealed multiple nodules in the left lower lobe and right upper lobe, the largest of which measured 1.0cm. Subcarinal and left hilar lymph nodes enlarged at 1.6cm and 1.4cm respectively (Figs. **2a-c**).

*Corresponding author Tay Chee Kiang Melvin: SingHealth Duke-NUS Lung Centre, Singapore; E-mail: melvin.tay.c.k@singhealth.com.sg

Intervention

Endobronchial ultrasound-guided transbronchial needle aspiration (EBUS-TBNA) of Station 7 lymph node was performed using 21G ViziShot 2 aspiration needle (NA-U401SX-4021-A, Olympus) (Fig. **3**). Rapid on-site cytologic examination (ROSE) of the first 3 passes yielded gross necrosis repeatedly. No cores were obtained.

Decision was made to employ the elastography "ELST" mode available on the Olympus EU-ME2 ultrasound processor to target the lymph node section demonstrating elastographic color pattern type 3 (predominantly blue). That pass yielded malignant cells. However, as the cytotechnologist commented that the number of tumor cells was not numerous, decision was made to change to a brand new needle as a substantial number of passes had been made. This step was merely precautionary against insufficient sampling on the operator's part as the 21G ViziShot 2 aspiration needle did yield cores on subsequent passes. The 22Ga Acquire Pulmonary Endobronchial Ultrasound Fine Needle Biopsy Device (M00552350, Boston Scientific) was used this time and also yielded cores (Fig. **3**).

Complications

Nil.

Post-Intervention

EBUS-TBNA Station 7 histopathological analysis revealed moderately differentiated adenocarcinoma arranged in a cribriform pattern, consistent with carcinoma of primary colorectal origin.

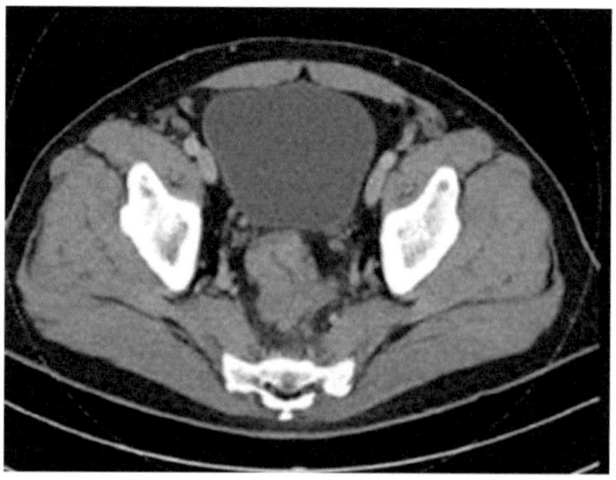

Fig. (1). Irregular mural thickening of rectum with luminal stenosis on CTAP.

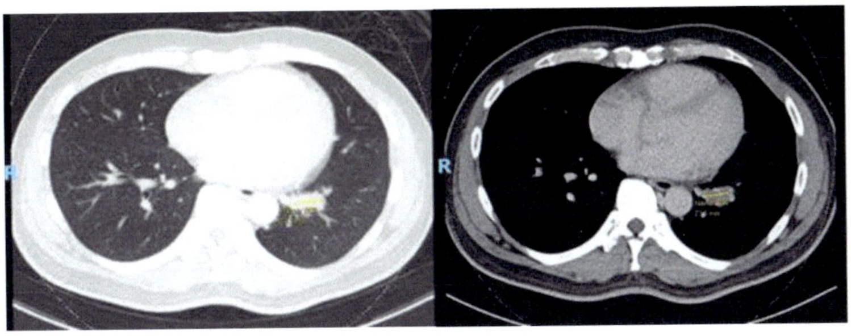

Fig. (2). (a) (Left) & **(b)** (Right). Left hilar node on axial cut of chest CT (lung and mediastinal windows).

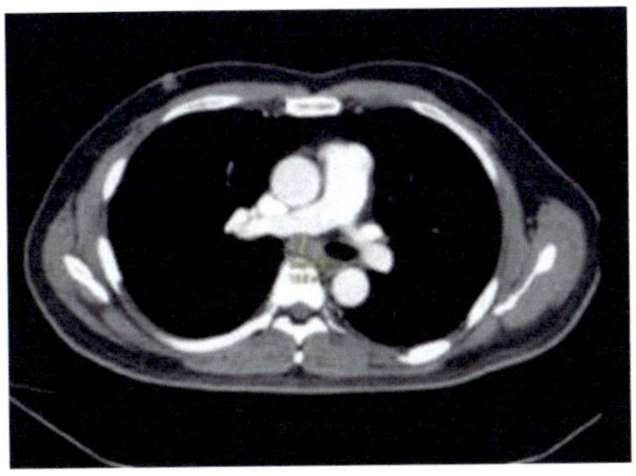

Fig. (2). (c) Subcarinal lymph node.

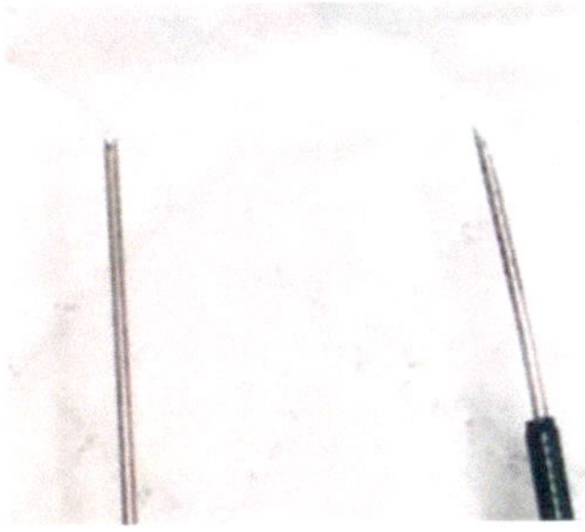

Fig. (3). (left) Acquire Pulmonary Endobronchial Ultrasound Fine Needle Biopsy Device 22G; (Right) ViziShot 2 aspiration needle 21G.

Learning Points

- EBUS-TBNA has a role in the evaluation of any mediastinal lymphadenopathy of uncertain etiology. In the presence of an extra-thoracic malignancy, mediastinal lymphadenopathy with lung nodule(s) could either represent distant metastasis or nodal metastasis from a synchronous primary lung cancer.
- EBUS-TBNA of lymph nodes with extensive necrosis may prove challenging and carry the risk of a non-diagnostic procedure. In such instances, ROSE

would be helpful to ensure adequacy of specimens, which may then potentially increase diagnostic accuracy.

- Although EBUS elastography has been largely studied as a diagnostic modality in differentiating malignant from benign lymph nodes, it is not unreasonable to use it to avoid sampling the "less stiff" or "low strain" parts of a lymph node, *i.e.*, the necrotic regions *via* the same reasoning. The classification of elastographic patterns follows the system described by Takehiro Izumo, which is based on the dominant colors and their distribution within the target lymph node [1]. The classification is as follows: Type 1, predominantly non-blue (green, yellow and red); Type 2, part blue, part non-blue; and Type 3, predominantly blue, with Type 1 representing the least and Type 3 the most in terms of tissue stiffness.

Video

EBUS-TBNA of station 7 lymph node with elastography.

CONSENT FOR PUBLICATION

Not applicable.

CONFLICT OF INTEREST

The authors declare no conflict of interest, financial or otherwise.

ACKNOWLEDGEMENT

Declared none.

REFERENCE

[1] Izumo T, Sasada S, Chavez C, Matsumoto Y, Tsuchida T. Endobronchial ultrasound elastography in the diagnosis of mediastinal and hilar lymph nodes. Jpn J Clin Oncol 2014; 44(10): 956-62.
[http://dx.doi.org/10.1093/jjco/hyu105] [PMID: 25121724]

Endoscopic Ultrasound with Bronchoscope-Guided Fine Needle Aspiration Case Series

Soo Chun Ian[1,*], **Tay Chee Kiang Melvin**[2] and **Anantham Devanand**[2]

[1] *University of Malaya Medical Center, Kuala Lumpur, Malaysia*

[2] *SingHealth Duke-NUS Lung Centre, Singapore*

Keywords: Transesophageal endobronchial ultrasound (EUS-B), Lung cancer, Mediastinal lymphadenopathy, Mediastinal lesion, EBUS.

Case A Presentation

A 69-year-old male presented with progressive dyspnoea and intermittent dry cough. He has a 100 pack-year smoking history. He also complained of non-specific mild headache and some sensation of dysphagia and had lost 15kg in 12 months. There were no night sweats, recent TB contact or family history of malignancy. On physical examination and lung auscultation, the patient had hyperinflated lungs and a prolonged expiratory phase. There was digital clubbing and a solitary deep-seated small right supraclavicular lymph node. Laboratory tests showed his corrected calcium was 2.8mmol/L and there was hyponatremia (130mmol/L).

Comorbidities

Nil.

Chest Imaging

CT thorax showed multiple large matted heterogenous mediastinal lymphadenopathy with some encasing the lower trachea, right pulmonary artery and main bronchi (Fig. **1**). In addition, there was pericardial effusion and an irregular and spiculated cavitary lesion at the periphery of the right upper lobe measuring 1.3 x 1.5 x 1.5cm. A CT brain showed multiple enhancing masses suggestive of metastatic lesions (Fig. **2**).

[*]**Corresponding author Soo Chun Ian:** University of Malaya Medical Center, Kuala Lumpur, Malaysia; E-mail: scianray@gmail.com

Jamalul Azizi Abdul Rahaman & Tinku Joseph (Eds.)

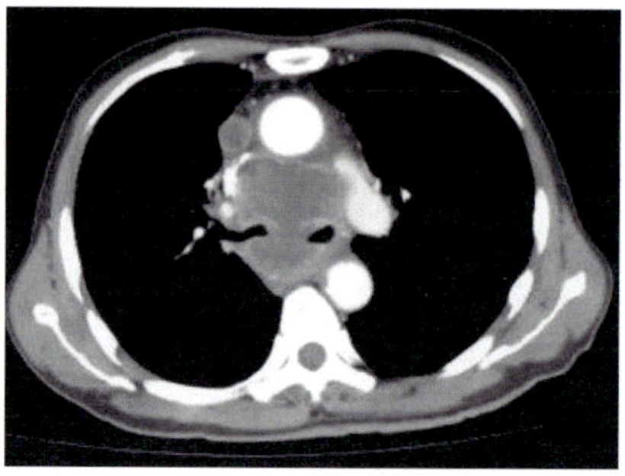

Fig. (1). Multiple bulky mediastinal lymph nodes.

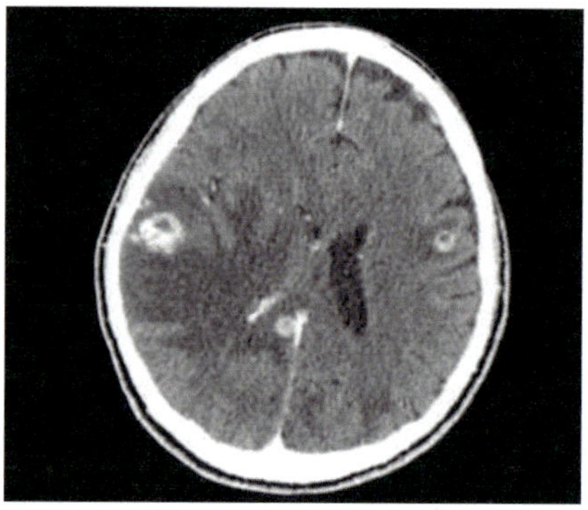

Fig. (2). Multiple enhancing lesions on CT brain.

Intervention

Endoscopic ultrasound with bronchoscope-guided fine needle aspiration (EUS-B-FNA) was preferred to the commonly performed EBUS-guided transbronchial needle aspiration (EBUS-TBNA). EUS-B-FNA was performed on the subcarinal lymph node (Station 7) (Fig. **3**). Procedure was performed under moderate sedation.

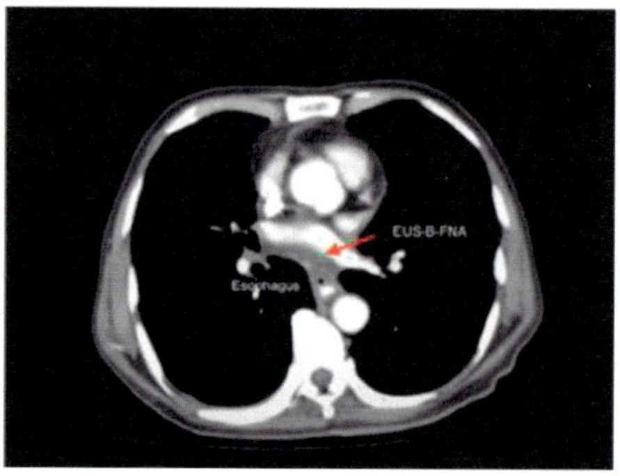

Fig. (3). EUS-B-FNA performed at subcarinal lymph node (station 7).

The Needle Used: EchoTip ProCore, Cook Medical 25G needle.

Sample:

Station 7 Lymph Node: Cytology smears on slides and liquid-based cell block (Cytolyt).

Complications

None.

Post-Intervention

Diagnosis –Squamous cell lung cancer.

Case B Presentation

A 70-year-old female with a background of asthma began to experience bouts of productive cough for eight months duration. She was treated as uncontrolled asthma by various general practitioners with no improvement in her symptoms. She denied hemoptysis, had no fever or any constitutional symptoms. There were no significant findings on physical examination.

Comorbidities

Hypertension.

Chest Imaging

Her CXR was suspicious of a left lower lobe collapse. Subsequently, a CT thorax demonstrated a retrocardiac left lower lobe mass with the presence of mediastinal lymphadenopathy.

Intervention

EBUS-TBNA was performed on the subcarinal lymph node (Station 7). EUS-B-FNA was performed on the left lower lobe mass (Fig. **4**). Procedure was performed under moderate sedation.

The Needle Used: EchoTip ProCore, Cook Medical 22G needle.

Samples:

- Station 7 Lymph Node: Cytology smears on slides and dry tissue clot cell block.
- Left Lower Lobe Mass: Cytology smears on slides and liquid-based cell block (Cytolyt).

Complications

Nil.

Post-Intervention

Diagnosis-Stage IIIb Lung adenocarcinoma.

EGFR +ve (Exon 19 deletion).

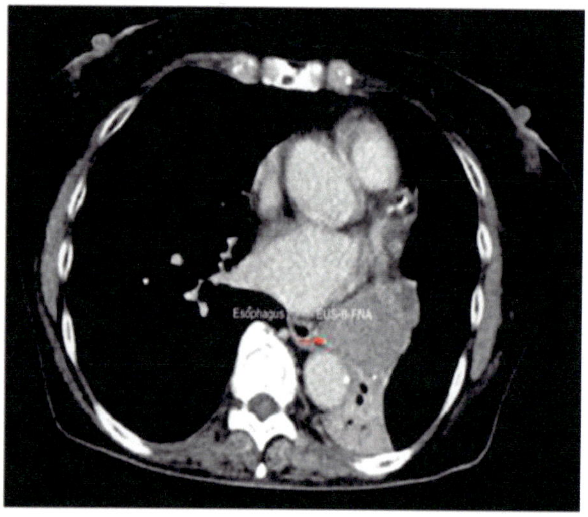

Fig. (4). EUS-B-FNA of the left lower lobe mass.

Case C Presentation

A 52-year-old male presented with chronic cough for 6 months duration. Occasionally, he also noticed some blood-streaked sputum. He had lost 10kg in 4 months despite normal diet. He had no family history of malignancy. He had a 20 pack-year cigarette smoking history. On physical examination, there was digital clubbing and bronchial breathing was heard on auscultation over the lower zone of his left lung.

Comorbidities

Diabetes, hyperlipidaemia and hypertension.

Chest Imaging

CXR showed an ill-defined lesion at the retrocardiac region. A CT thorax demonstrated a left hilar to retrocardiac mass with the presence of multiple mediastinal lymphadenopathies (Fig. **5**).

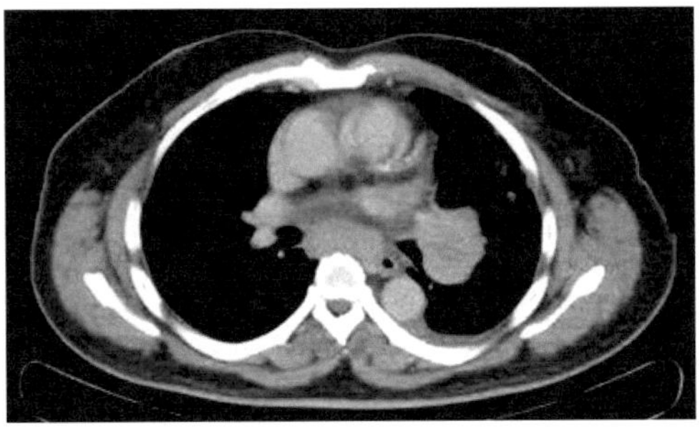

Fig. (5). Left hilar to retrocardiac mass with the presence of multiple mediastinal lymphadenopathy.

Intervention

EBUS-TBNA was performed on the right lower paratracheal lymph node (station 4R) followed by the subcarinal lymph node (station 7). EUS-B-FNA was performed on the left lower paratracheal lymph node (station 4L) (Fig. **6**). Endobronchial biopsy was performed at the narrowed left lower lobe segment. The procedure was performed under moderate sedation.

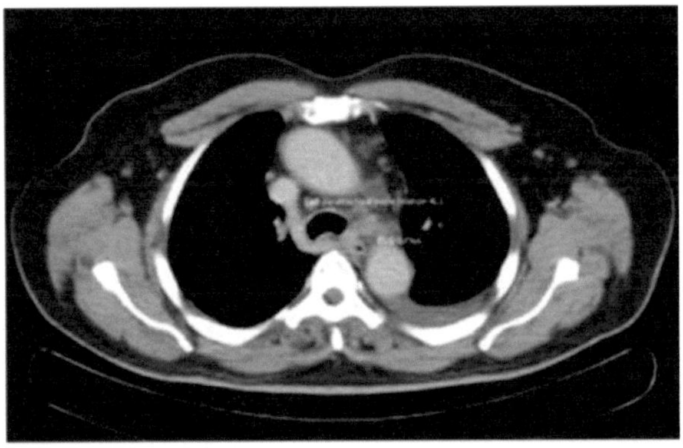

Fig. (6). EUS-B-FNA of left lower paratracheal lymph node (station 4L).

The Needle Used: EchoTip ProCore, Cook Medical 22G needle.

Samples:

- Station 4R, 7 & 4L Lymph Nodes: Cytology smears on slides and separate liquid-based cell block (Cytolyt).
- Left hilar to Retrocardiac Lesion: Histology specimen.

Complications

Nil.

Post-Intervention

Diagnosis-Locally advanced squamous cell lung carcinoma (minimum of stage IIIb). Station 4R was negative for malignant cells.

Learning Points

- The rationale for EUS-B-FNA in these three cases was to have a better procedure tolerance. EUS-B-FNA was performed in the first case as it required lower doses of sedation and had a lower risk of hypoxaemia in high-risk individuals (especially in a patient with emphysaema, multiple brain metastases, and the presence of pericardial effusion). EUS-B-FNA is also an option especially when patients desaturate during EBUS-TBNA. It also provides more flexibility in sampling, especially when dealing with lesions near the segmental bronchus.
- When combined, EBUS and EUS-B increase the diagnostic yields in the diagnosis and staging of lung cancer and have been recommended in the guidelines [1].
- The combined technique enables the augmentation of diagnostic potentials all under one sitting by a single operator [2].

Video

EUS-B-FNA was performed on subcarinal lymph node (Station 7) for Case A and

EUS-B- FNA of the left lower lobe mass for Case B.

CONSENT FOR PUBLICATION

Not applicable.

CONFLICT OF INTEREST

The authors declare no conflict of interest, financial or otherwise.

ACKNOWLEDGEMENT

Declared none.

REFERENCES

[1] Vilmann P, Clementsen P, Colella S, *et al.* Combined endobronchial and esophageal endosonography for the diagnosis and staging of lung cancer: European Society of Gastrointestinal Endoscopy (ESGE) Guideline, in cooperation with the European Respiratory Society (ERS) and the European Society of Thoracic Surgeons (ESTS). Endoscopy 2015; 47(6): 545-59.

[http://dx.doi.org/10.1055/s-0034-1392040] [PMID: 26030890]

[2] Soo CI, Kho SS, Ng BH, Tie ST. Endobronchial and endoscopic ultrasound: it only takes an echobronchoscope to tango. Respirol Case Rep 2019; 7(8): e00482.

[http://dx.doi.org/10.1002/rcr2.482] [PMID: 31467678]

Case 6

Linear EBUS Guided Trans-Vascular Needle Aspiration (EBUS-TVNA)

Tinku Joseph[1,*] and **Sathish C. Reddy**[1]

[1]*Division of Interventional Pulmonology, Amrita Institute of Medical Sciences, Kochi, India*

Keywords: CECT, Linear EBUS, EBUS-TVNA, Mediastinal lymphadenopathy, Transpulmonary.

Presentation

A 64-year-old lady was initially evaluated in the gastrosurgery department for anorexia and abdominal pain of 1 month duration and for associated weight loss. Upper gastrointestinal endoscopy showed mild gastritis. Later, she was evaluated with CECT abdomen which was normal with lower chest cuts showing a soft tissue density lesion measuring 19x16mm seen in the anteromedial segment of the left lower lobe, adjacent to the pericardium. She was further evaluated with whole body PET CT which showed abnormally increased FDG uptake in the soft tissue density lesion in the anteromedial basal segment of left lower lobe. Hence, she was referred to our department for further evaluation.

Comorbidities

No known comorbidities.

Chest Imaging

CXR showed a retrocardiac lesion (Fig. **1**).

CECT abdomen with lower chest cuts.

A soft tissue density lesion measuring 19x16mm is seen in the anteromedial segment of the left lower lobe, adjacent to the pericardium (Fig. **2**). No significant abnormality in the abdomen.

*__Corresponding author Tinku Joseph:__ Division of Interventional Pulmonology, Amrita Institute of Medical Sciences, Kochi, India; E-mail: tinkujoseph2010@gmail.com

Jamalul Azizi Abdul Rahaman & Tinku Joseph (Eds.)

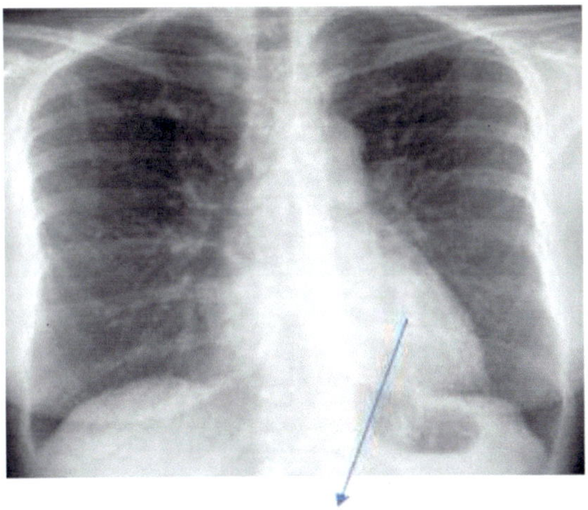

Fig. (1). CXR: Retrocardiac lesion.

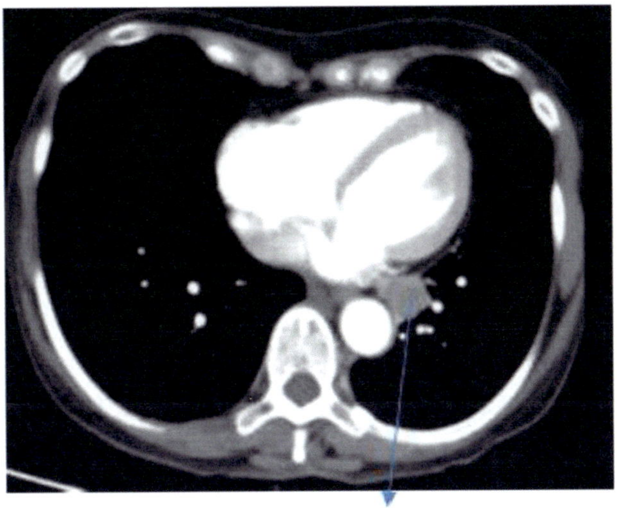

Fig. (2). CECT Chest: Mass lesion in left lower lobe.

Whole Body PET CT:

- Abnormal increased FDG uptake noted in soft tissue density lesion in anteromedial basal segment of left lower lobe (Fig. **3**).

- Abnormal increased FDG uptake seen in hypodense nodule in lower pole of left lobe of thyroid gland.

- Abnormal increased focal FDG uptake seen in following sites at the level of D10, at D11 vertebral level, crural thickening at the level of L1 vertebra.

- Abnormal increased FDG uptake seen in lytic lesion involving glenoid of left scapula and left iliac bone.

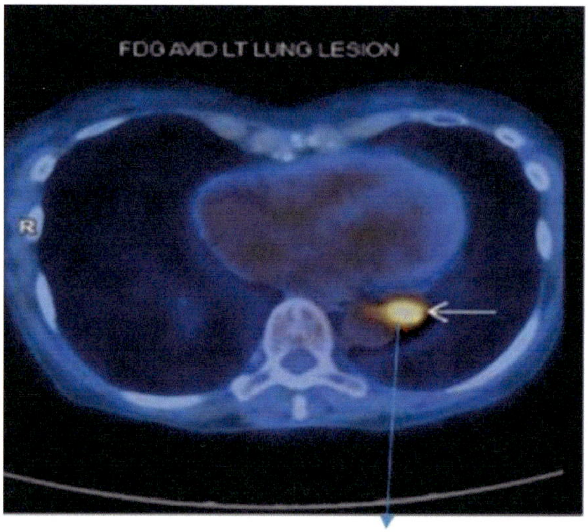

Fig. (3). FDG avid mass lesion in left lower lobe.

Intervention

Under general anaesthesia, she was intubated with 8.5F endotracheal tube and flexible bronchoscopy was done, which showed mucosal irregularity at the medial basal segment of left lower lobe. Linear EBUS showed mass lesion (24x18mm) at left hilar region behind the left main pulmonary artery (Fig. **4**). No other mediastinal lymph nodes were detected. In view of absence of other mediastinal lymph nodes to sample and the presence of pulmonary artery between the airway and mass lesion, a transvascular approach (EBUS-TVNA) was used to sample the mass lesion (Fig. **5**). Multiple TBNA samples were taken from the mass lesion through transpulmonary artery approach. 21G EBUS needle was used for the procedure. Once the site of entry was finalized, the needle was advanced into the lesion traversing the pulmonary artery. Once the needle was in the lesion, the stylet was removed and the needle was moved back and forth for 5 times with application of suction. After each pass, the airway was examined for bleeding and vessel was examined for haematoma. Adequate haemostasis was achieved with cold saline and adrenaline.

Complications

No immediate or delayed post-procedure complications.

Post-Intervention

EBUS-TVNA cytology showed the presence of malignant cells favoring adenocarcinoma.

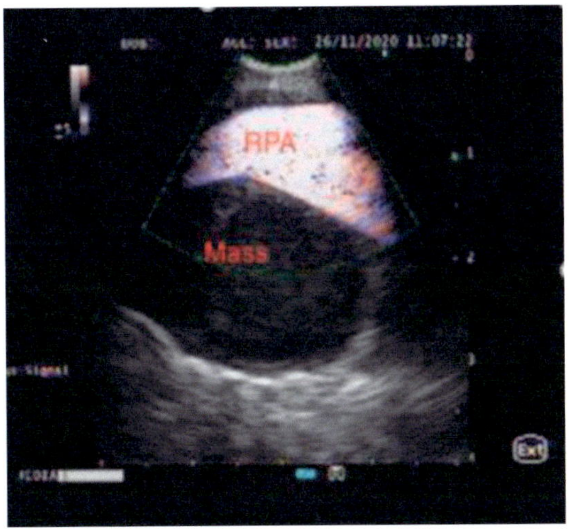

Fig. (4). Linear EBUS (Doppler mode) showing a lesion beyond the right main pulmonary artery.

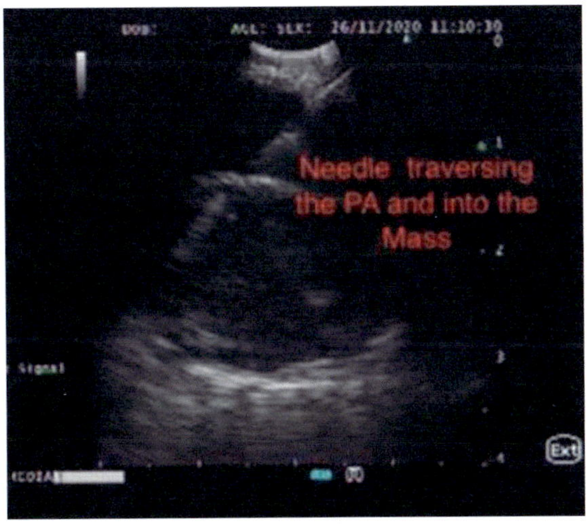

Fig. (5). EBUS-TVNA.

Learning Points

- Using transvascular approach expands the stations and areas in the mediastinum amenable to biopsy during EBUS.
- EBUS-TVNA appears to be a relatively safe procedure in skilled hands, but safety precautions with strict adherence to protocols and patient selection are advised [1].

CONSENT FOR PUBLICATION

Not applicable.

CONFLICT OF INTEREST

The authors declare no conflict of interest, financial or otherwise.

ACKNOWLEDGEMENT

Declared none.

REFERENCE

[1] Perathur AM, Joseph T, Nair SR, Varma U. To Do or Not to Do—That Is the Question". transvascular needle aspiration during EBUS (EBUS-TVNA) with review of the literature. Adv Respir Med 2021; 89(4): 386-91.

Case 7

Radial EBUS

Novel Flexible Ultrathin Cryoprobe in the Biopsy of SPN under Radial Endobronchial Ultrasound Guidance

Kho Sze Shyang[1,*], **Mona Zaria Nasaruddin**[1] and **Jamalul Azizi Abdul Rahaman**[1]

[1] *Department of Pulmonology, Serdang Hospital, Selangor, Malaysia*

Keywords: Radial endobronchial ultrasound, cryobiopsy, Ultrathin cryoprobe, solitary pulmonary nodule, Bronchoscopy.

Presentation

A 65-year-old gentleman with intermittent cough for one-month duration. No constitutional symptoms or family history of malignancy. Flexible bronchoscopy at the referring centre did not reveal endobronchial lesions. CT guided transthoracic needle aspiration only revealed necrotic tissue.

Comorbidities

Active smoker of 20 pack years.

Chest Imaging

Plain CXR and CECT thorax demonstrated a spiculated SPN measuring 2.20 x 2.09cm (Figs. **1a** and **b**). 18F-FDG PET/ CT scan confirmed hypermetabolic activity. Primary lung cancer was suspected.

Intervention

Flexible bronchoscopy showed no intraluminal lesion (Fig. **2a**). Under rigid bronchoscopy and total intravenous anaesthesia (propofol and remi-fentanyl), the target lesion was localized to RB2biα (anterior subsegment of the posterior segment

*Corresponding author Kho Sze Shyang:** Department of Pulmonology, Serdang Hospital, Selangor, Malaysia; E-mail: khosze@moh.gov.my

Jamalul Azizi Abdul Rahaman & Tinku Joseph (Eds.)

of RUL) (Fig. **2b**). Radial endobronchial ultrasound (rEBUS) and guide sheath (GS) examination confirmed an eccentrically orientated lesion with no significant vascularity (Figs. **3a** and **b**). Transbronchial biopsy (TBB) was performed with a 2.0mm flexible forceps (FB231-D, Tokyo, Japan). Target lesion was then re-localized with rEBUS/GS followed by the insertion of 1.1mm novel flexible ultrathin cryoprobe (ERBE, Medizintechnik, Tübingen, Germany) *via* the GS into the lesion under fluoroscopic guidance. The cryoprobe was activated for 5 seconds and the bronchoscope-GS-cryoprobe were removed en bloc to retrieve the tissue. The specimen was thawed in normal saline and measured around 4mm macroscopically. It was preserved in formalin solution immediately and sent for histopathological analysis. The GS was flushed with normal saline and sent for microbiological analysis.

Complications

Minimal bleeding at the ostium of RB2 which resolved spontaneously. The patient was extubated post-procedure and discharged the following day. No pneumothorax.

Post-Intervention

HPE showed necrotizing granulomatous inflammation from both forceps and cryobiopsies (Fig. **4**). The cryobiopsy specimen measured 4x2x1mm with minimal fragmentation compared to the forceps biopsy specimen. Mycobacterium tuberculosis was detected through PCR assay from the GS flushed specimen. The patient was initiated on standard anti-TB therapy.

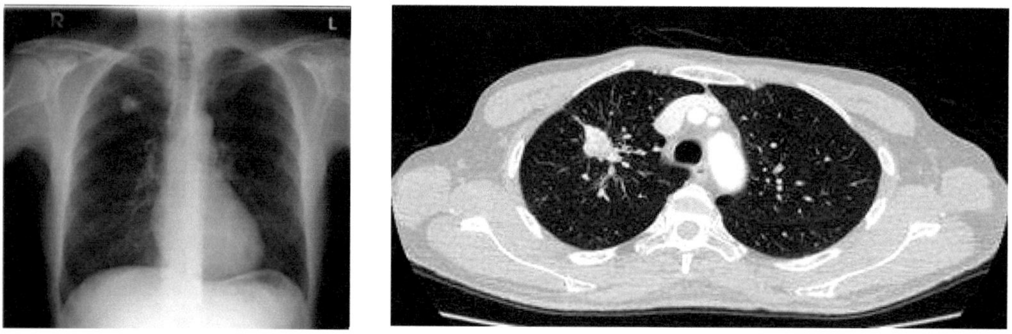

Fig. (1). (**a**) (Left) Plain CXR & (**b**) (Right) CECT thorax showing RUL spiculated SPN measuring 2.20 x 2.09cm.

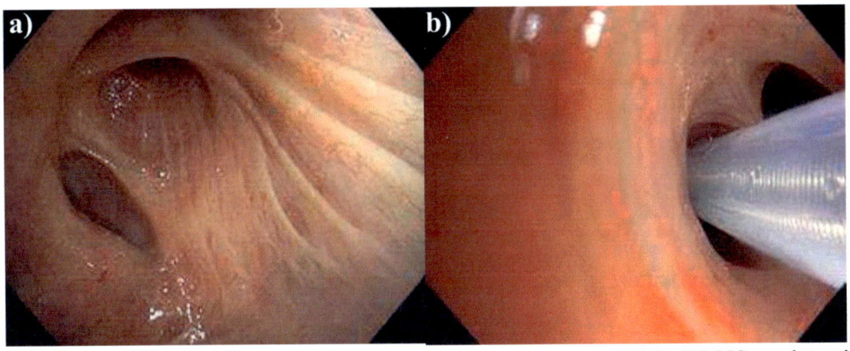

Fig. (2). (a) No intraluminal lesion was seen during bronchoscopy. (**b**) rEBUS probe with GS was inserted into anterior subsegment of RB2.

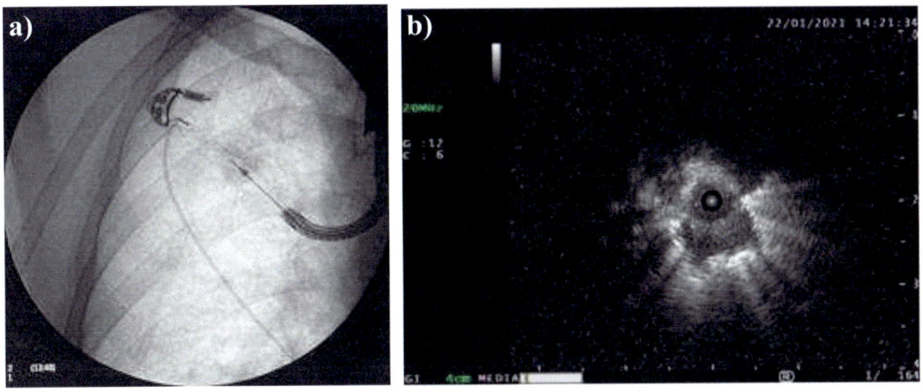

Fig. (3). (a) The lesion was successfully localized with single planar fluoroscopy. (**b**) rEBUS demonstrated an eccentrically orientated lesion.

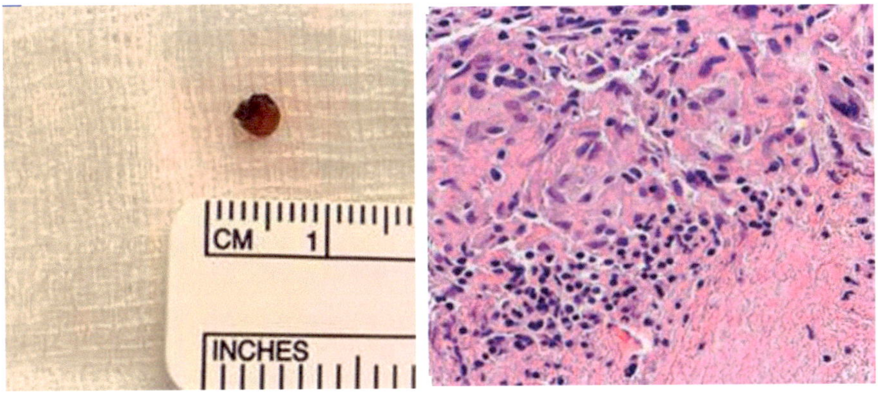

Fig. (4). Gross cryobiopsy specimen measuring around 4mm. HPE (hematoxylin and eosin stain, x 40 magnification) revealed chronic necrotizing granulomatous inflammation with epithelioid histiocytes and area of necrosis.

Learning Points

- The ability of the flexible cryoprobe to acquire larger specimens is frequently hindered by its stiffness to reach the highly angulated regions of the lungs. Our early experience demonstrated the ability of this ultrathin flexible cryoprobe in acquiring adequate tissue for the diagnosis of SPN [1]. Flexible ultrathin cryoprobe is a promising biopsy tool in the approach of peripheral pulmonary lesion. It may be particularly useful when the initial biopsy attempt was non-representative as demonstrated in our case by acquiring larger representative specimens. Further study to establish its diagnostic yield and safety is required. The patient was initially suspected to have lung cancer, but this was proven to be TB underscoring the importance of tissue diagnosis.

CONSENT FOR PUBLICATION

Not applicable.

CONFLICT OF INTEREST

The authors declare no conflict of interest, financial or otherwise.

ACKNOWLEDGEMENTS

The authors acknowledge the support received from Dr. Amizatul Aini Salleh, Department of Pathology, Serdang Hospital, Selangor, Malaysia.

REFERENCE

[1] Kho SS, Chai CS, Nyanti LE, Ismail AM, Tie ST. Combination of 1.1 mm flexible cryoprobe with conventional guide sheath and therapeutic bronchoscope in biopsy of apical upper lobe solitary pulmonary nodule. BMC Pulm Med 2020; 20(1): 158.
[http://dx.doi.org/10.1186/s12890-020-01199-3] [PMID: 32493437]

Case 8

Radial Endobronchial Ultrasound Guided Transbronchial Biopsy of SPN

Kho Sze Shyang[1,*], **Suhashini Ganapaty**[2], **Mona Zaria Nasaruddin**[1] and **Jamalul Azizi Abdul Rahaman**[1]

[1] *Department of Pulmonology, Serdang Hospital, Selangor, Malaysia*

[2] *Department of Pathology, Serdang Hospital, Selangor, Malaysia*

Keywords: Radial endobronchial ultrasound, cryobiopsy, transbronchial lung biopsy, solitary pulmonary nodule, bronchoscopy.

Presentation

A 59-year-old gentleman with significant weight loss over 3 months associated with a non-productive cough. He denied any fever or haemoptysis.

Comorbidities

End-stage renal failure on regular hemodialysis. Type 2 diabetes mellitus and essential hypertension.

Chest Imaging

CT thorax was grossly abnormal with diffuse perilymphatic nodules and a dominant spiculated lung nodule measuring 2.09 x 1.8cm at the lateral basal segment of left lower lobe (LB9) with a direct bronchus sign (Figs. **1a** and **b**). As it was a centrally located lesion adjacent to the heart, the patient was deemed unsuitable for a percutaneous approach.

Intervention

Under total intravenous anaesthesia, the patient was intubated with a 12mm rigid tracheoscope for airway access. Flexible bronchoscopy ruled out the presence of an endobronchial lesion (Fig. **2**). The target lesion was mapped beforehand to be at LB9b (medial subsegment of LB9) (Fig. **3**) which was confirmed by rEBUS/GS system demonstrating a concentrically orientated lesion (Figs. **4a** and **b**). Forceps biopsy was performed under fluoroscopic guidance through the GS. After forceps biopsy, an 8Fr endobronchial blocker was placed prophylactically at the ostium of LB9 through the

*Corresponding author Kho Sze Shyang: Department of Pulmonology, Serdang Hospital, Selangor, Malaysia; E-mail: khosze@moh.gov.my

Jamalul Azizi Abdul Rahaman & Tinku Joseph (Eds.)

suction port of the rigid bronchoscope. A 1.1mm flexible cryoprobe was then inserted into LB9b and activated for 5 seconds after placement was confirmed by fluoroscopy. The bronchoscope-cryoprobe unit was removed en bloc and the endobronchial blocker was inflated immediately (Figs. **5a** and **b**). The specimen was fixed in a formalin solution and sent to the laboratory immediately for analysis. The total procedure time was 45 minutes.

Complications

No bleeding or pneumothorax was encountered. The patient was discharged home well the following day.

Post-Intervention

HPE revealed fibrous tissue infiltrated by malignant cells which were arranged in solid clusters and focal acinar patterns. Immunohistochemistry examination showed positivity towards TTF-1 and p40 consistent with adenocarcinoma of the lung (Fig. **6**). A sensitizing mutation on exon 19 was detected on the epidermal growth factor receptor (EGFR). The patient was referred to the oncologist for consideration of TKI therapy.

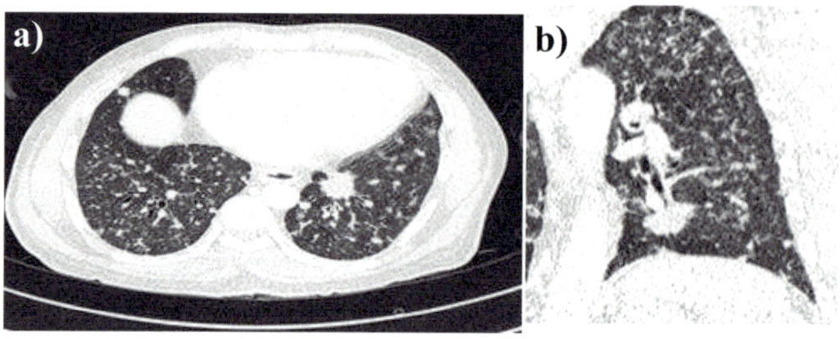

Fig. (1). (**a**) Axial CT Thorax. (**b**) Sagittal CT thorax.

CT thorax demonstrated a lung nodule measuring 2.09 x 1.8cm in LB9 with direct bronchus sign.

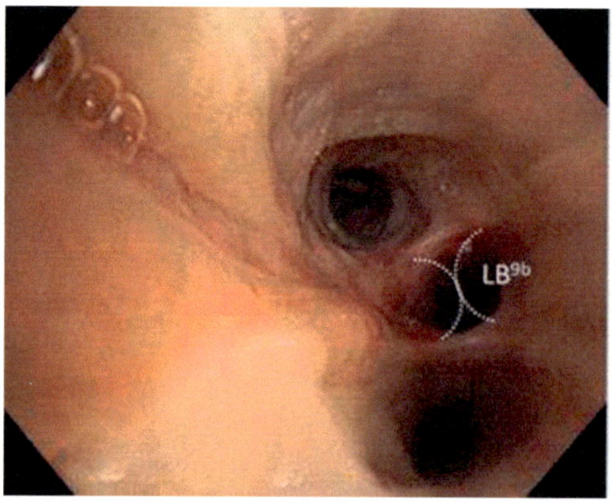

Fig. (2). No intraluminal lesion was encountered during airway examination.

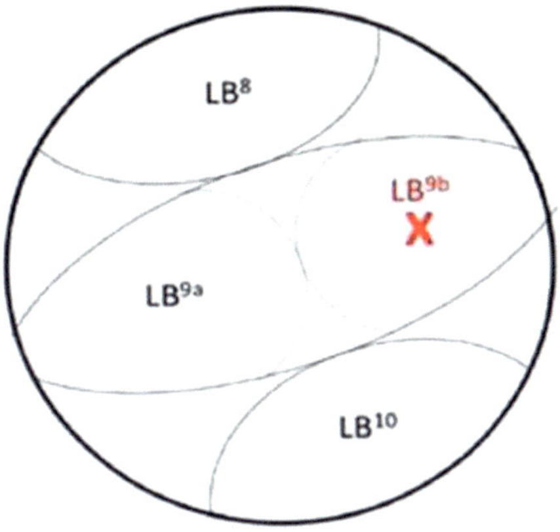

Fig. (3). The target lesion was mapped to LB9b (medial subsegment of LB9).

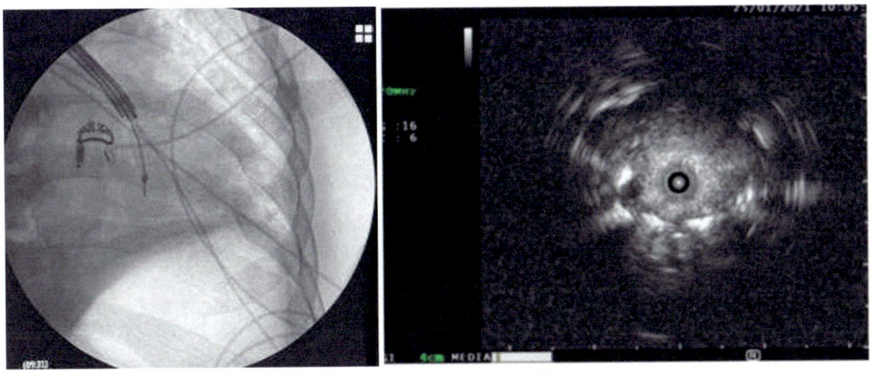

(a) **(b)**

Fig. (4). (a and b). A concentric target was localized by rEBUS and GS at the pre-planned subsegment under fluoroscopic guidance.

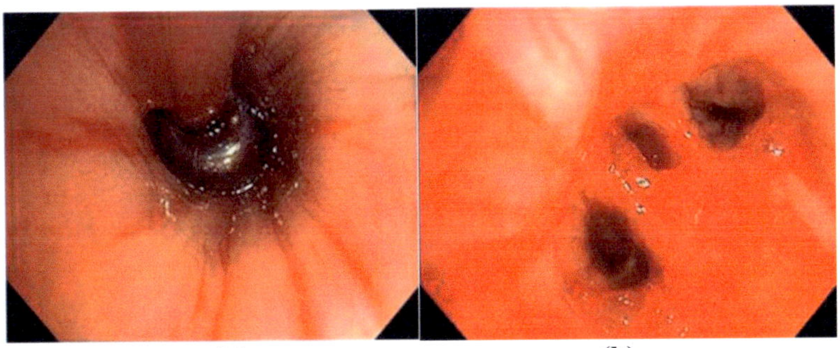

(a) **(b)**

Fig. (5). (**a** and **b**) Prophylactic endobronchial blocker was inflated immediately when the cryo-probe was retracted. No active bleeding was observed upon deflation of the endobronchial blocker.

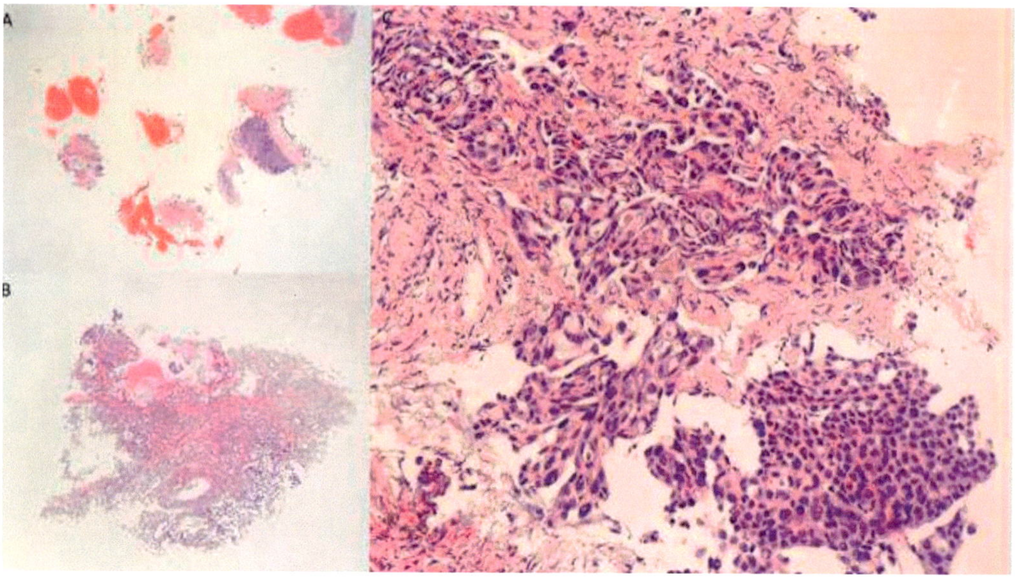

Fig. (6). Panel A demonstrated fragmented specimen from forceps biopsy. Panel B showed high quality specimen from cryobiopsy with preserved architecture on low power view. Panel C showed fibrous tissue infiltrated by malignant cells arranged in solid clusters and focal acinar pattern. The malignant cells were moderately pleomorphic with desmoplastic stromal reaction (hematoxylin & eosin stain).

Learning Points

- EBUS guided transbronchial biopsy is a feasible technique for biopsy of SPN. In recent years, cryobiopsy is gaining popularity among bronchoscopists due to its ability to obtain adequate tissue for diagnosis and profiling of lung cancer, as demonstrated in our case. Cryobiopsy may be useful for a lesion which is orientated eccentrically or adjacently to the airway due to the ability to do lateral biopsy by obtaining a spherical core of tissue surrounding the tip of the cryoprobe when activated [1]. However, as bleeding remains a concern with cryobiopsy, prophylactic endobronchial blocker should be placed prior to cryobiopsy to allow effective control of bleeding. Performing rEBUS guided transbronchial cryobiopsy *via* rigid bronchoscopy allows the operator to place an endobronchial blocker at the same time to control bleeding after cryobiopsy.

CONSENT FOR PUBLICATION

Not applicable.

CONFLICT OF INTEREST

The authors declare no conflict of interest, financial or otherwise.

ACKNOWLEDGEMENTS

The authors acknowledge the support received from Dr. Suhashini Ganapaty, Department of Pathology, Serdang Hospital, 43000 Serdang, Selangor, Malaysia.

REFERENCE

[1] Kho SS, Chan SK, Yong MC, Tie ST. Performance of transbronchial cryobiopsy in eccentrically and adjacently orientated radial endobronchial ultrasound lesions. ERJ Open Res 2019; 5(4): 00135-2019.
[http://dx.doi.org/10.1183/23120541.00135-2019] [PMID: 31649952]

Case 9

Manual Bronchial Branch Reading Technique in the Localization of Peripheral Pulmonary Lesion

Kho Sze Shyang[1,2,*] and **Tie Siew Teck**[1]

[1] *Division of Respiratory Medicine, Sarawak General Hospital, Kuching, Malaysia*

[2] *Department of Pulmonology, Serdang Hospital, Selangor, Malaysia*

Keywords: Radial endobronchial ultrasound, Bronchoscopy, Bronchial branch reading, Navigational bronchoscopy, Airway mapping.

Presentation

A 64-year-old gentleman was referred by the oncology team for the evaluation of an enlarging SPN noted during a surveillance scan.

Comorbidities

A known case of stage IA right middle lobe adenocarcinoma of the lung in which curative right middle lobectomy was performed 12 months prior to the current presentation.

Chest Imaging

CT thorax showed a solid, spiculated 1.97 x 1.80cm SPN in the anterior segment of the right upper lobe (Fig. **1**). The target lesion demonstrated a direct bronchus sign and was situated in the middle third of the right hemithorax. 18F-FDG PET/CT demonstrated hypermetabolic activity (Fig. **2**).

Intervention

The CT scan was analysed using a free open-source DICOM software (Radiant DICOM viewer version 5.0.0; Medixant, Poznań, Poland). The CT thorax in axial reconstruction was rotated 90° counterclockwise to simulate the standard

***Corresponding author Kho Sze Shyang:** Division of Respiratory Medicine, Sarawak General Hospital, Kuching, Malaysia and Department of Pulmonology, Serdang Hospital, Selangor, Malaysia; E-mail: khosze@moh.gov.my bronchoscopic view. The bronchus leading into the target lesion was traced proximally from the origin of RB3 (anterior segment of right upper lobe) and followed through until it entered the target lesion. All the bifurcations were identified sequentially and hand drawn into representative schematic diagrams, taking special consideration into the angle of bifurcation and size of the bronchus (Fig. **3**).

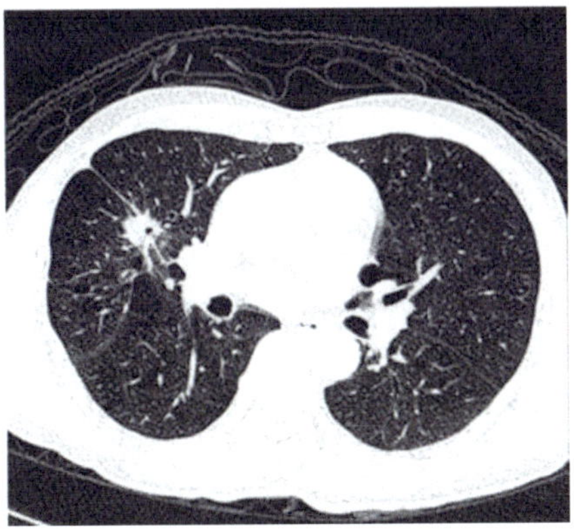

Fig. (1). Axial CT thorax - a right upper lobe SPN.

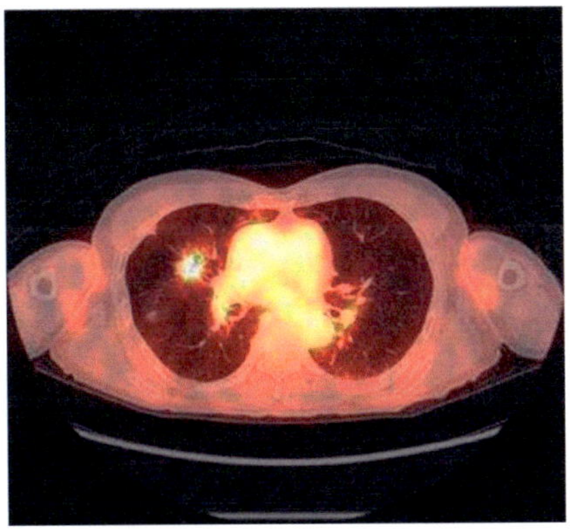

Fig. (2). PET scan – hypermetabolic activity.

Under conscious sedation (intravenous boluses of midazolam and fentanyl), no abnormalities were seen in the right middle lobe stump and the rest of the airway using a standard diagnostic flexible bronchoscope (BF-Q180, Olympus, Japan). A concentric lesion was localized to RB3bi (antero-lateral subsegment of RB3) using the 1.7mm radial endobronchial ultrasound probe (rEBUS UM-S20-17S, Olympus, Japan) following the pre-planned airway map (Fig. **4**). Transbronchial biopsy was then performed using a 2.0mm flexible forceps under fluoroscopic guidance (Fig. **5**).

Complications

Procedure was uneventful with no occurrence of pneumothorax or bleeding. The patient was discharged well six hours post-procedure.

Post-Intervention

Transbronchial lung biopsy confirmed adenocarcinoma of the lung. The immunohistochemistry and molecular profile (negative for EGFR and ALK) were similar to the initial malignancy; a decision of metastatic disease was made after a tumor board multidisciplinary discussion and the patient was managed by the oncology team subsequently.

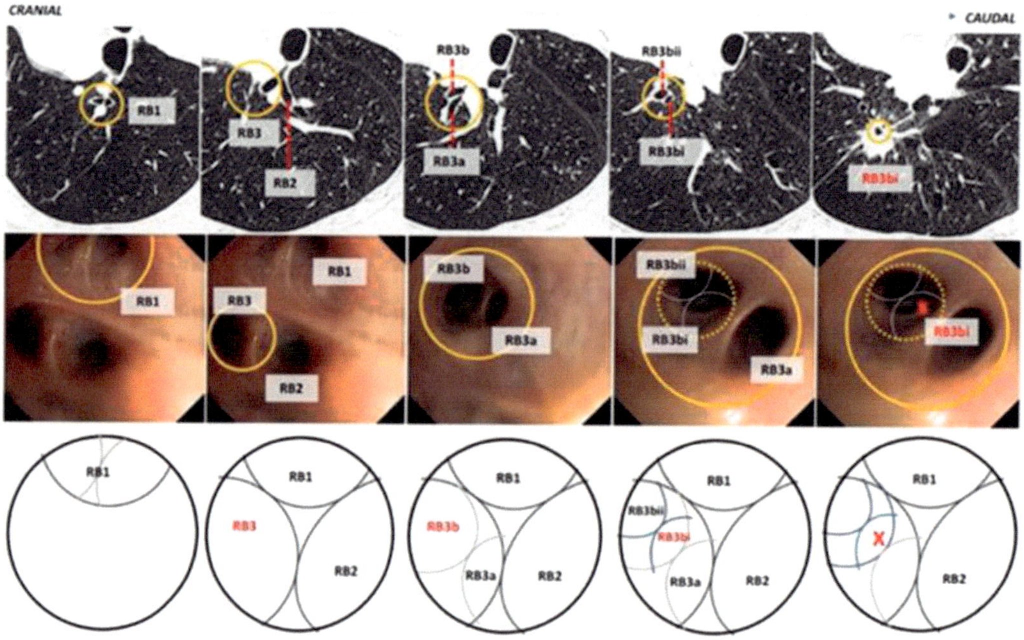

Fig. (3). CT thorax in axial reconstruction rotated in 90° counterclockwise direction. All bifurcations leading to the target lesion were analyzed and marked and hand-drawn into a schematic airway map which was comparable to the actual bronchoscopic view.

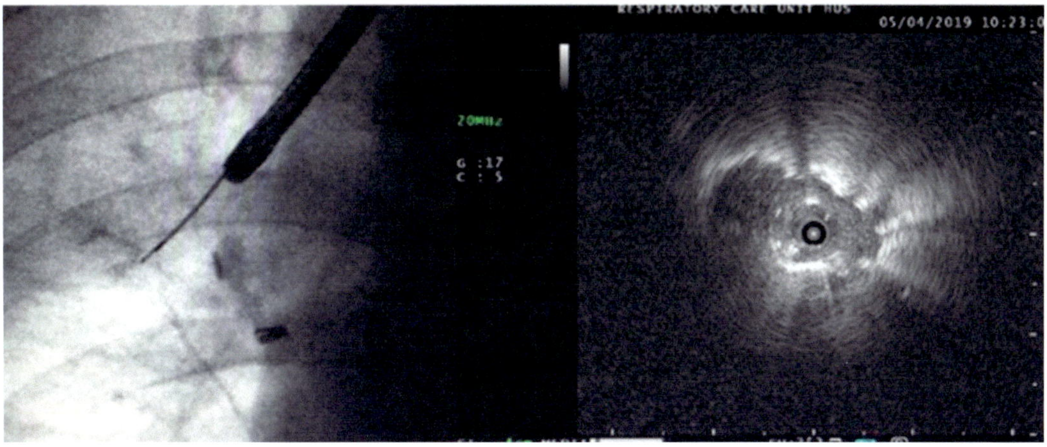

Fig. (4). Concentric rEBUS lesion was identified at the pre-planned subsegment under fluoroscopic guidance using a standard diagnostic flexible bronchoscope.

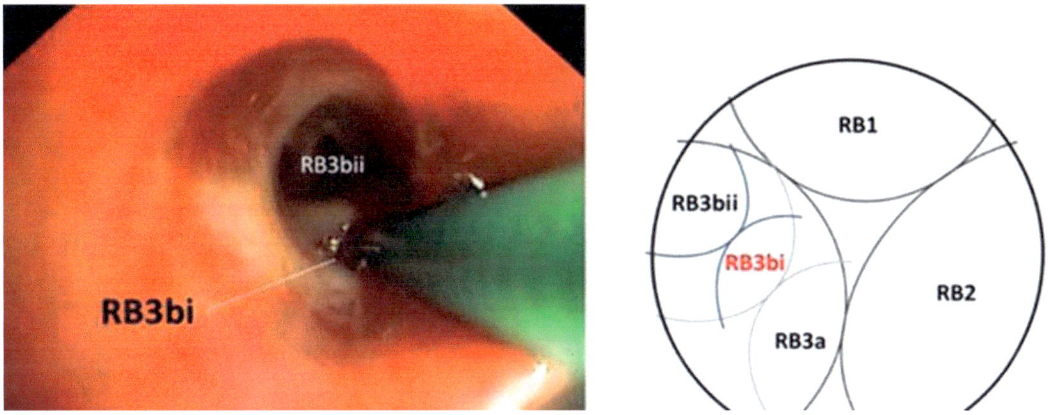

Fig. (5). Transbronchial lung biopsy was performed using a flexible forceps through RB3bi.

Learning Points

- Manual bronchial branch reading technique which was pioneered by Professor Dr. Noriaki Kurimoto is a feasible technique for SPN localization [1]. Our early experience with this technique demonstrated 98.9% navigational success rate with a diagnostic yield of 88.8% especially for target lesion within five airway generations [2]. Our case demonstrated the feasibility of this technique even in a patient with a history of major anatomical resection. Further prospective randomised studies are needed to validate manual bronchial branch reading technique as a sole navigational tool in the evaluation of SPN.

CONSENT FOR PUBLICATION

Not applicable.

CONFLICT OF INTEREST

The authors declare no conflict of interest, financial or otherwise.

ACKNOWLEDGEMENT

Declared none.

REFERENCES

[1] Kurimoto N, Morita K. Bronchial Branch Tracing. Singapore: Springer Nature Singapore Pte. Ltd. 2020.

[http://dx.doi.org/10.1007/978-981-13-9905-3]

[2] Kho SS, Nyanti LE, Chai CS, *et al.* Feasibility of manual bronchial branch reading technique in navigating conventional rEBUS bronchoscopy in the evaluation of peripheral pulmonary lesion. Clin Respir J 2020; 2020 online ahead of print.

[http://dx.doi.org/10.1111/crj.13297] [PMID: 33113256]

Case 10

USG Chest & Guided Procedures

Peripheral Lung Mass with Ultrasound Assisted Percutaneous Lung Biopsy

Muhammad Redzwan S. Rashid Ali[1,*]

[1] *KPJ Johor Specialist Hospital, Johor Bahru, Malaysia*

Keywords: Chronic obstructive pulmonary disease (COPD), Computerized Tomography (CT), Percutaneous biopsy, Squamous cell cancer, Ultrasonography (USG).

Presentation

A 52-year-old man. Active smoker. Cough associated with loss of appetite and weight for 2 months.

Comorbidities

Chronic obstructive pulmonary disease (COPD) with persistent wheezing and bronchospasm.

Chest Imaging

CXR showed an LUL mass with consolidation. CT Thorax demonstrated a left hilar mass with adjacent collapse consolidation (Fig. **1**).

Flexible bronchoscopy was planned but was canceled in view of persistent bronchospasm despite on optimal medical and inhaler therapy.

Intervention

The patient underwent USG assisted percutaneous biopsy for histological confirmation and mutation testing.

* **Corresponding author Muhammad Redzwan S. Rashid Ali:** KPJ Johor Specialist Hospital, Johor Bahru, Malaysia; E-mail: redzwanrashid@gmail.com

Jamalul Azizi Abdul Rahaman & Tinku Joseph (Eds.)

Complications

None.

Post-Intervention

HPE confirmed squamous cell carcinoma with mutation testing for EGFR, ALK, ROS and PD-L1 being negative (Fig. **2**). Referred to the thoracic oncologist for chemoradiotherapy.

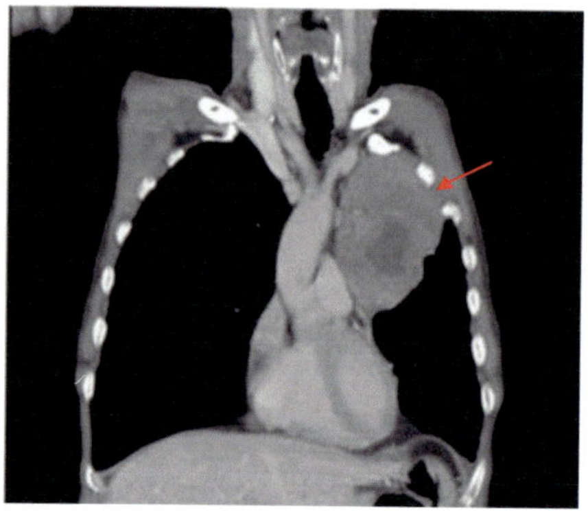

Fig. (1). Coronal CT thorax showing a large left hilar mass with compression of the left upper lobe and chest wall (red arrow).

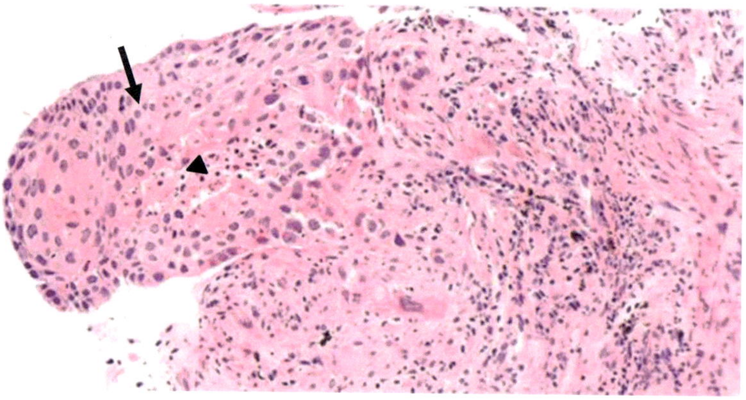

Fig. (2). The cells display moderately pleomorphic hyperchromatic nuclei with occasional prominent nucleoli and moderate eosinophilic cytoplasm. Individual cell keratinization (arrowhead) and intercellular bridges (arrow) are appreciated (Haematoxylin and eosin stain, original magnification x 400).

Learning Points

- Patients with persistent bronchospasm due to severe COPD may present with peripheral lung masses with collapse consolidation. The risk of bronchoscopic biopsy aggravating the bronchospasm is significant and frequently such patients are deemed not fit for bronchoscopy. A less risky option especially if the lesion is peripherally located is USG guided percutaneous biopsy to obtain tissue diagnosis [1].

Video

USG assisted biopsy of the consolidated lung and mass was performed using an 18G x 11cm biopsy needle.

CONSENT FOR PUBLICATION

Not applicable.

CONFLICT OF INTEREST

The authors declare no conflict of interest, financial or otherwise.

ACKNOWLEDGEMENTS

The author acknowledges the support received from Dr. Ikmal Hisyam Bakrin, Department of Pathology, Faculty of Medicine and Health Sciences, Universiti Putra Malaysia, 43400 Serdang, Selangor, Malaysia and Dr. Sanveer Singh Dhillon, KPJ Johor Specialist Hospital, Johor, Malaysia.

REFERENCE

[1] DiBardino DM, Yarmus LB, Semaan RW. Transthoracic needle biopsy of the lung. J Thorac Dis 2015; 7(Suppl. 4): S304-16.
[http://dx.doi.org/10.3978/j.issn.2072-1439.2015.12.16] [PMID: 26807279]

Case 11

Chest Wall and Pleural Lesion with Ultrasound Assisted Percutaneous Biopsy

Muhammad Redzwan S. Rashid Ali[1,*]

[1] *KPJ Johor Specialist Hospital, Johor Bahru, Malaysia*

Keywords: Lung entrapment, Indwelling pleural catheter (IPC), Adenocarcinoma, Trapped lung, Percutaneous biopsy, Chest wall nodule.

Presentation

A 46-year-old non-smoker, Indonesian lady presented with progressive cough, loss of weight and loss of appetite for 3 months. She was treated as recurrent left-sided pleural effusion with lung entrapment. She had been on prolonged pleural pigtail drainage and was referred for an indwelling pleural catheter (IPC) with suspected malignant pleural effusion and trapped lung. Pleural fluid cytology was suspicious of atypical malignant cells possibly adenocarcinoma. Repeat pleural fluid cytology confirmed adenocarcinoma noma but it was not adequate for mutation testing. IPC was inserted uneventfully.

Comorbidities

None.

Chest Imaging

CXR showed a trapped left lung with IPC *in situ* (Fig. **1**). CT thorax revealed a large loculated left pleural effusion with a mass seen in the collapsed left lower lobe (Fig. **2**).

Subsequent PET CT was done for staging and this revealed hypermetabolic FDG avid pleural thickening and irregularity, FDG avid mass within the collapsed left lower lobe and small foci of FDG avid nodule in the chest wall corresponding to

*Corresponding author Muhammad Redzwan S. Rashid Ali: KPJ Johor Specialist Hospital, Johor Bahru, Malaysia; E-mail: redzwanrashid@gmail.com

the previous pigtail drainage site. IPC was *in situ* with large loculated effusion and trapped lung.

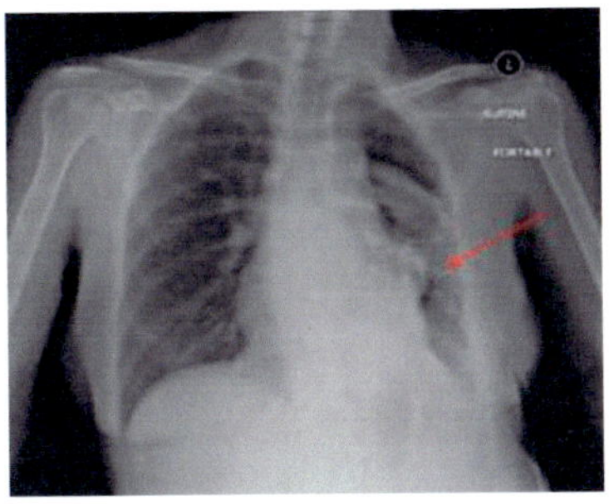

Fig. (1). CXR - IPC *in situ* (red arrow) with trapped left lung despite adequate pleural drainage.

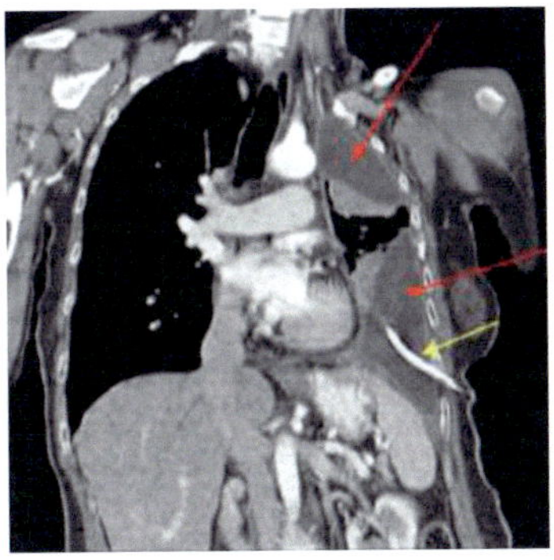

Fig. (2). Coronal CT Thorax: Large loculated pleural effusion (red arrows) with parietal pleural thickening and collapse of left upper lobe and left lower lobe. IPC *in situ* (yellow arrow).

Intervention

Chest wall nodule biopsy under USG guidance was performed to confirm the histology and for mutation testing.

Complications

None.

Post-Intervention

HPE confirmed metastatic adenocarcinoma. Mutation testing confirmed ALK gene rearrangement. She was referred for consideration of anaplastic lymphoma kinase (ALK) inhibitor (Alectinib) and was on periodic drainage of IPC for the malignant pleural effusion.

Learning Points

- In certain cases where the diagnosis of malignant pleural effusion or metastases has not been confirmed histologically, it may be necessary to repeat the pleural fluid cytology. If this is still inconclusive or the tissue is inadequate for mutation driver testing analysis, USG-guided percutaneous needle biopsy of any abnormal pleural nodules, thickening or chest wall nodules (metastases) is recommended especially if the patient is not fit for invasive medical thoracoscopy [1].

Video

Imaging shows complex hypoechoic chest wall nodule. USG-guided biopsy done with 18G X 9cm needle.

CONSENT FOR PUBLICATION

Not applicable.

CONFLICT OF INTEREST

The authors declare no conflict of interest, financial or otherwise.

ACKNOWLEDGEMENTS

The author acknowledges the support received from Dr. Sanveer Singh Dhillon, KPJ Johor Specialist Hospital, Johor, Malaysia.

REFERENCE

[1] Koegelenberg CFN, Diacon AH. Image-guided pleural biopsy. Curr Opin Pulm Med 2013; 19(4): 368-73.

[http://dx.doi.org/10.1097/MCP.0b013e32835f4c23] [PMID: 23719295]

Case 12

Lung Mass with Ultrasound Guided Percutaneous Biopsy

Muhammad Redzwan S. Rashid Ali[1,*]

[1] *KPJ Johor Specialist Hospital, Johor Bahru, Malaysia*

Keywords: Squamous cell carcinoma, Positron-emission tomography (PET), fluorodeoxyglucose (FDG), Ultrasonography USG), Percutaneous biopsy, Neoadjuvant chemotherapy.

Presentation

A 52-year-old smoker presented with progressive cough, loss of appetite and loss of weight for 4 months.

Comorbidities

Nil.

Chest Imaging

CXR revealed a left lung mass.

PET and CT Thorax showed a large well defined encapsulated cystic/necrotic mass occupying almost the entire left lower lobe (Fig. **1**), peripheral irregular rim of soft tissue with FDG avidity (SUVmax 14.62) measuring 13.35 x 9.90 x 15.58cm and multiple FDG avid mediastinal lymph nodes (Fig. **2**).

Intervention

USG-guided percutaneous biopsy (Fig. **3**).

[*]**Corresponding author Muhammad Redzwan S. Rashid Ali:** KPJ Johor Specialist Hospital, Johor Bahru, Malaysia; E-mail: redzwanrashid@gmail.com

Jamalul Azizi Abdul Rahaman & Tinku Joseph (Eds.)

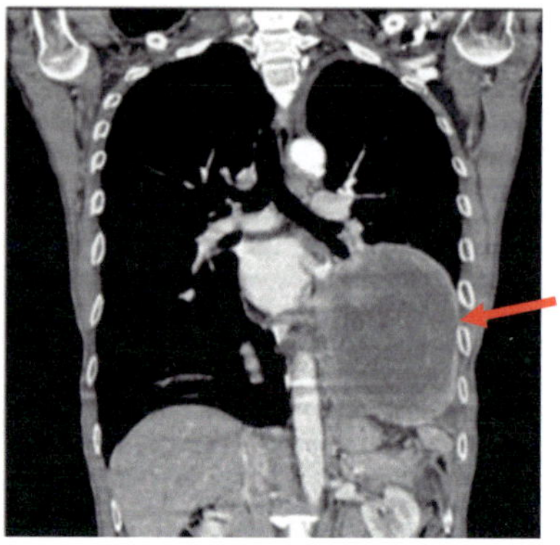

Fig. (1). Coronal CT Thorax showing a large left lower lobe mass with cystic and necrosis features (red arrow).

Complications

None.

Post-Intervention

HPE confirmed squamous cell carcinoma and the patient subsequently was referred to oncology for consideration of neoadjuvant chemotherapy and radiotherapy with possible surgical resection if deemed fit.

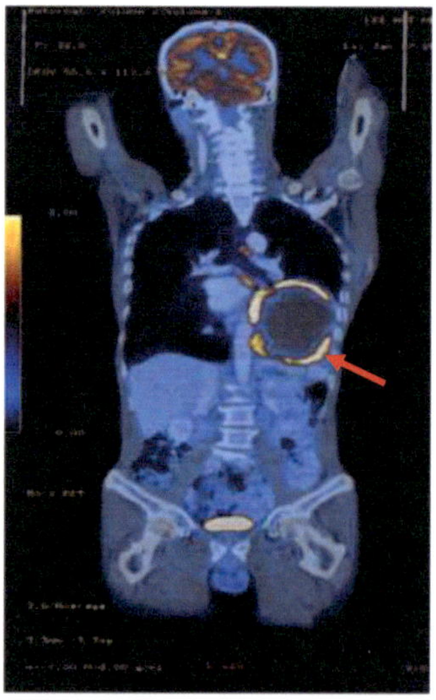

Fig. (2). PET CT thorax showing a large left lower lobe mass with irregular rim of FDG avidity (red arrow).

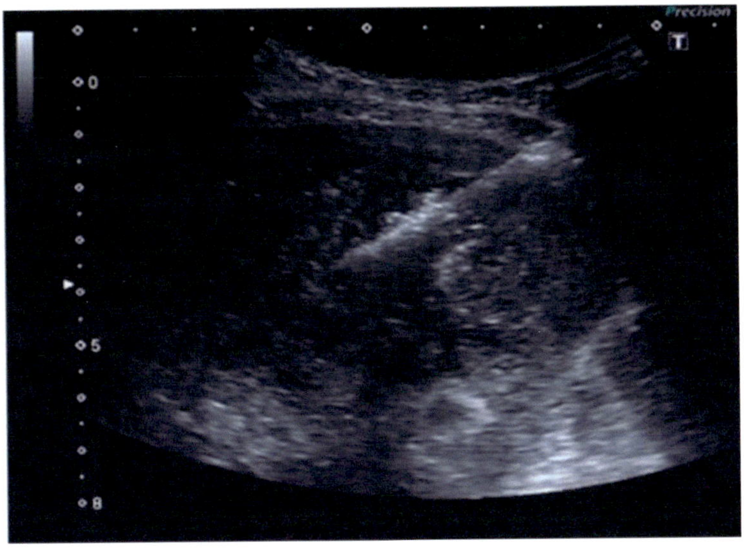

Fig. (3). Video image showing the left lower lobe mass and 18G x 10cm needle in the mass for biopsy.

Learning Points

- Transthoracic ultrasound guided percutaneous biopsy can be attempted if the patient is unable to undergo bronchoscopy or EBUS-guided evaluation of mediastinal nodes. Large lung masses located peripherally and abutting the pleura are usually easily accessible by USG and suitable for biopsy as illustrated in this case [1].

Video

The video shows real time biopsy of the left lower lobe mass with 18G x 10cm needle.

CONSENT FOR PUBLICATION

Not applicable.

CONFLICT OF INTEREST

The authors declare no conflict of interest, financial or otherwise.

ACKNOWLEDGEMENTS

The author acknowledges the support received from Dr. Sanveer Singh Dhillon, KPJ Johor Specialist Hospital, Johor, Malaysia.

REFERENCE

[1] Anzidei M, Porfiri A, Andrani F, *et al.* Imaging-guided chest biopsies: Techniques and clinical results. Insights Imaging 2017; 8(4): 419-28. [https://doi.org/10.1007/s13244-017-0561-6]

Case 13

Ultrasound Guided Percutaneous Biopsy of Mediastinal Mass

Muhammad Redzwan S. Rashid Ali[1,*]

[1] *KPJ Johor Specialist Hospital, Johor Bahru, Malaysia*

Keywords: Mediastinal mass, Thymoma, Percutaneous biopsy, Ultrasonography (USG), Neoplastic.

Presentation

A 46-year-old man, a social smoker with unexplained loss of weight, loss of appetite and focal left chest pain for 2 months. Clinical examination revealed focal percussive dullness over the left upper chest.

Comorbidities

Nil.

Chest Imaging

CXR showed a large left parahilar mass (Fig. **1**). CT Thorax showed a large solid well defined enhancing mass lesion in the left anterior mediastinum measuring 8.0x7.5x8.3cm (Fig. **2**). A few small specks of calcification seen within the mass. The suspicion was either teratoma or thymoma.

Intervention

USG-guided percutaneous biopsy (Fig. **3**).

Complications

None.

*****Corresponding author Muhammad Redzwan S. Rashid Ali:** KPJ Johor Specialist Hospital, Johor Bahru, Malaysia; E-mail: redzwanrashid@gmail.com

Jamalul Azizi Abdul Rahaman & Tinku Joseph (Eds.)

Post-Intervention

HPE revealed features in 2 strips of tumor tissues composed of neoplastic cells arranged in solid sheets and nesting pattern accompanied by variable amount of fibrotic stroma. The cells are mainly round to oval shape displaying mild to moderately pleomorphic vesicular nuclei with occasional small prominent nuclei and indistinct eosinophilic cytoplasm. The neoplastic cells were immunoreactive for CK AE1/ AE3 P63 and PAX8 suggestive of thymoma type AB (Fig. **4**).

He was referred to an oncologist for further assessment in view of chemoradiation and possible resection later.

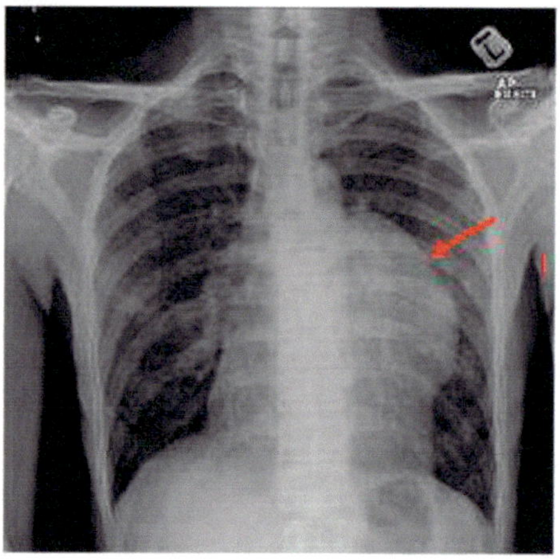

Fig. (1). CXR showing a large left parahilar mass (red arrow) with suspicion of anterior mediastinal mass.

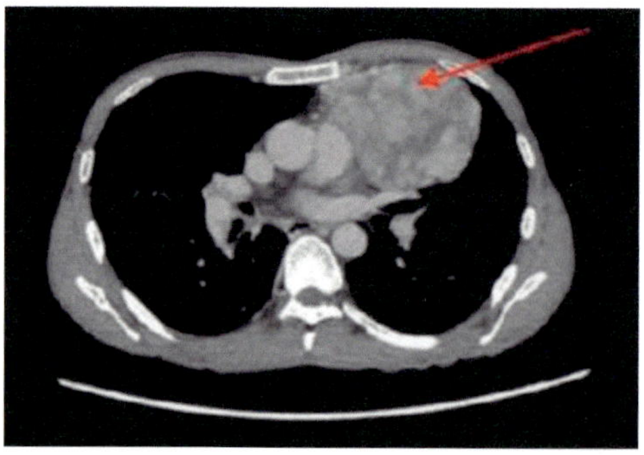

Fig. (2). Axial CT Thorax showing a large anterior well defined enhancing mass (red arrow) with suspicion of either teratoma or thymoma.

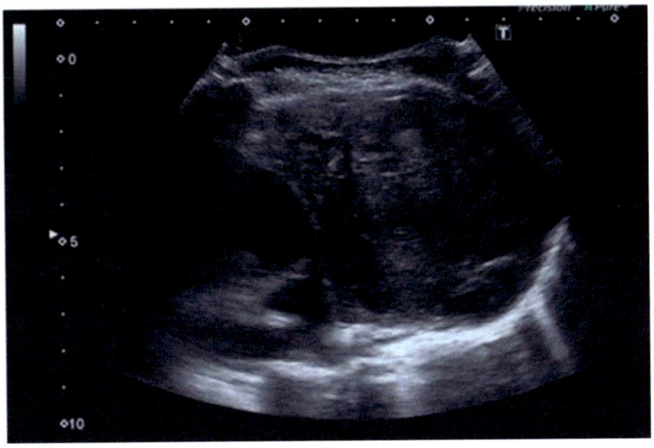

Fig. (3). USG guided biopsy image showing the mediastinal mass and 18G X 10cm biopsy needle subsequently inserted for sampling.

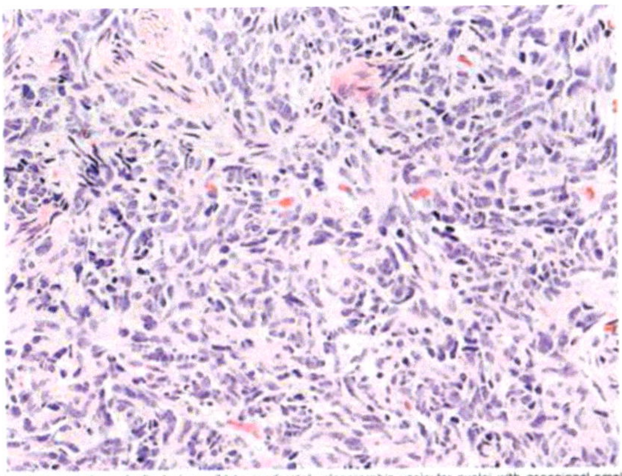

The cells are mainly round to oval shaped, displaying mild to moderately pleomorphic vesicular nuclei with occasional small prominent nuclei and indistinct eosinophilic cytoplasm . Occasional spindle shaped cells with normochromic nuclei are also appreciated. (Haematoxylin and eosin stain original magnification x 400)

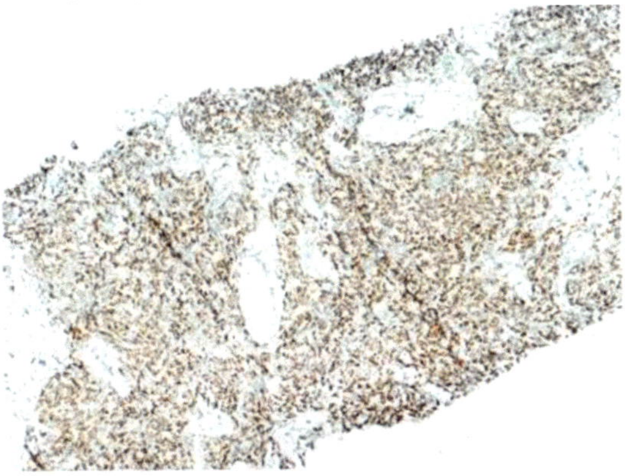

PAX8 nuclear positivity further support thymic in origin
(Immunohistochemistry study, original magnification x 100)

Fig. (4). The HPE.

Learning Points

- Large anterior mediastinal mass which are abutting the chest wall can be accessed for biopsy *via* USG guided percutaneous approach with good accuracy and adequate tissue for histological confirmation [1]. This obviates the need for more invasive biopsy methods such as mediastinoscopy or VATS.

Video

USG-guided biopsy of the mediastinal mass and 18G X 10cm biopsy needle inserted for sampling.

CONSENT FOR PUBLICATION

Not applicable.

CONFLICT OF INTEREST

The authors declare no conflict of interest, financial or otherwise.

ACKNOWLEDGEMENTS

The author acknowledges the support received from Dr. Ikmal Hisyam Bakrin, Department of Pathology, Faculty of Medicine and Health Sciences, Universiti Putra Malaysia, 43400 Serdang, Selangor, Malaysia and Dr. Sanveer Singh Dhillon, KPJ Johor Specialist Hospital, Johor, Malaysia.

REFERENCE

[1] Gupta S, Seaberg K, Wallace MJ, *et al.* Imaging-guided Percutaneous Biopsy of Mediastinal Lesions: Different Approaches and Anatomic Considerations. RadioGraphics 2005; 25(3): 763-86.
[http://dx.doi.org/10.1148/rg.253045030] [PMID: 15888624]

Case 14

Ultrasound Guided Percutaneous Trucut Biopsy of Chest Wall Mass

Tie Siew Teck[1,*] and **Chai Chan Sin**[1]

[1] *Division of Respiratory Medicine, Sarawak General Hospital, Kuching, Malaysia*

Keywords: Lung mass, Real time ultrasound guidance, Chest wall, Trucut biopsy, Complication.

Presentation

A 67-year-old gentleman, recently diagnosed with Stage 4 adenocarcinoma presented with liver, bone and dry pleural metastasis. Initial CT guided biopsy was not adequate for mutation analysis, hence the oncologist requested additional tissue sampling.

Comorbidities

A smoker with COPD, hypertension and old pulmonary TB 25 years ago.

Chest Imaging

CT thorax showed a solid mass at the left lower lobe abutting the chest wall (Fig. **1**).

Intervention

USG-guided percutaneous trucut biopsy using standard equipments (Figs. **2** and **3**). The step-by-step procedure is explained (Figs. **4** and **6**). Good cores were obtained (Fig. **7**).

*__Corresponding author Tie Siew Teck:__ Division of Respiratory Medicine, Sarawak General Hospital, Kuching, Malaysia; E-mail: tiest@moh.gov.my

Complications

Procedure was uneventful with no occurrence of pneumothorax or bleeding. The patient was discharged well six hours post procedure.

Post-Intervention

Trucut biopsy revealed lung adenocarcinoma. The patient was followed up by the oncology team.

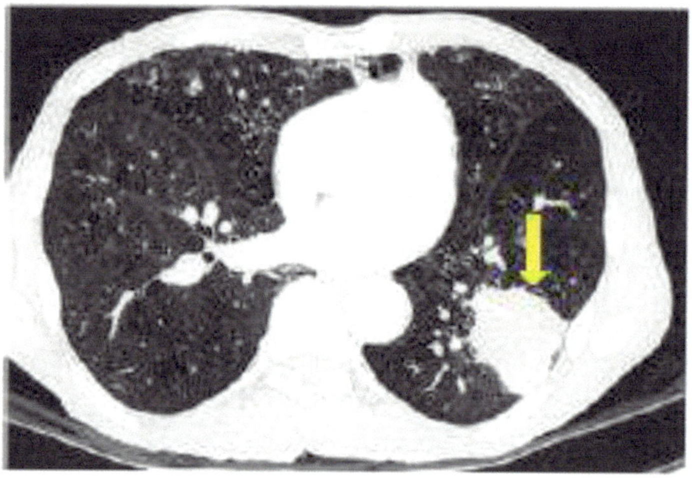

Fig. (1). Axial CT thorax showing a solid mass at the left lower lobe abutting the chest wall (yellow arrow).

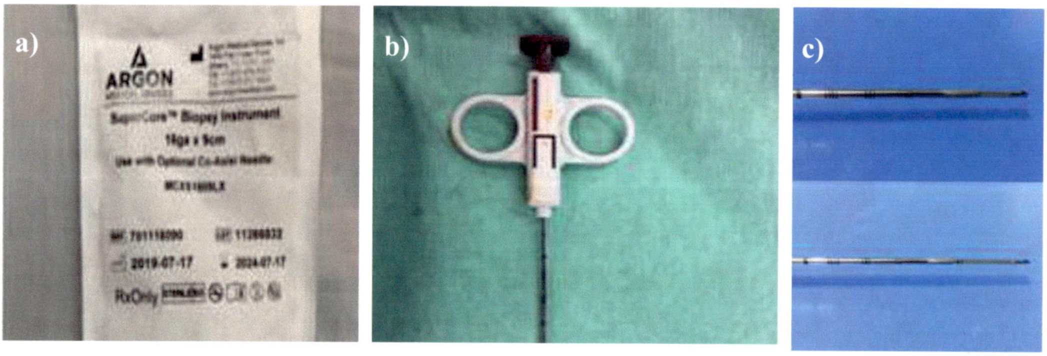

Fig. (2). Equipments for trucut biopsy. **a**) Semi-automatic trucut biopsy needle (Supercore^{TM} Argon Medical Devices Inc., USA). **b**) 18G, 9cm long trucut needle. **c**) Operator can choose a cutting length of 1cm or 2cm.

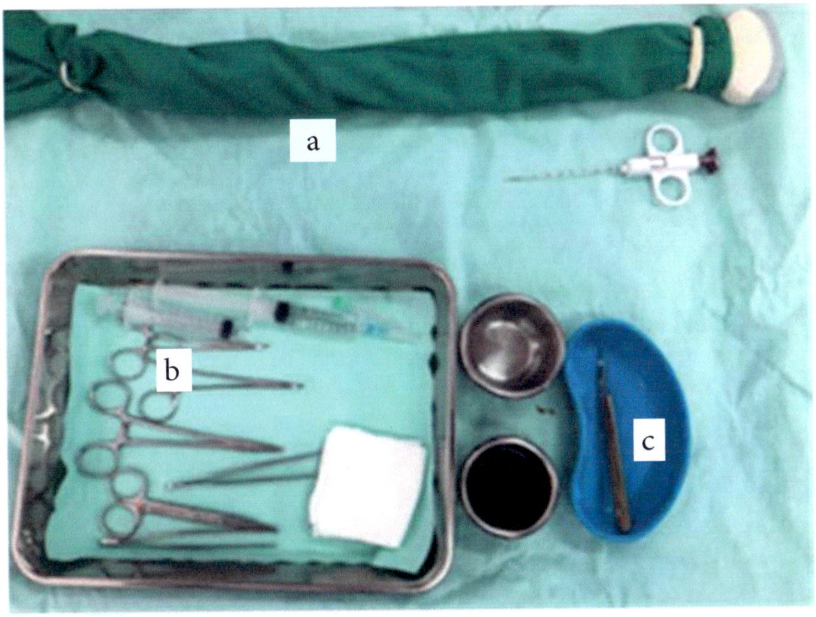

Fig. (3). The ultrasound probe is draped with sterile glove and sterile towel (**a**) Other instruments include injection needle, 10cc syringe (**b**) and a blade (**c**).

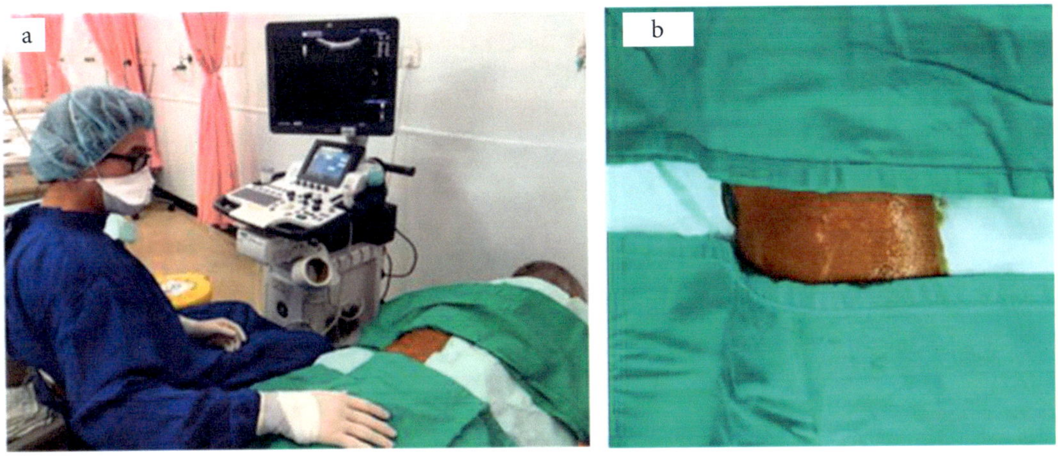

Fig. (**4**). (**a**) (Left) The procedure is performed in the thoracic endoscopy room, with the patient lying in a prone position. The operator sits on the right side of the patient. A small dose of midazolam and pethidine is given. Patient's heart rate, oxygen saturation and blood pressure are monitored continuously. (**b**) (Right) The biopsy site is cleaned with alcohol and iodine povidone and draped.

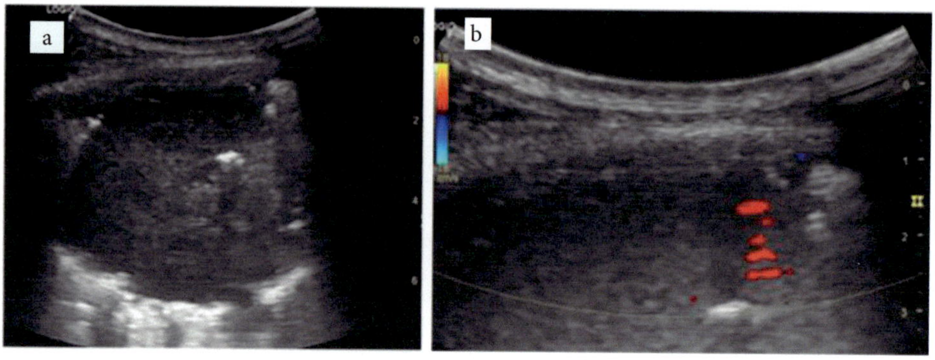

Fig. (5). (a) (Left) Initial ultrasound is performed to assess the size and vascularity. The operator also determines the point of entry and the needle trajectory. (**b**) (Right) Special attention is made to assess the intercostal artery at the point of entry by using ultrasound colour mode.

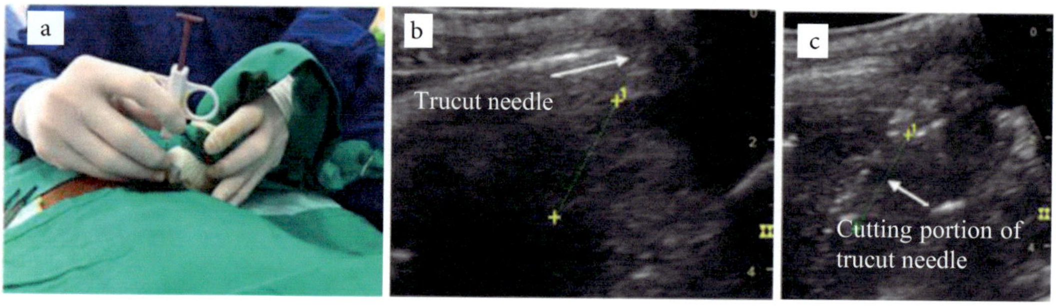

Fig. (6). (a) Once the point of entry is decided, the skin and the needle path are infiltrated with 5-10 ml of 1% lignocaine under ultrasound guidance. In this case, an "in-plane"method is deemed to be most appropriate. A small cut is subsequently made using a sharp blade at the site of entry. The trucut needle is inserted in a similar fashion. (**b**) The trucut needle is advanced until the tumor is reached. (**c**) The cutting portion of the needle is advanced (2cm in length in this case) and biopsy is taken.

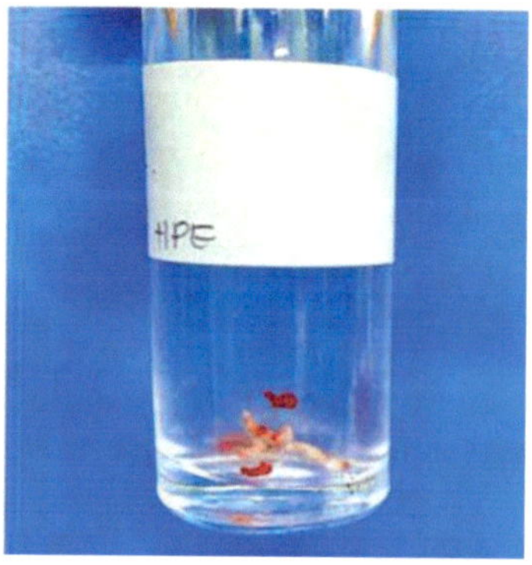

Fig. (7). 3-5 good cores of tissue are obtained.

Learning Points

- Ultrasound guided transthoracic trucut biopsy is a simple and fast method of tissue sampling for chest wall, pleural and lung lesion that is abutting the pleura. It also has a high diagnostic accuracy of 88.7% and safe with a pneumothorax risk of 4.4% [1].
- The advantage of ultrasound over CT guidance lies in the fact that ultrasound provides a continuous real-time guidance during the whole biopsy process. Therefore, avoidance of large vessels and necrotic areas as well as the accurate placement of biopsy needle becomes easier compared to CT guidance. The disadvantage is that it cannot detect biopsy lung lesion that is not in contact with the pleura.

CONSENT FOR PUBLICATION

Not applicable.

CONFLICT OF INTEREST

The authors declare no conflict of interest, financial or otherwise.

ACKNOWLEDGEMENT

Declared none.

REFERENCE

[1] DiBardino DM, Yarmus LB, Semaan RW. Transthoracic needle biopsy of the lung. J Thorac Dis 2015; 7(Suppl 4): S304-16.
[http://dx.doi.org/10.3978/j.issn.2072-1439.2015.12.16] [PMID: 26807279]

Case 15

Navigation Bronchoscopy (Biopsy, Dye Marking, Fiducial Marking)

One-Stop Lung Nodule Biopsy and Fiducial Marker Placement with Electromagnetic Navigation Bronchoscopy

Joyce W.Y. Chan[1], **Rainbow W.H. Lau**[1] and **Calvin S.H. Ng**[1,*]

[1] *Department of Surgery, The Chinese University of Hong Kong, N.T., Hong Kong SAR*

Keywords: Biopsy, Cone-Beam CT, Electromagnetic Navigation Bronchoscopy, Fiducial, Lung Nodule, Radiotherapy.

Presentation

Radiologically suspicious right lower lobe lung mass (4.4cm, SUVmax 4.3 on PET/CT). Biopsy *via* EBUS was insufficient for diagnosis. Patient was a poor surgical candidate due to poor lung function and advanced age.

Comorbidities

An 82-year-old lady, ex-smoker, GOLD Stage 3 COPD, diabetes, peripheral vascular disease.

Chest Imaging

CT scan showed a right lower lobe lung mass (Fig. **1**).

Intervention

Electromagnetic navigation bronchoscopy (ENB) biopsy of lesion was performed in the hybrid theatre with cone-beam CT [1]. Following ENB navigation, the tip of catheter reached within 1.3cm from the centre of lesion and pointing directly at it. Multiple FNA, triple-needle brush and biopsy with forceps were performed (Fig. **2**). Frozen section revealed adenocarcinoma.

*__Corresponding author Calvin S.H. Ng:__ Department of Surgery, The Chinese University of Hong Kong, N.T., Hong Kong SAR; E-mail: calvinng@surgery.cuhk.edu.hk

Subsequently, 3 Superlock™ fiducial markers (Nitinol Coil 4x7mm) were delivered to the lesion in 3 different positions to mark the lesion for SBRT (Fig. **3**).

Complications

None. Patient was discharged on post-operative day 1.

Post-Intervention

The intra-operative samples were adequate to perform EGFR sequencing (del19 +ve). She subsequently received SBRT with fiducial marker guidance.

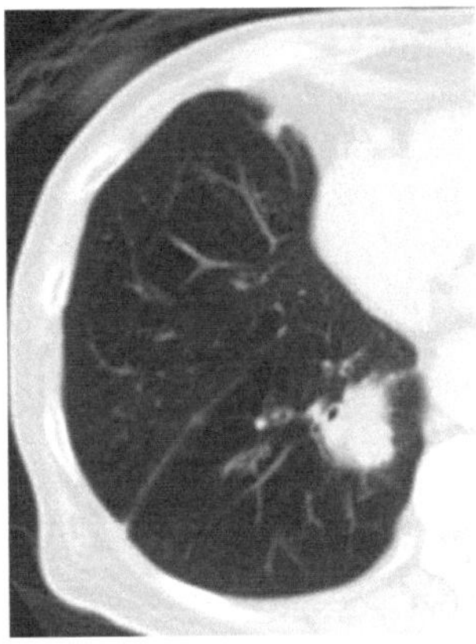

Fig. (1). Obvious bronchus sign leading into the solid right lower lobe lung mass, indicating high chance of successful navigation to the mass with ENB.

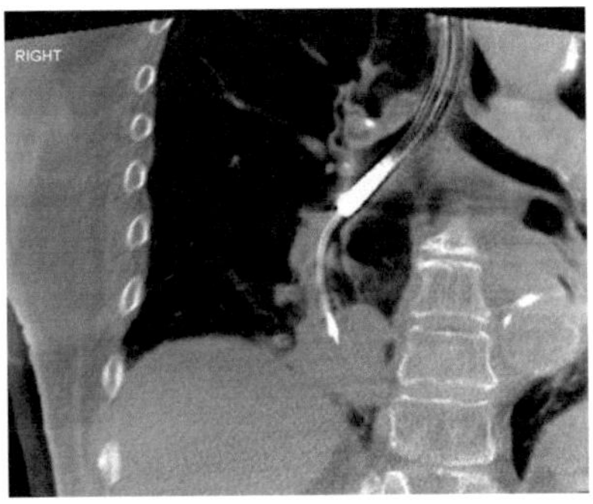

Fig. (2). Intra-operative CT scan: Lung mass was successfully punctured with FNA needle within the extended working channel (EWC) of the electromagnetic navigation bronchoscope.

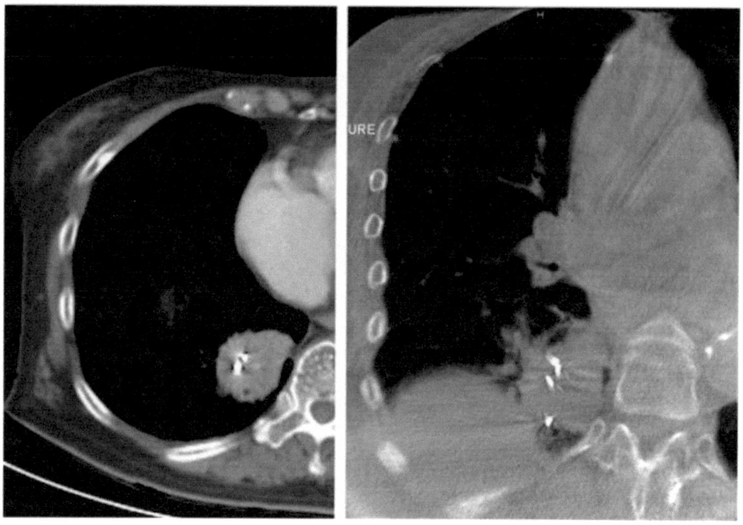

Fig. (3). Post-operative CT scan: 3 fiducial markers were seen located in different parts of the lung mass to aid subsequent SBRT.

Learning Points

- ENB in the hybrid operating room is able to provide one-stop diagnosis of lung lesion and fiducial marker placement to aid future SBRT. ENB has relatively high yield in lesions with bronchus sign [2].

Video

The video shows real-time fluoroscopy during the intra-tumoral implantation of the first (00:00), second (00:15) and third (00:35) fiducial markers through the extended working channel of the ENB bronchoscope.

CONSENT FOR PUBLICATION

Not applicable.

CONFLICT OF INTEREST

The authors declare no conflict of interest, financial or otherwise.

ACKNOWLEDGEMENT

Declared none.

REFERENCES

[1] Ng CSH, Yu SCH, Lau RWH, Yim APC. Hybrid Dyna-CT Guided Electromagnetic Navigational Bronchoscopic Biopsy. Eur J Cardiothorac Surg 2016; 48(S1): i87-88. [http://dx.doi.org/10.1093/ejcts/ezv405] [PMID: 26604298]

[2] Lau WH, Chow CYS, Ho YKJ, *et al*. Hybrid operating room dynaCT real-time image guided electromagnetic navigation bronchoscopic biopsy (iENB) – the initial experience. Respirology 2016; 21: (Suppl. 3): 74.

Case 16

Electromagnetic Navigation Bronchoscopy Lung Nodule Dye-Marking for Re-Do Thoracoscopic Surgery

Joyce W.Y. Chan[1], **Rainbow W.H. Lau**[1] and **Calvin S.H. Ng**[1,*]

[1] *Department of Surgery, The Chinese University of Hong Kong, N.T., Hong Kong SAR*

Keywords: Cone-Beam CT, Dye-marking, Electromagnetic Navigation Bronchoscopy, Lung metastasis, Methylene blue, Surgery.

Presentation

A 71-year-old man had primary thigh leiomyosarcoma resection in addition to right upper lobe wedge resection for isolated lung metastasis a few years ago. In his latest PET/CT, two new and growing right upper lobe nodules (12mm and 3mm) were found. There were no other distant metastases.

Comorbidities

Diabetes, hypertension, previous minor stroke.

Chest Imaging

Pre-operative CT scan showed 2 right upper lobe lesions (Fig. **1**).

Intervention

Electromagnetic navigation bronchoscopy (ENB) dye-marking of both lesions were performed in the hybrid theatre with cone-beam CT [1, 2]. Successful navigation to both lesions was followed by injection of dye near pleural surface and close to the lesions respectively (Figs. **2a** and **b**) [3]. During re-do 2-port VATS in the same general anaesthetic session, extensive adhesiolysis was required. However, methylene blue dye was still discernible and guided successful wedge resection of both lesions (Fig. **3**) [4].

*__Corresponding author Calvin S.H. Ng:__ Department of Surgery, The Chinese University of Hong Kong, N.T., Hong Kong SAR; E-mail: calvinng@surgery.cuhk.edu.hk

Jamalul Azizi Abdul Rahaman & Tinku Joseph (Eds.)

Complications

None.

Post-Intervention

The pathology reports of both specimens confirmed metastatic leiomyosarcoma with clear margins.

In this re-do VATS case, we expect difficulty in palpating and localizing small lung nodules, especially after adhesiolysis and lung manipulation. The blue dye near pleural surface guides intra-operative localization.

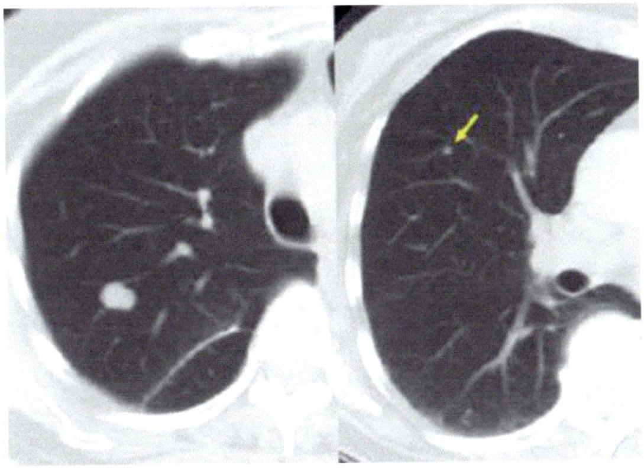

Fig. (1). Pre-operative: Two right upper lobe lesions measuring 12mm (left) and 3mm (right; yellow arrow).

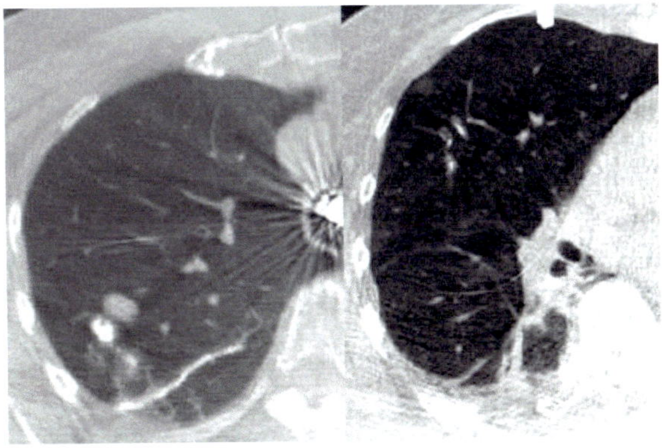

Fig. (2). (a) Intra-operative: Dye (0.2ml methylene blue-Visipaque solution in 3:1 ratio) was injected in close proximity to lesions. The iodixanol contrast dye confirms accurate dye placement with cone-beam CT, while the methylene blue aid thoracoscopic visualization of dye.

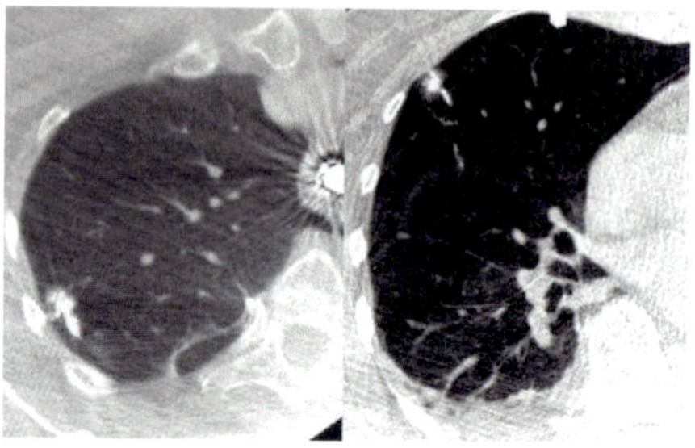

Fig. (2). (b) Intra-operative: Dye was also injected near pleural surface to aid localization of lung nodules during thoracoscopic surgery.

Learning Points

- ENB dye-marking is a useful adjunct for accurate localization of deep, small, or sub-solid lung lesions for subsequent VATS resection [5, 6].

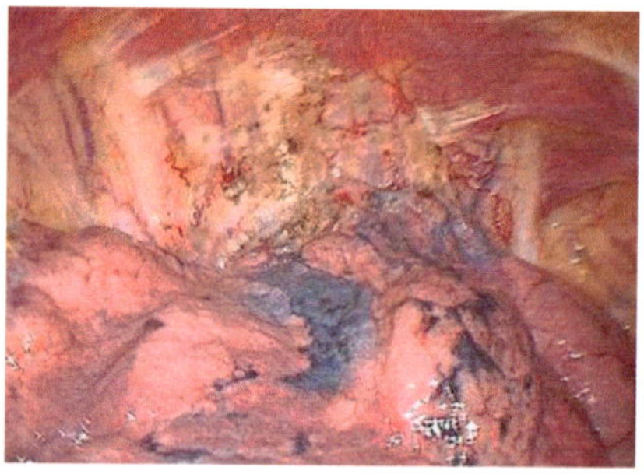

Fig. (3). Patch of blue dye visible on the lung surface of right upper lobe during VATS. The lung is densely adhered to posterior chest wall.

Video

The first part of the video shows the real-time fluoroscopy during the injection of dye near pleural surface for the two right upper lobe lesions respectively (00:00 and 00:16). The second part is an intra-operative video showing meticulous adhesiolysis with blue-dyed patch of lung in the foreground (00:27), careful digital palpation of one of the lung nodules within the dyed lung (00:41), followed by wedge resection of the lung nodule with staplers (01:01).

CONSENT FOR PUBLICATION

Not applicable.

CONFLICT OF INTEREST

The authors declare no conflict of interest, financial or otherwise.

ACKNOWLEDGEMENT

Declared none.

REFERENCES

[1] Zhao Z, Lau RWH, Ng CSH. Hybrid theatre & alternate localization techniques in conventional and single-port video assisted thoracoscopic surgery. J Thorac Dis 2016; 8(Suppl 3): S319-27.
[http://dx.doi.org/10.3978/j.issn.2072-1439.2016.02.27] [PMID: 27014480]

[2] Zerui Z, Ng CSH. Image Guided Uniportal VATS in the Hybrid Operating Room. In: Gonzalez-Rivas D, Ng CSH, Rocco G, A D'Amico T, Eds. Atlas of Uniportal Video Assisted Thoracic Surgery. Springer 2019.
[http://dx.doi.org/10.1007/978-981-13-2604-2_39]

[3] Zhao ZR, Lau RWH, Ng CSH. Hybrid theatre and uniportal VATS: the perfect match for lung nodule localization. Thorac Surg Clin 2017; 27(4): 347-55.
[http://dx.doi.org/10.1016/j.thorsurg.2017.06.003] [PMID: 28962707]

[4] Ng CSH, Chu CM, Lo CK, Lau RWH. Hybrid operating room Dyna-computed tomography combined image-guided electromagnetic navigation bronchoscopy dye marking and hookwire localization video-assisted thoracic surgery metastasectomy. Interact Cardiovasc Thorac Surg 2018; 26(2): 338-40.
[http://dx.doi.org/10.1093/icvts/ivx313] [PMID: 29049613]

[5] Zhao ZR, Lau RWH, Yu PSY, Ng CSH. Devising the guidelines: the techniques of pulmonary nodule localization in uniportal video-assisted thoracic surgery—hybrid operating room in the future. J Thorac Dis 2019; 11(Suppl 16): S2073-78.
[http://dx.doi.org/10.21037/jtd.2019.01.82] [PMID: 31637041]

[6] Ng CSH, Zhao Z, Long H, Lau RWH. Electromagnetic Navigation Bronchoscopy Triple Contrast Dye Marking for Lung Nodule Localization. Thorac Cardiovasc Surg 2020; 68(3): 253-55.
[http://dx.doi.org/10.1055/s-0038-1676964] [PMID: 30634186]

Case 17

Robotic Bronchoscopy

Robotic Bronchoscopy for Peripheral Pulmonary Nodule

Kyle Potts[1] and **D. Kyle Hogarth**[1,*]

[1] *University of Chicago, Chicago, USA*

Keywords: Single pulmonary nodule, Robotic bronchoscopy, Navigation bronchoscopy, Lung cancer, Abnormal CT of the chest.

Presentation

5mm left upper lobe nodule initially seen on low-dose CT chest for lung cancer screening. Lost to follow-up and repeat CT chest was performed for chronic cough 2 years later, which demonstrated enlarging nodule concerning for malignancy.

Comorbidities

A 72-year-old, moderate COPD with severe emphysematous changes, prior CVA history with returned function is presented.

Chest Imaging

Interval increase in LUL solitary pulmonary nodule from 5mm x 5mm to 18mm x 15mm and an associated increase in subaortic lymphadenopathy were observed (Fig. **1**). PET demonstrated hypermetabolic LUL nodule (SUV max 14.2).

Intervention

Robotic bronchoscopy performed with direct visualization of the tumor in the airway (Fig. **2**). Peripheral tumor aspiration and forceps biopsy were performed under direct visualization. EBUS staging performed afterwards.

[*]**Corresponding author D. Kyle Hogarth:** University of Chicago, Chicago, USA; E-mail: Hogarth2.5@me.com

Complications

None.

Post-Intervention

Successful robotic bronchoscopy. The patient was diagnosed with pT3N2M0 squamous cell carcinoma of the lung (Fig. **3**). He underwent LUL tri-segmentectomy followed by radiation therapy and adjuvant chemotherapy.

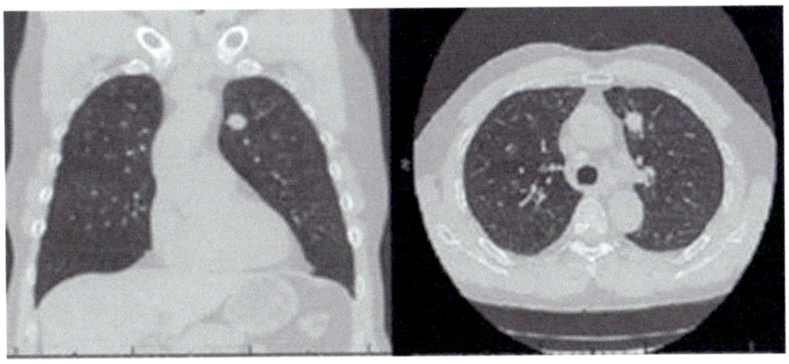

Fig. (1). A high-resolution coronal and axial CT chest demonstrates a spiculated, left upper lobe 18mm by 15mm solitary pulmonary nodule.

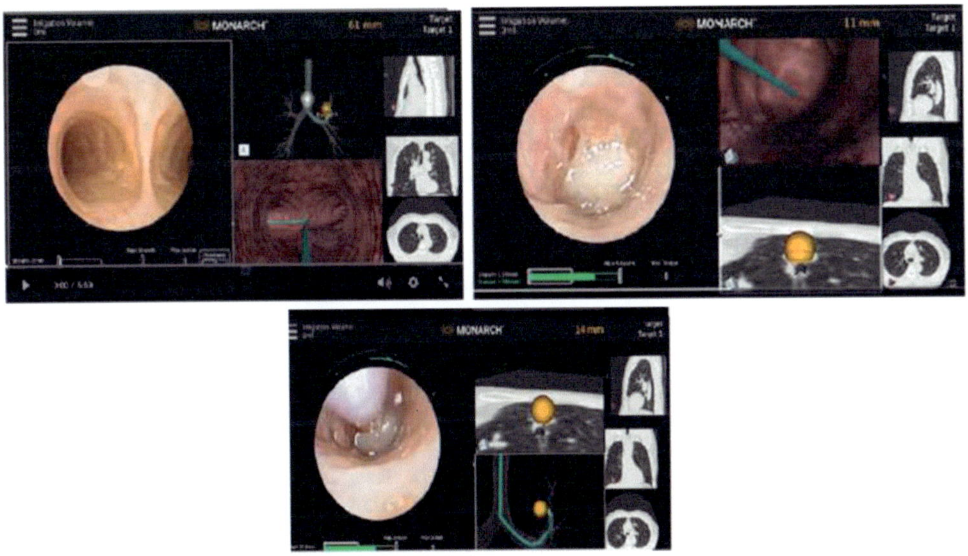

Fig. (2). A sequence of bronchoscopy images acquired. The first image demonstrates the main carina, the bronchoscopic navigation and target lesion on CT scan. The second image demonstrating the bronchoscopic view of the endobronchial mass. The third image demonstrates direct visualization of tumor aspiration.

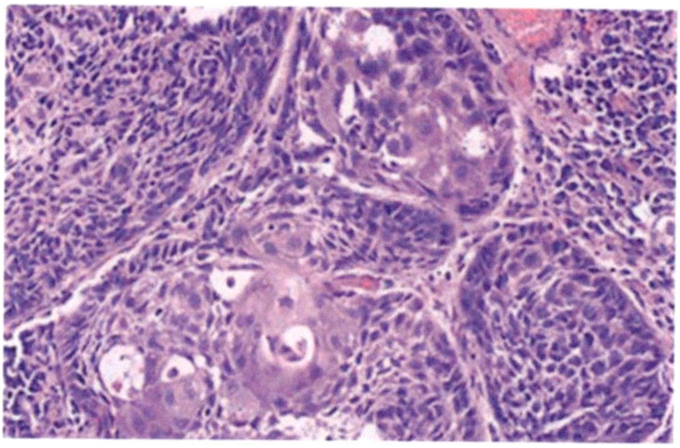

Fig. (3). Histopathology demonstrating squamous cell carcinoma.

Learning Points

- Robot-assisted bronchoscopy (RAB) is a safe, effective and feasible way to navigate to the periphery of the lung. The successful utilization of RAB in addition to EBUS-TBNA allows for the physician to diagnose and stage lung cancer in a single procedure [1, 2].

Videos

The 4 videos show robotic bronchoscopy to biopsy the LUL solitary pulmonary nodule.

1

2

3

4

CONSENT FOR PUBLICATION

Not applicable.

CONFLICT OF INTEREST

The author is a consultant for Auris Health/Johnson & Johnson.

ACKNOWLEDGEMENT

Declared none.

REFERENCES

[1] Chaddha U, Kovacs SP, Manley C, *et al*. Robot-assisted bronchoscopy for pulmonary lesion diagnosis: results from the initial multicenter experience. BMC Pulm Med 2019; 19(1): 243. [http://dx.doi.org/10.1186/s12890-019-1010-8]

[2] Agrawal A, Hogarth DK, Murgu S. Robotic bronchoscopy for pulmonary lesions: a review of existing technologies and clinical data. J Thorac Dis 2020; 12(6): 3279-86. [http://dx.doi.org/10.21037/jtd.2020.03.35] [PMID: 32642251]

Case 18

Evaluation of Cough and Left Lower Lobe "Pneumonia"

Christopher Manley[1,*]

[1] *Department of Pulmonary and Critical Care, Fox Chase Cancer Center, Philadelphia, USA*

Keywords: Robotic bronchoscopy, Interstitial lung disease, Lung cancer, Biopsy, Adenocarcinoma, Organizing pneumonia.

Presentation

A 60-year-old female presented with shortness of breath and nonproductive cough. She had been empirically treated with antibiotics. CT guided biopsy was then performed which was nondiagnostic and patient was then referred to pulmonology for evaluation.

Comorbidities

None. Never smoker.

Chest Imaging

CT thorax showed diffuse fibrotic lung disease and a 7cm area of consolidation *vs* mass in the left lower lobe (Fig. **1**).

Initial Testing

BD glucan normal. ANA, Rheumatoid factor, ANCA negative. Patient had a normal white blood cell count. CT guided needle aspirate showed bronchial cells and alveolar cells.

*__Corresponding author Christopher Manley:__ Department of Pulmonary and Critical Care, Fox Chase Cancer Center, Philadelphia, USA; E-mail: Christopher.Manley@fccc.edu

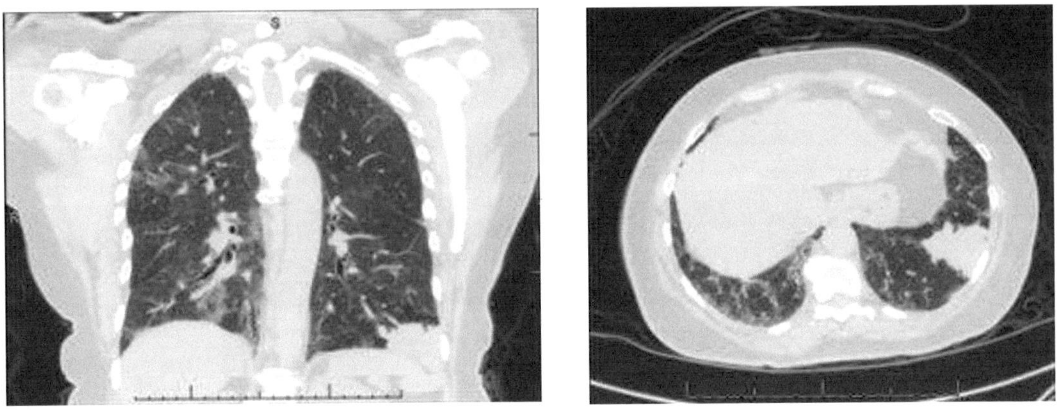

Fig. (1). Coronal and axial CT scan of LLL lung mass.

Intervention

The patient underwent robotic assisted navigational bronchoscopy (Monarch Bronchoscope, Auris Health Inc, Redwood City, CA) under general anesthesia. The patient was intubated with an 8.5 endotracheal tube (ETT) with the tube's distal tip secured 40 mm from the patient's main carina. The robot was docked and scope was introduced through the ETT. The robotic sheath was positioned in the LLL takeoff and the internal bronchoscope was advanced in the LLL lateral basal segment. The LLL was filled with thick fibropurulent mucus (Figs. **2** and **3**). Secretions were lavaged and therapeutically aspirated. Examination of the airways upon clearance of mucus revealed a small partially obstructing lesion in the LLL lateral basal airway (Fig. **4**). The lesion was biopsied with a 24G TBNA needle. ROSE revealed tumor cells. Final cytology revealed adenocarcinoma (Fig. **5**).

Linear EBUS was performed and all lymph nodes were negative.

Complications

None.

Post-Intervention

The patient was then taken for curative LLL lobectomy. Final pathology showed a small area of tumor surrounded by organizing pneumonia.

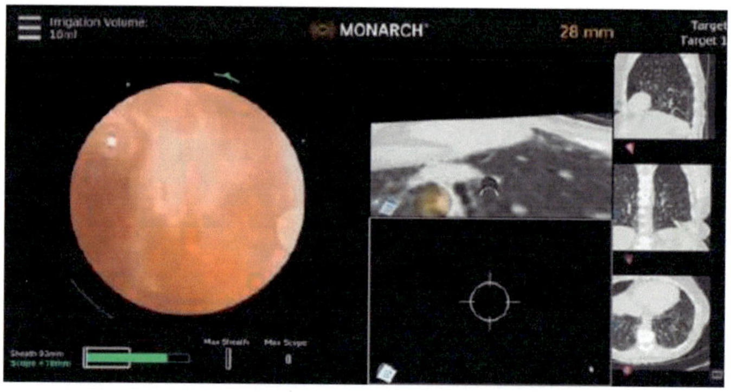

Fig. (2). Bronchoscopic view of airways impacted with mucus.

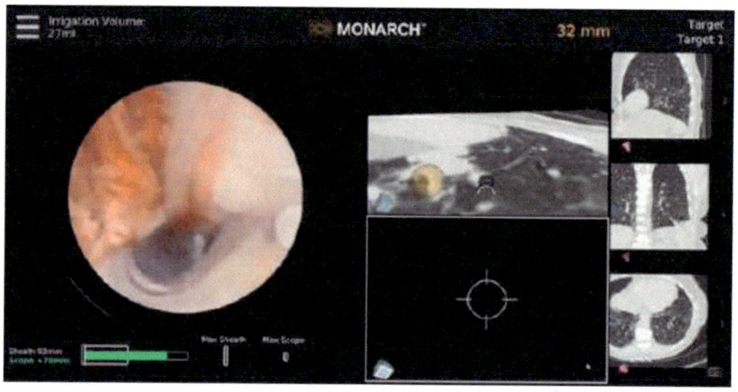

Fig. (3). Bronchoscopic view of partially cleared airways.

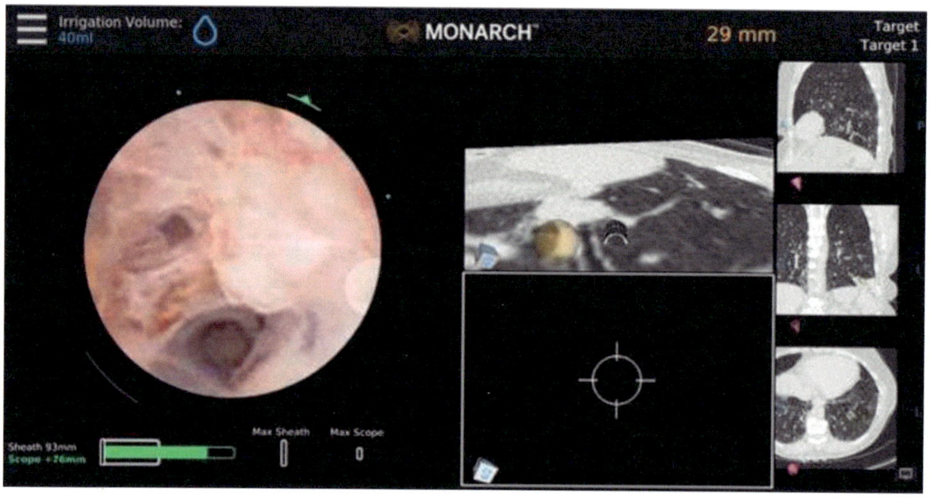

Fig. (4). Bronchoscopic view of endobronchial lesion, clearly visible after clearance of mucus.

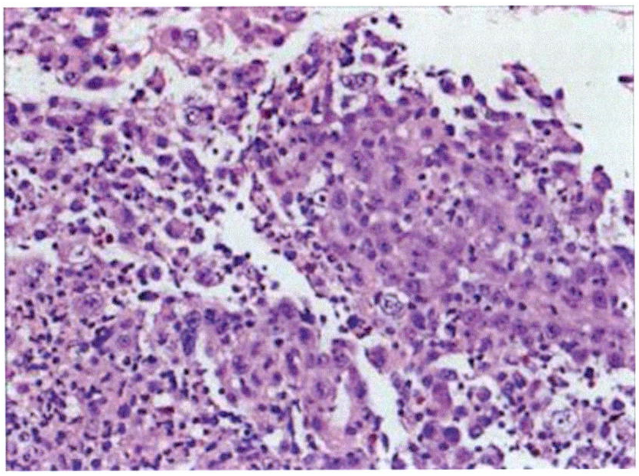

Fig. (5). TBNA of LLL endobronchial lesion showing adenocarcinoma.

Learning Points

- Robotic bronchoscopy is a safe and effective modality for diagnosis of suspicious lung lesions [1].
- A small obstructing lung lesion may cause post-obstructive changes which obscure the lesion and make targeting by CT guided biopsy difficult.

CONSENT FOR PUBLICATION

Written informed consent was obtained from the patient for publication of this case report and any accompanying images.

CONFLICT OF INTEREST

The author serves as a consultant and educational speaker for Johnson and Johnson (including Ethicon/ Auris Health). He has worked with Galvanize therapeutics as an advisory board member.

ACKNOWLEDGEMENTS

The author acknowledges the research grant (funding) received from Mauna Kea, Aquyre Bioscience, and Johnson and Johnson.

REFERENCE

[1] Chaddha U, Kovacs SP, Manley C, *et al*. Robot-assisted bronchoscopy for pulmonary lesion diagnosis: results from the initial multicenter experience. BMC Pulm Med 2019; 19: 243. [http://dx.doi.org/10.1186/s12890-019-1010-8] [PMID: 31829148]

Case 19

Cone Beam CT

Cone Beam CT for the Diagnosis of Small Peripheral Pulmonary Nodules: It's Not Always Lung Cancer

Michael Pritchett[1,*]

[1] *FirstHealth of the Carolinas and Pinehurst Medical Clinic, Pinehurst, North Carolina, USA*

Keywords: Cone-beam CT (CBCT), Robotic bronchoscopy, Lung metastasis, Pulmonary nodule, Augmented fluoroscopy.

Presentation

A 63-year-old female referred for evaluation of an abnormal CT scan of the chest. The CT showed a right upper lobe nodule measuring 6mm.

Comorbidities

Patient started smoking cigarettes at 13-years-old and continues to smoke 1½ packs per day. She has chronic obstructive pulmonary disease. She has symptoms of chronic bronchitis with daily mucus production in the morning. She has a remote history of cervical dysplasia and had a partial hysterectomy in the 1980s. More recently she was diagnosed with vaginal carcinoma in 2011 and underwent radiation therapy for this.

Chest Imaging

Multiplanar CT imaging shows a 6mm nodule in the right upper lobe (RUL) (Fig. **1**).

Intervention

The patient underwent shape-sensing robotic navigational bronchoscopy (Ion, Intuitive). The procedure was done under general anesthesia, including the use of paralytics, based on a specific protocol developed for guided bronchoscopy to

*Corresponding author **Michael Pritchett:** FirstHealth of the Carolinas and Pinehurst Medical Clinic, Pinehurst, North Carolina, USA; E-mail: Mpritchett@pinehurstmedical.com prevent atelectasis. After a brief registration process, we navigated to the lesion in the right upper lobe (Fig. **2**). Attempts were made to localize the lesion with radial endobronchial ultrasound but this was unsuccessful. A CBCT spin was performed (Philips Allura Xper FD20 with Lung Suite). Minor adjustments in positioning of the robotic catheter were made based on the CBCT spin and with the use of augmented fluoroscopy in multiple planes (Fig. **3**). After adjustments, we began the biopsy process with brushings, then FNA with 21G needle followed by transbronchial forceps biopsies. On-site pathologic examination showed evidence of malignancy on the FNA and forceps biopsies. Additional material was obtained for cell block. Another CBCT scan was performed to confirm tool-in-lesion with the 21G needle deployed (Fig. **4**). The images confirmed the presence of the needle in the center of the 6mm lesion, in multiple orthogonal planes. The total radiation dose for the CBCT spins was only 1.18 mSv (0.59 mSv per spin). This was using a low dose protocol proprietary to Philips Lung Suite.

Complications

There were no complications. Post-procedure CXR showed no evidence of pneumothorax. The patient was discharged home 2 hours after the procedure.

Post-Intervention

Brushings from the RUL lesion were non-diagnostic. The forceps biopsies and FNA were diagnostic. These biopsies showed a squamous cell carcinoma (Fig. **5**). The squamous cells show focal mitotic activity and diffusely express p16 antigen. The patient's prior vaginal carcinoma was reviewed for comparison and had similar morphology and p16 expression. The final diagnosis was metastatic squamous cell carcinoma from vaginal primary.

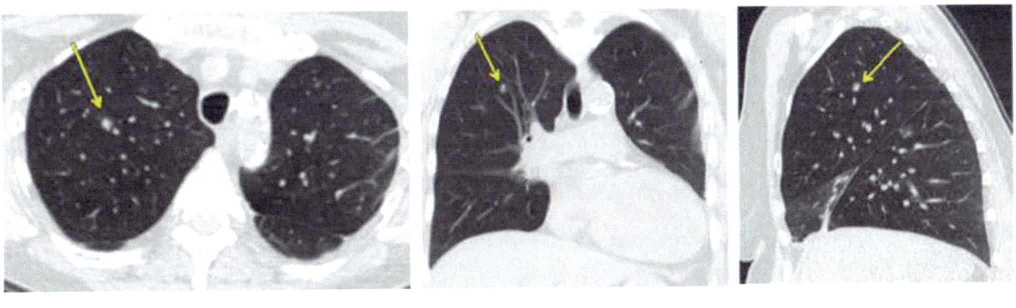

Fig. (1). Multiplanar CT imaging shows a 6mm nodule in the right upper lobe.

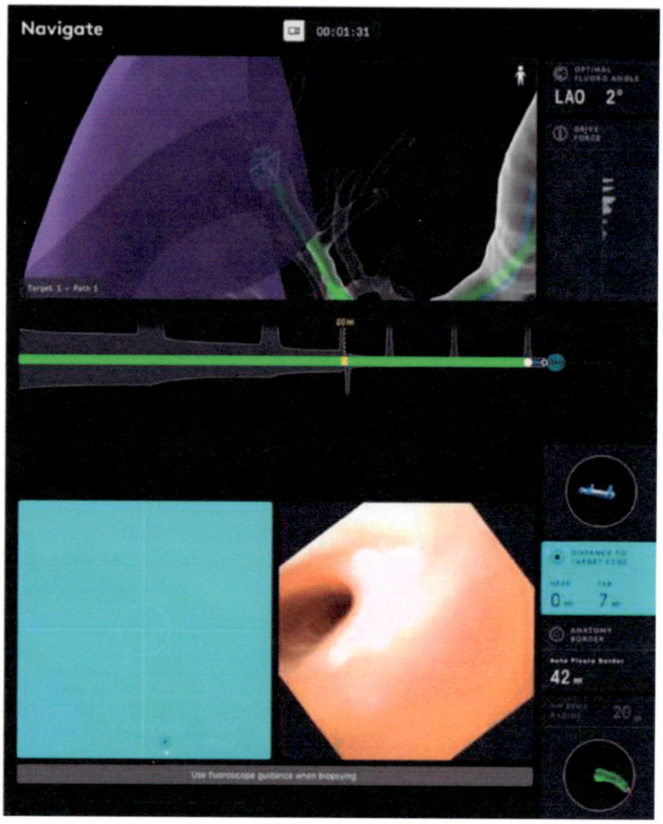

Fig. (2). Navigation system images (Ion endoluminal robotic system by Intuitive). Time showing 1 min 31 seconds. This is total time for registration and navigation to the lesion.

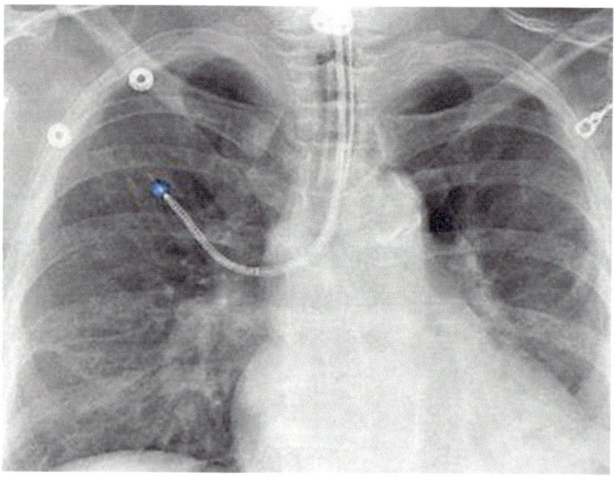

Fig. (3). Augmented fluoroscopic image with robotic catheter in place at the lesion with 21G needle deployed.

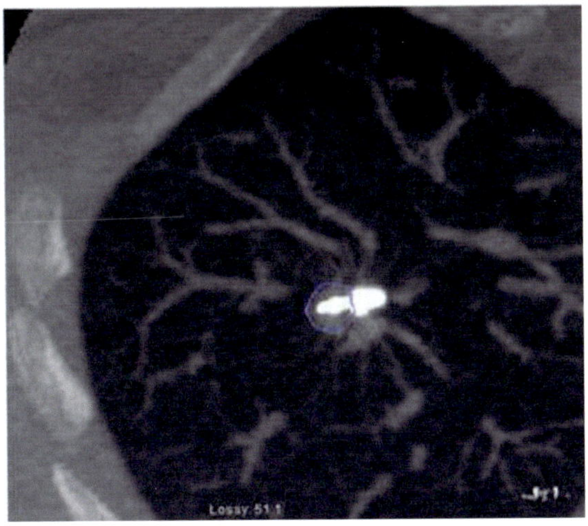

Fig. (4). Tool-in-lesion CBCT image in axial plane showing 21G needle in the center of the 6mm RUL lesion.

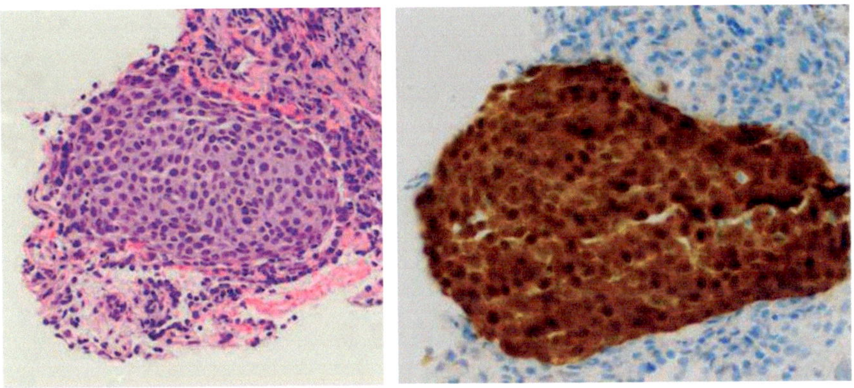

Fig. (5). An H & E stained slide showing a small focus of well differentiated squamous cell carcinoma (left). P16 stain (right) showing strong expression. P16 is not expressed in atypical squamous metaplasia but it is positive in HPV-related squamous cell carcinoma of the uterine cervix.

Learning Points

- This case highlights the advantages that CBCT has to offer with real-time intraprocedural imaging, augmented fluoroscopy and the ability to confirm tool-in-lesion [1]. The spatial resolution of CBCT is close to that of conventional CT scanning, and offers excellent image quality, even when using a dose saving protocol as in this case. Not all lesions will be visualized with rEBUS due to a variety of factors (user error, small or ground glass lesions, lesions far outside the airway) and there also can be false rEBUS signals secondary to atelectasis or blood clot. These limitations are largely overcome with the use of CBCT (although atelectasis or local hemorrhage after biopsy can obscure a small lesion). This highlights the importance of using a specific anesthesia protocol to eliminate atelectasis [2]. Additionally, if biopsying a pure ground glass lesion, it's often helpful to do an initial CBCT scan before biopsy attempts. This will enable the use of augmented fluoroscopy (currently only possible on fixed systems, this is not available on mobile systems). When combined with robotic bronchoscopy, CBCT is even more valuable with the ability to make precise adjustments and the stability which enables biopsy of eccentric lesions, outside of the airway, without any deflection of the catheter while passing biopsy tools [3].

Video

The video shows the first ever cone-beam CT master class. Hosted at FirstHealth Moore Regional Hospital on January 15th and 17th, 2020. This event was sponsored by Philips and the Society for Advanced Bronchoscopy. Procedures performed by Dr. Michael Pritchett at FirstHealth of the Carolinas. This event was meant to increase the awareness of this effective tool in diagnosing small peripheral lung nodules with high diagnostic accuracy.

CONSENT FOR PUBLICATION

Not applicable.

CONFLICT OF INTEREST

The author declares no conflict of interest, financial or otherwise.

ACKNOWLEDGEMENTS

The author acknowledges the support received from Dr. Charles Schirmer, Department of Pathology, FirstHealth of the Carolinas, USA.

REFERENCES

[1] Pritchett MA, Schampaert S, de Groot JAH, *et al.* Cone-beam CT with augmented fluoroscopy combined with electromagnetic navigation bronchoscopy for biopsy of pulmonary nodules . J Bronchology Interv Pulmonol 2018; 25(4): 274-82.
[http://dx.doi.org/10.1097/LBR.0000000000000536]

[2] Pritchett MA, Lau K, Skibo S, *et al.* Anesthesia considerations to reduce motion and atelectasis during advanced guided bronchoscopy. BMC Pulm Med 2021; 21; 240.
[http://dx.doi.org/10.1186/s12890-021-01584-6 PMID: 34273966]

[3] Reisenauer J, Simoff MJ, Pritchett MA, *et al.* Ion: technology and techniques for shape-sensing robotic-assisted bronchoscopy. Ann Thorac Surg 2022; 113(1): 308-15.
[http://dx.doi.org/10.1016/j.athoracsur.2021.06.086] [PMID: 34370981]

Case 20

Two for the Price of One

Michael Pritchett[1,*]

[1] *FirstHealth of the Carolinas and Pinehurst Medical Clinic, Pinehurst, North Carolina, USA*

Keywords: CT-to-body-divergence, Cone-beam CT (CBCT), Robotic bronchoscopy, Pulmonary nodule, Lung cancer.

Presentation

A 75-year-old female underwent lung cancer screening.

Comorbidities

She has smoked 1 pack per day since the age of 15. She is still an active smoker.

Chest Imaging

On the CT, she was noted to have bilateral lung lesions. In the left upper lobe, there was a spiculated 18mm lesion and in the right lower lobe, there was a smooth rounded density measuring 11mm (Figs. **1a** and **b**).

Intervention

We began using robotic navigation bronchoscopy to the left upper lobe lesion. Upon arrival to the virtual target, a search for the lesion with rEBUS was unsuccessful at localizing the lesion. CBCT scan was performed which showed we were not on target due to significant CT-to-body divergence (Fig. **2**). There was no evidence of atelectasis on the scan. We renavigated using augmented fluoroscopy and arrived at the lesion *via* a different path than what was initially planned with the navigation software. A search with rEBUS at this location confirmed localization with a concentric signal. Tool-in-lesion CBCT scan was taken and confirmed the tool inside the lesion (Fig. **3**). Biopsies were taken with a 21G needle. ROSE confirmed malignancy and additional biopsies were taken for creation of a cell block.

[*]**Corresponding author Michael Pritchett:** FirstHealth of the Carolinas and Pinehurst Medical Clinic, Pinehurst, North Carolina, USA; E-mail: Mpritchett@pinehurstmedical.com

We then navigated to the RLL lesion. A very faint eccentric signal was noted on rEBUS. Adjustments were made based on augmented fluoroscopy which was provided by the previous CBCT scan for the LUL lesion. Again some degree of CT-to-body divergence was noted. A 23G needle was deployed based on the augmented fluoroscopic image and a CBCT scan was performed. This scan confirmed the biopsy needle in the lesion in multiple orthogonal planes (Fig. **4**). Initial ROSE interpretation felt this could be a hamartoma.

Additional biopsies were taken for cell block. Linear EBUS staging was then performed. ROSE showed no evidence of metastatic disease.

Complications

There were no complications. Pneumothorax was ruled out with intraprocedural CBCT as well as with a 1-hour post-procedure CXR.

Post-Intervention

The left upper lobe lesion was consistent with squamous cell carcinoma on the final pathology report. The right lower lobe lesion (initially thought to be a hamartoma during the procedure) was found to be a matrix producing epithelial neoplasm. Final pathology from linear EBUS staging showed no evidence of metastatic disease from either lesion.

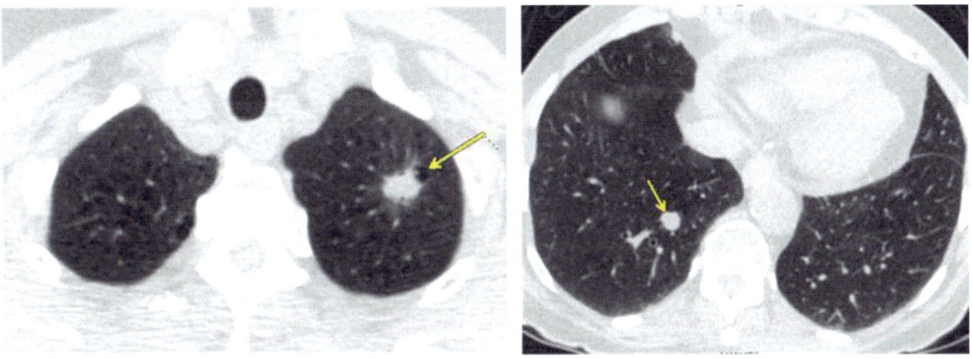

Fig. (1). (**a**) (Left) In the left upper lobe, there was a spiculated 18mm lesion. (**b**) (Right) In the right lower lobe there was a smooth rounded density measuring 11mm.

Procedural Images

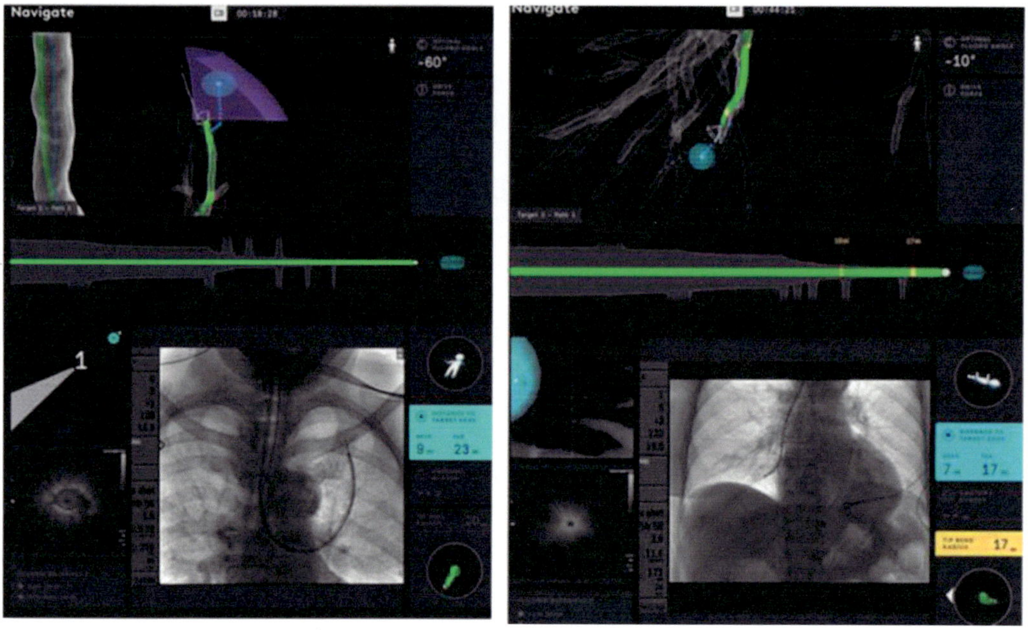

Fig. (2). Screen shots from the Ion robotic navigation system. Navigation to the LUL lesion (left), note the divergence (top left image). Navigation to the RLL lesion (top right image), again with mild divergence.

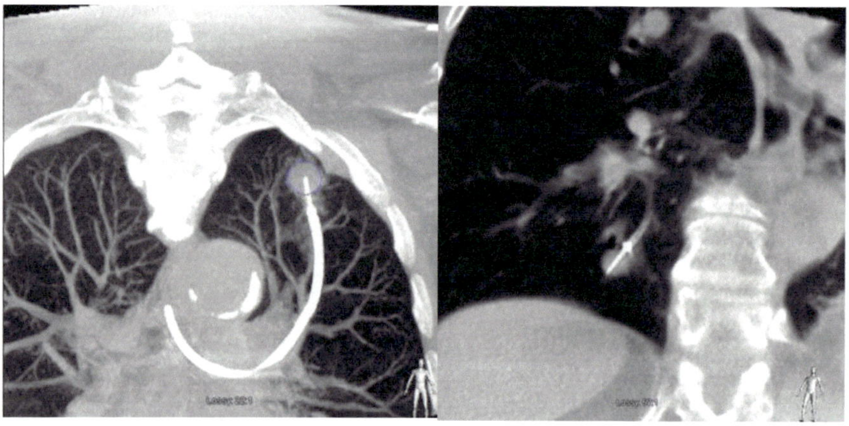

Fig. (3). Tool-in-lesion confirmation for LUL (left) and RLL (right) lesions.

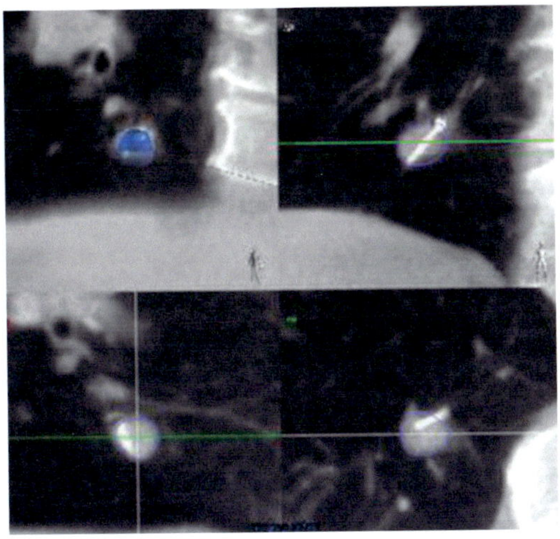

Fig. (4). Tool-in-lesion should always be confirmed in 3 orthogonal planes, as is shown for the RLL lesion.

Learning Points

- It's important to remember that any navigation procedure that is based solely from a preoperative CT scan can be subject to CT-to-body divergence [1]. The use of CBCT scan can overcome any divergence by always showing the ground truth, as it relates to the position of the catheter, tool and lesion. Additionally, performing a CBCT scan allows one to evaluate for pneumothorax, which is of particular importance if performing bilateral lung biopsies.

Video

This video highlights Dr. Michael Pritchett's recent experience with augmented CBCT and electromagnetic navigation bronchoscopy (ENB).

CONSENT FOR PUBLICATION

Not applicable.

CONFLICT OF INTEREST

The author declares no conflict of interest, financial or otherwise.

ACKNOWLEDGEMENT

Declared none.

REFERENCE

[1] Pritchett MA, Bhadra K, Calcutt M, Folch E. Virtual or reality: divergence between preprocedural computed tomography scans and lung anatomy during guided bronchoscopy. J Thorac Dis 2020; 12(4): 1595-1611.
[http://dx.doi.org/10.21037/jtd.2020.01.35] [PMID: 32395297]

Case 21

One View is Not Enough

Michael Pritchett[1,*]

[1] *FirstHealth of the Carolinas and Pinehurst Medical Clinic, Pinehurst, North Carolina, USA*

Keywords: Cone-beam CT (CBCT), Augmented fluoroscopy, Robotic bronchoscopy, Pulmonary nodule, Lung cancer.

Presentation

A 67-year-old male underwent lung cancer screening with low-dose CT scan.

Comorbidities

Smoked 1 pack per day for 45 years. Quit 1 year prior to procedure. Moderate COPD with an FEV1 of 59% of predicted.

Chest Imaging

The scan identified two right-sided nodules of concern. There was a 14mm cavitary lesion in the RUL and additionally there was a 7mm pleural based lesion, also in the RUL (Figs. **1a** and **b**).

Intervention

Robotic navigation bronchoscopy was used to navigate first to the spiculated cavitary lesion. rEBUS was used for localization. An eccentric view was initially noted. We then performed brushings, fine needle aspiration and forceps biopsies. ROSE was consistent with malignancy. We then navigated to the smaller more apical lesion. We were unable to localize the lesion with rEBUS at the site of the virtual target so a CBCT scan was performed. The catheter was directly posterior to the lesion (Fig. **2**). Augmented fluoroscopy was used to make precise adjustments with the robotic catheter to move in an anterior direction (Fig. **3**). An additional CBCT scan was performed which confirmed tool-in-lesion (Fig. **4**). Brushings,

*Corresponding author Michael Pritchett: FirstHealth of the Carolinas and Pinehurst Medical Clinic, Pinehurst, North Carolina, USA; E-mail: Mpritchett@pinehurstmedical.com

Jamalul Azizi Abdul Rahaman & Tinku Joseph (Eds.)

FNA and forceps biopsies were taken at this lesion. On-site evaluation showed atypical cells suspicious for malignancy. Linear EBUS staging was performed after the navigation procedure. There was no evidence of nodal metastasis.

Complications

No complications were observed. The patient was discharged home several hours after the procedure.

Post-Intervention

Brushings from the RUL lesion were non-diagnostic. The forceps biopsies and FNA were diagnostic. Both lesions were confirmed to be squamous cell carcinoma on final pathology report. There was no chance of cross contamination, as new tools were used for each lesion.

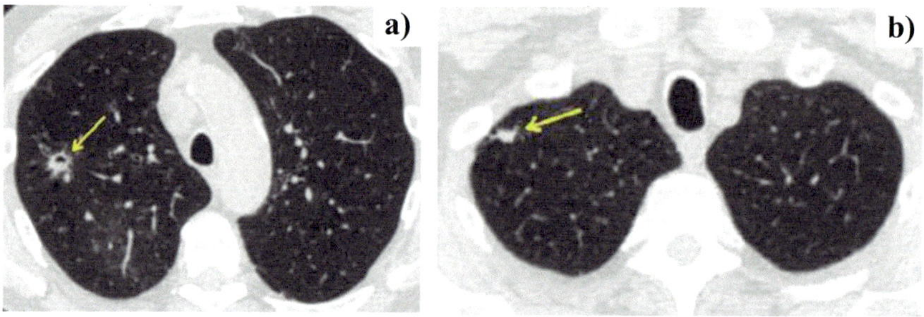

Fig. (1). (**a**) (Left) There is a 14mm cavitary lesion in the RUL. (**b**) (Right) Additionally there is 7mm pleural based lesion, also in the RUL.

Procedural Images

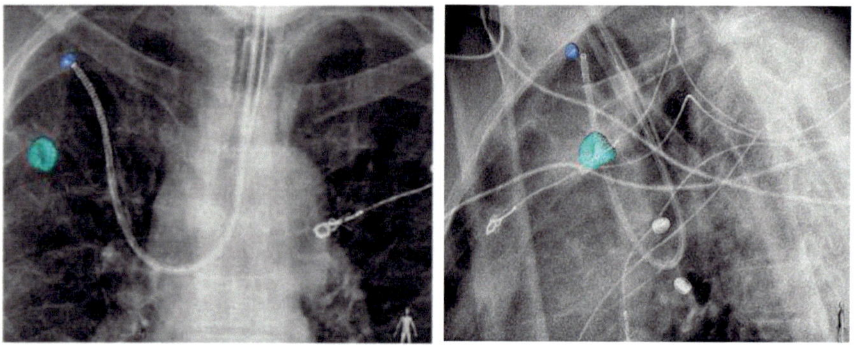

Fig. (2). AP view with augmented fluoroscopy (left) showing perfect alignment to the target. A 70-degree LAO view showing the catheter is actually posterior to the lesion (right).

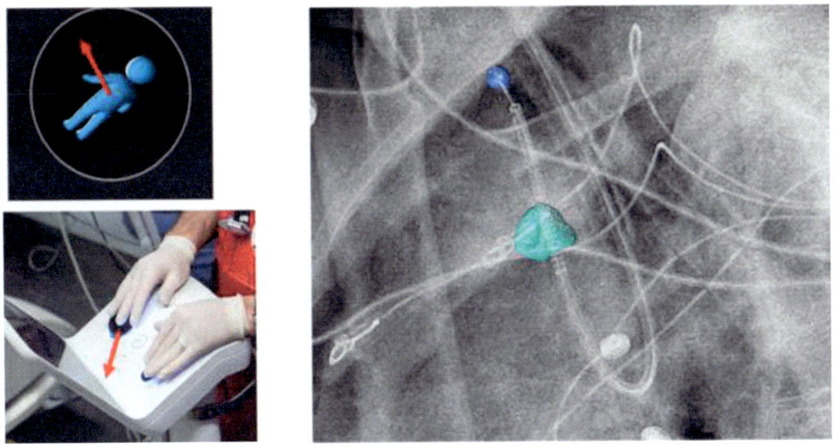

Fig. (3). Making minor adjustments with the Ion endoluminal robotic catheter (left). First looking at the orientation guide (top left). The red arrow is pointing the direction of anterior, which is the direction the catheter needs to be moved to be on target. Moving the scroll wheel (bottom left) in that 11 O'clock direction results in the catheter moving anteriorly, while watching with augmented fluoroscopy until on target (70-degree LAO view shown on the right). Now on target, brushings are performed.

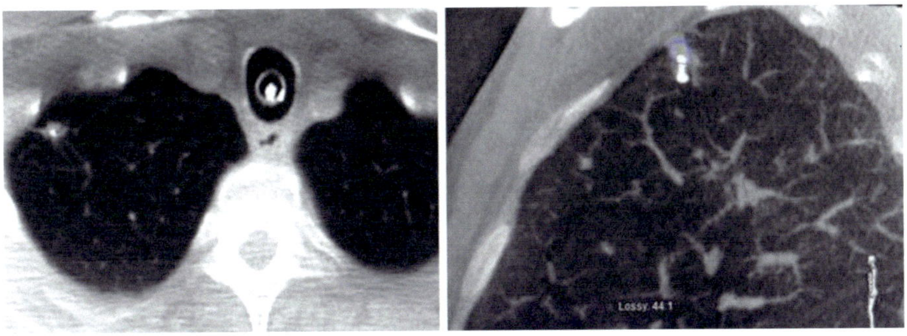

Fig. (4). Axial image (left) and sagittal image (right) show tool-in-lesion confirmation for the 7mm RUL nodule.

Learning Points

- This case highlights the importance of checking your location in multiple planes. If we had trusted only the AP view, we would have biopsied in the wrong location. CBCT enabled us to see that we were off target and gave us the ability to use augmented fluoroscopy to make the necessary corrections. The precision of the robotic system combined with CBCT imaging makes these minor adjustments relatively easy, even with very small lesions [1].

CONSENT FOR PUBLICATION

Not applicable.

CONFLICTS OF INTEREST

The author declares no conflict of interest, financial or otherwise.

ACKNOWLEDGEMENT

Declared none.

REFERENCE

[1] Reisenauer J, Simoff MJ, Pritchett MA, *et al.* Ion: technology and techniques for shape-sensing robotic-assisted bronchoscopy. Ann Thorac Surg 2022; 113(1): 308-15. [http://dx.doi.org/10.1016/j.athoracsur.2021.06.086] [PMID: 34370981]

Case 22

Cellvizio

Optical Lung Biopsy

Anantham Devanand[1,*] and **Tay Chee Kiang Melvin**[1]

[1] *Sing Health Duke-NUS Lung Centre, Singapore*

Keywords: Confocal imaging, Endomicroscopy, Optical biopsy, *In vivo* imaging, Non-invasive diagnosis.

Presentation

Our patient was a 49-year-old Indian male, non-smoker, who presented with a four-month history of non-productive cough. There was no fever or loss of weight. He had no known medical co-morbidities or occupational/recreational exposures. There was neither clinical nor radiological response to an antibiotic course of amoxicillin/clavulanic acid and Clarithromycin.

Comorbidities

None.

Chest Imaging

CXR showed bilateral lower zone infiltrates (Fig. **1**). CT thorax reported thickened interlobular septa, atelectasis, ground glass opacities and distortion (Fig. **2**). Autoimmune serological testing was negative.

Intervention

The patient consented to confocal endomicroscopy prior to the transbronchial lung biopsy and the acquired images showed no evidence of lung fibrosis.

Probe-based confocal laser endomicroscopy All procedures were performed with a diagnostic flexible bronchoscope (4.9mm outer diameter) that had a 2.0mm

***Corresponding author Anantham Devanand:** SingHealth Duke-NUS Lung Centre, Singapore; E-mail: anantham.devanand@singhealth.com.sg working channel. The small field of view rendered systematic examination of the entire airways impractical with confocal endomicroscopy. Therefore, white light bronchoscopy was performed first before a target area was scanned. Secretions were suctioned out to provide a clear field and the air ways were adequately anaesthetized with topical lidocaine. Confocal images were obtained by gentle perpendicular application of the endomicroscope probe directly against the mucosa. Subsequent processing of video sequences was done with an algorithm that combined successive images, as well as canceled movement-induced artifacts. This reconstituted a widened field of view.

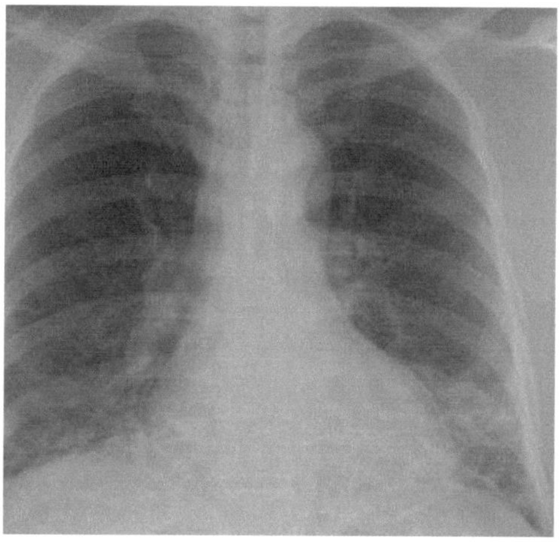

Fig. (1). CXR 2 months after completion of antibiotics.

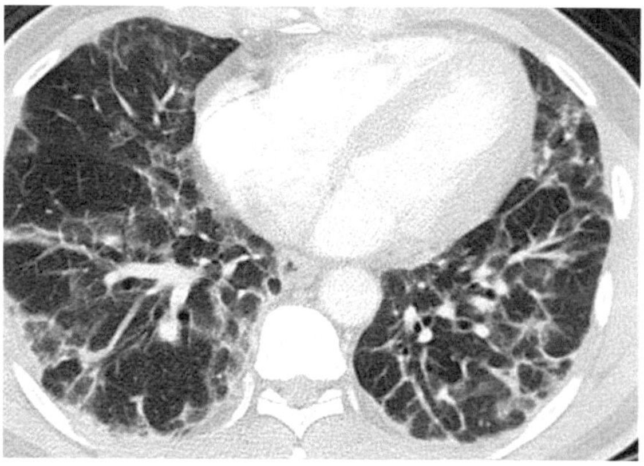

Fig. (2). CT thorax.

Only unilateral examination of distal airspaces was attempted because of the potential for pneumothorax. Once the bronchoscope was placed in the smallest accessible bronchus, the probe was gently advanced until it passed through the bronchiolar walls. Best results were obtained by withdrawing the probe when acini were first seen and analyzing the last image before contact was lost. At this point, alveolar deformation was minimized and reproducible measurements were possible. When clear images were seen, video clips of up to 30 seconds were recorded in each bronchopulmonary segment for subsequent analysis.

Image Interpretation

The predominant fluorescence emission originates from elastin in the lungs while collagen and intracellular flavins cannot be seen. Elastin is a component of the subepithelial layer of the airways and the scaffolding of alveolar duct rims. Elastin is also a component of the external sheath of small blood vessels. In addition, fluorescence is seen in the alveolar macrophages of smokers. Minor trauma can be expected because of the relative size of the probe compared to the terminal bronchioles. Therefore, free swaying septal walls and severing of small vessels may be detected even in normal lungs.

Complications

The reported complication rate is low with occasional cases of pneumothorax that do not usually require chest tube insertion. This can potentially be minimized by using fluoroscopic guidance. Other reported complications are minor bleeding and transient desaturations. It is estimated that when up to eight bronchopulmonary segments are examined, confocal endomicroscopy adds approximately 10 minutes to the duration of the procedure.

Post-Intervention

Transbronchial lung biopsy revealed organizing pneumonia with pneumonitis and the patient was successfully treated with systemic steroids.

Learning Points

- Confocal endomicroscopy utilizes point illumination and a pinhole apparatus to block out-of-focus rays of light, thereby enabling the generation of high-resolution images. Cellvizio® (Mauna Kea Technologies, Paris, France) utilizes a semi-flexible probe. A 600 × 600μm field of view is obtained under the illumination of a laser source with an excitation wavelength of 488nm. The lateral resolution is 3.5μm [1].

- Bronchoscopic lung biopsy can be complicated by pneumothorax or bleeding. Forceps biopsies are subject to crush artifact and the histological processing of specimens can alter the nature of sampled tissue. *In vivo* optical biopsies *via* probe-based confocal laser endomicroscopy address these limitations by facilitating non-invasive diagnosis.
- Examination of distal airspaces should be attempted only after detailed review of computed tomography imaging to identify likely target bronchopulmonary segments. Scanning of the apical and posterior segment of the upper lobes is not always possible because of the stiffness of the probe and the angulation of the airways [2].
- There are several emerging diagnostic applications of confocal endomicroscopy. In chronic obstructive pulmonary disease, alveolar diameter is inversely related to measures of airflow limitation such as the forced expiratory volume in 1 second. The combination of the auto fluorescent cell count, intensity of cellular fluorescence and vascularity has been used in diagnosing acute rejection post lung transplantation. In pulmonary fibrosis, elastin fibres have been found to be thickened and densely packed and there may be an indistinct alveolar architecture.
- The presence of at least one alveolar area with large (>20μm) and strongly fluorescent cells has a reported sensitivity of 100% and a specificity of 88% in the diagnosis of pneumonitis due to amiodarone. These cells correspond to foamy macrophages, although their presence may not only be restricted to only amiodarone related lung disease.

In patients with pulmonary alveolar proteinosis, fluorescent floating complexes (100-450 μm) have been seen. Bronchoalveolar lavage shows globular lipoproteinaceous material that corresponded in size and morphology to these images. Needle based versions of this technology have also been tested in cancer diagnosis [3].

- Despite these promising developments, there is currently no clear consensus on standardization of procedure, image acquisition and analysis. Therefore, all diagnoses on confocal endomicroscopy still require conventional methods before clinical action is taken.

Video

Probe-based Confocal Laser Endomicroscopy of the lateral segment of the right lower lobe. Initial images are taken of the central airways before advancing the probe through the terminal bronchioles to visualise alveolar duct rims and small vessels.

CONSENT FOR PUBLICATION

Not applicable.

CONFLICT OF INTEREST

The authors declare no conflict of interest, financial or otherwise.

ACKNOWLEDGEMENT

Declared none.

REFERENCES

[1] Thiberville L, Salaün M, Lachkar S, *et al*. Human *in vivo* fluorescence microimaging of the alveolar ducts and sacs during bronchoscopy. Eur Respir J 2009; 33: 974-85. [http://dx.doi.org/10.1183/09031936.00083708] [PMID: 19213792]

[2] Meng P, Tan GL, Low SY, *et al*. Fibred confocal fluorescence microscopy in the diagnosis of interstitial lung diseases. J Thorac Dis. 2016 Dis 2016; 8(12): 3505-14. [http://dx.doi.org/10.21037/jtd.2016.12.60] [PMID: 28149543]

[3] Peng M, Liang TG, Anantham D. Probe-based confocal laser endomicroscopy of the lungs. J Pulm Respir Med 2016; 6: 373. [http://dx.doi.org/10.4172/2161-105X.1000373]

Case 23

Incidental Finding of Latent Tuberculosis in the Evaluation of Locally Advanced Colon Cancer

Christopher Manley[1,*], **Shuanzeng Wei**[2], **Tess Kramer**[3] and **Jouke Annema**[3]

[1] *Department of Pulmonary and Critical Care, Fox Chase Cancer Center, Philadelphia, PA, USA*

[2] *Department of Pathology, Fox Chase Cancer Center, Philadelphia, PA, USA*

[3] *Department of Respiratory Medicine, Amsterdam UMC, Amsterdam, Netherlands*

Keywords: TB, Confocal microscopy, Bronchoscopy, Robotic bronchoscopy, Lung malignancy.

Presentation

A 64-year-old male with newly diagnosed adenocarcinoma status post right hemicolectomy revealing T4b N2b (Stage IIIC) disease. Staging CT thorax revealed a group of small right upper lobe (RUL) lung nodule concerning for metastatic disease. The patient reported no pulmonary symptoms.

Comorbidities

He previously worked as a seaman on a ship transporting crude oil in China. He is a former smoker of 15 years, quit 30 years ago. Initial Testing: Quantiferon gold was positive.

Chest Imaging

Staging CT thorax revealed a group of small right upper lobe (RUL) lung nodules concerning for metastatic disease. Positron emission tomography (PET) scan demonstrated avidity within the RUL nodular infiltrate (SUV of 6 and 6.5 for the early and late phase of the scan, respectively) (Fig. **1**).

***Corresponding author Christopher Manley:** Department of Pulmonary and Critical Care, Fox Chase Cancer Center, Philadelphia, USA; E-mail: Christopher.Manley@fccc.edu

Jamalul Azizi Abdul Rahaman & Tinku Joseph (Eds.)

Intervention

The patient underwent robotic assisted navigational bronchoscopy (Monarch Bronchoscope, Auris Health Inc, Redwood City, CA) under general anesthesia. The patient was intubated with an 8.5 endotracheal tube (ETT) with the tube's distal tip secured 40mm from the patient's main carina. The robot was docked and scope was introduced through the ETT. The robotic sheath was positioned in the RUL takeoff and the internal bronchoscope was advanced in the RUL apical segment. Airway evaluation of the apical segment just proximal to the lung lesion showed anthracotic pigment staining the airways and small firm endobronchial lesions (Fig. **2**). Using radial ultrasound, the RUL nodule was localized (Fig. **3**). Prior to the procedure, the CLE-miniprobe (AQ-flex, Mauna Kea, Paris) was preloaded into the 18G-Flex needle (Bronchus Medical Inc, San Jose, USA), positioning the tip of the probe 3mm past the needle tip using a locking device as previously described [1]. Before advancing the needle into the working channel of the bronchoscope, the locking device was unscrewed from the needle and the CLE-miniprobe was retracted inside the needle tip. The preloaded needle was introduced through the working channel of the bronchoscope and lesion puncture was performed under fluoroscopic guidance (Fig. **4**). Right before CLE-imaging, fluorescein (2.5mg of 10% fluoresceindinatrium) was infused through a peripheral IV. Imaging was performed in real time which revealed dense clumping of pleomorphic material consistent with a dense lung lesion.

The confocal fiber was removed from the needle and transbronchial needle aspirates (TBNA) were performed with the 18g needle. The lesion was very firm and yielded little tissue. Without changing robot position, transbronchial biopsies (TBBX) were performed with flexible forceps. Final pathology confirmed granulomatous inflammation. Ziehl-Neelson stain is negative for acid fast bacilli (Fig. **5**).

Complications

None.

Post-Intervention

The patient was started on Rifampin for treatment of latent TB prior to starting adjuvant FOLFOX chemotherapy for locally advanced colonic adenocarcinoma.

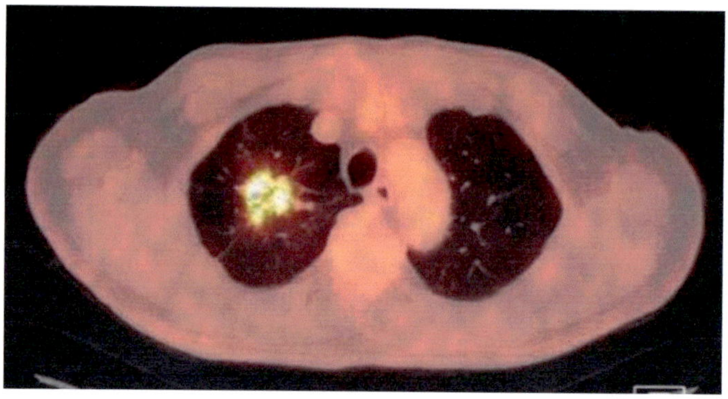

Fig. (1). PET CT.

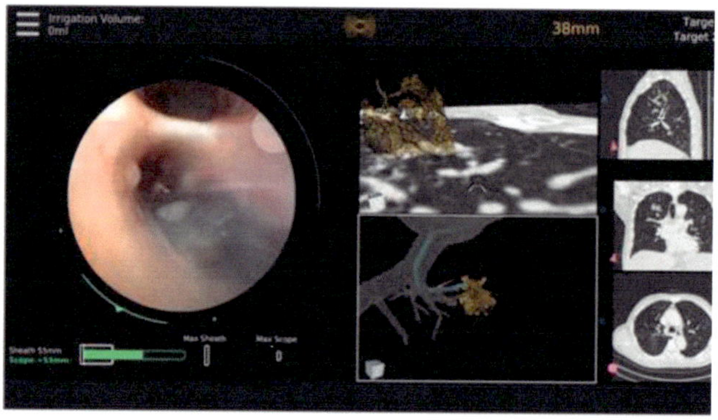

Fig. (2). Robotic bronchoscopy view of anthracotic pigment and endobronchial studding in airway leading to lung nodule.

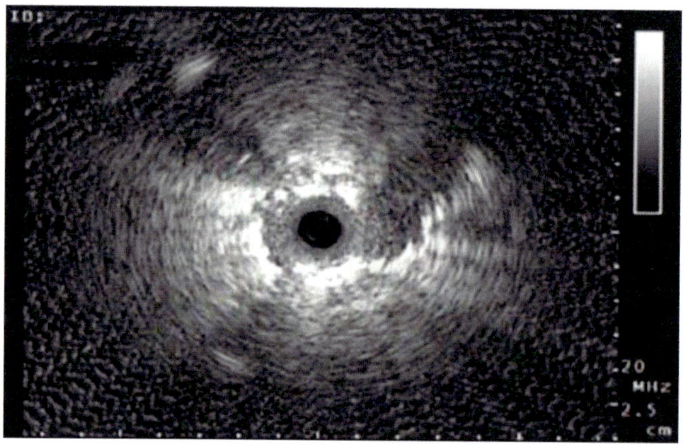

Fig. (3). Radial EBUS of the RUL lung lesion.

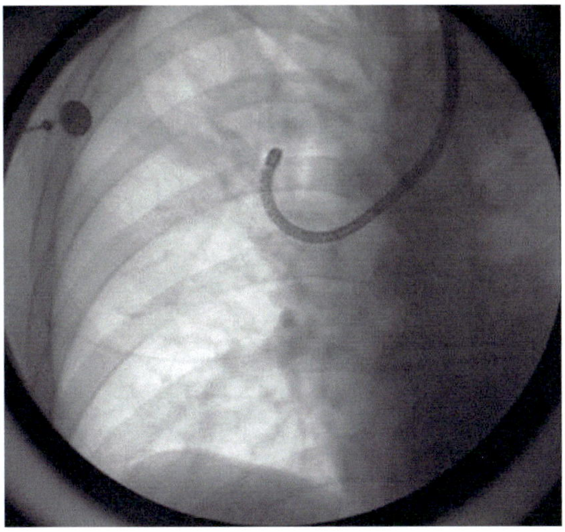

Fig. (4). Robotic bronchoscopy with bronchoscope tip just inferior to nodular density.

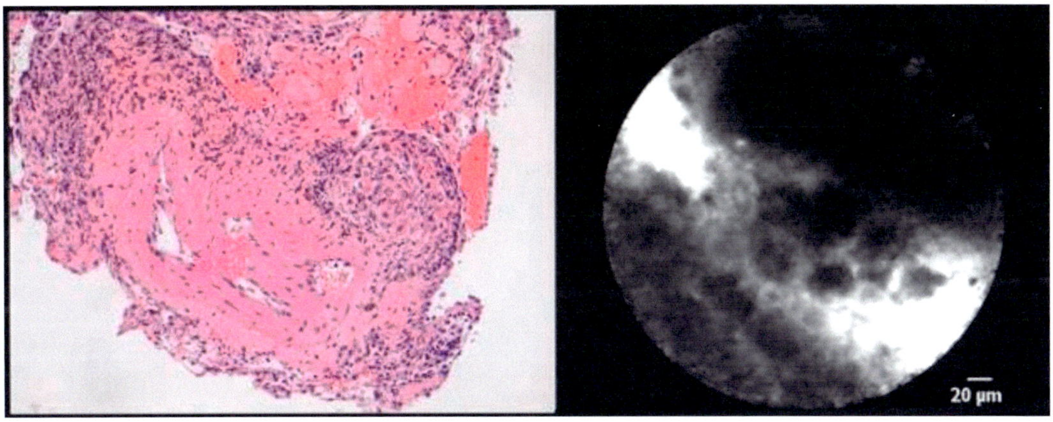

Fig. (5). Transbronchial biopsy showing granulomas and corresponding confocal image of the lung lesion.

Learning Points

- There are many etiologies for PET avid lung lesions. Even in patients with known malignancy, lesions suspicious for metastatic disease should be confirmed by tissue diagnosis.
- Robotic navigational bronchoscopy provides excellent reach, dexterity, and stability for localization and biopsy of lung lesions.

- Real-time imaging with needle based confocal endomicroscopy allows for visualization of tissue to discern between airway mucosa, lung parenchyma, and lung lesions.

CONSENT FOR PUBLICATION

Written informed consent was obtained from the patient for publication of this case report and any accompanying images.

CONFLICT OF INTEREST

The author serves as a consultant and educational speaker for Johnson and Johnson (including Ethicon/Auris Health). He has worked with Galvanize therapeutics as an advisory board member. Other authors report no conflicts of interest.

ACKNOWLEDGEMENTS

The author acknowledges the research grant (funding) received from Mauna Kea, Aquyre Bioscience, and Johnson and Johnson.

REFERENCE

[1] Kramer T, Wijmans L, de Bruin D, *et al.* Bronchoscopic needle based confocal laser endomicroscopy (nCLE) as a real-time detection tool for pe ripheral lung cancer. Thorax 2021; 1-8.
[PMID: 34172559]

Case 24

Cryobiopsy in DPLD

Transbronchial Lung Cryobiopsy to Diagnose Chronic Hypersensitivity Pneumonitis

Wong Soo Fen[1], **Mona Zaria Nasaruddin**[1] and **Jamalul Azizi Abdul Rahaman**[1,*]

[1] *Department of Pulmonology, Serdang Hospital, Selangor, Malaysia*

Keywords: Transbronchial lung cryobiopsy (TBLC), Chronic hypersensitivity pneumonitis, Latex, Pneumothorax, Surgical lung biopsy.

Presentation

55-year-old lady with chronic cough for one year. History of latex exposure for two years while working in a glove factory.

Comorbidities

Nil

Chest Imaging

HRCT thorax showed bilateral upper lobe predominant subpleural and bronchocentric reticulation with air trapping (mosaic attenuation), presence of traction bronchiectasis and bronchiolectasis (Figs. **1a** and **b**).

Intervention

Transbronchial lung cryobiopsy (TBLC) *via* rigid bronchoscopy. Biopsy specimens were taken from RB7, RB9 and RB10 using a 2.4mm ERBE flexible cryoprobe.

[*]**Corresponding author Jamalul Azizi Abdul Rahaman:** Department of Pulmonology, Serdang Hospital, Selangor, Malaysia; E-mail: jamalulazizi@gmail.com

Complications

Right-sided pneumothorax requiring tube thoracostomy. After 3 days, the air leak did not resolve and hence she was sent back to the referring hospital on a Heimlich valve. The air leak resolved after several days and the chest tube was removed.

Post-Intervention

HPE from TBLC showed bronchiolocentric fibrosis with peribronchiolar metaplasia and bronchiolitis, suggestive of chronic hypersensitivity pneumonitis (CHP) despite the absence of granuloma or interstitial giant cells (Figs. **2a** and **b**). She was treated with prednisolone with symptomatic improvement. Her FVC and DLCO remained stable within the next 12 weeks. However, she became symptomatic again when prednisolone was reduced to 20mg daily and therefore Azathioprine was added as a steroid-sparing drug.

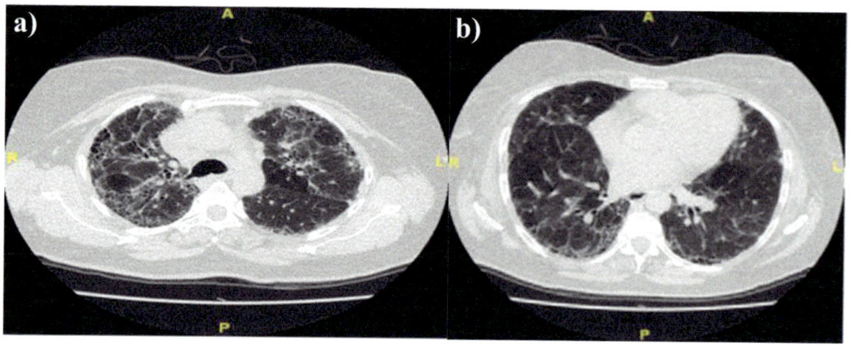

Fig. (1). (**a** and **b**) Axial HRCT thorax shows subpleural and bronchocentric reticulation with traction bronchiolectasis and associated mosaic attenuation.

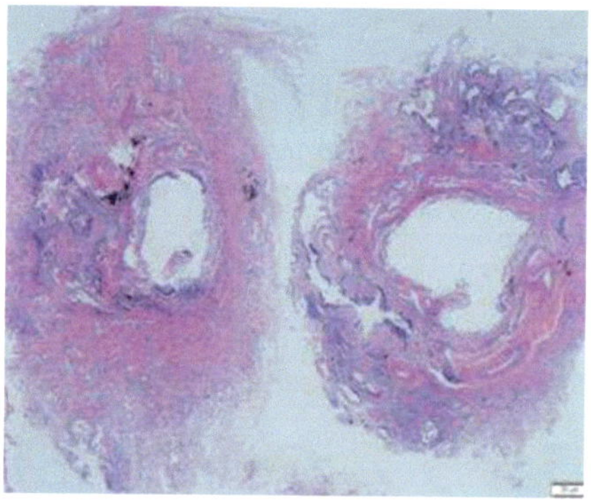

Fig. (2). (**a**) Fragments of fibrotically thickened bronchioles and peribronchiolar walls (H & E x20).

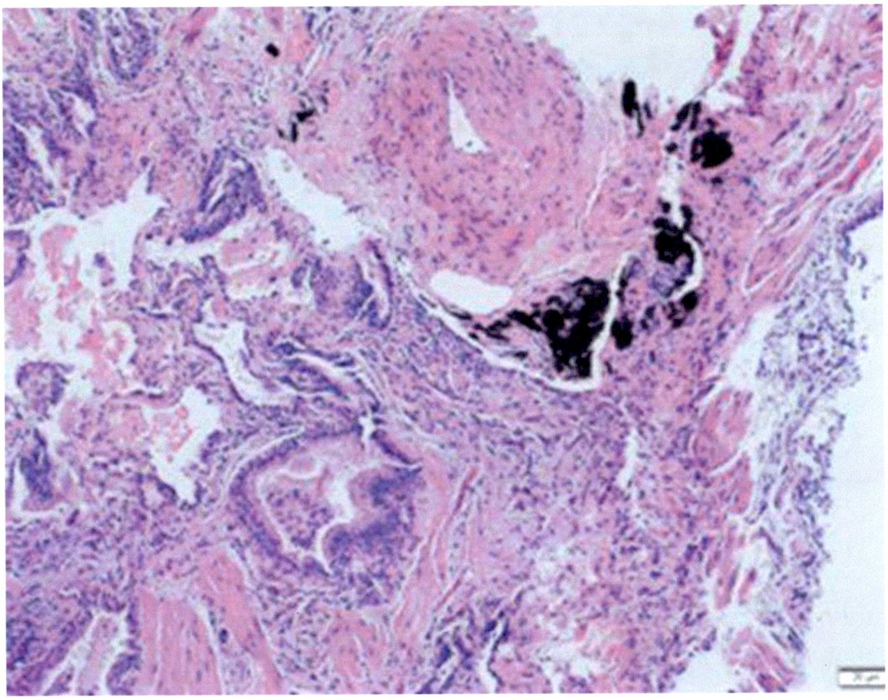

Fig. (2). (**b**) Focal epithelial erosion with bronchiolitis and peribronchiolar metaplasia. Peribronchiolar stroma infiltrated by chronic inflammatory cells (H & E x200).

Learning Points

- TBLC is a novel technique for sampling lung tissue for interstitial lung disease (ILD) diagnosis. In the presence of typical HRCT findings coupled with exposure history and multidisciplinary discussion, a confident diagnosis of CHP can be achieved even though the TBLC is only suggestive of CHP.
- TBLC is less invasive than surgical lung biopsy in obtaining lung biopsy and data support its clinical utility in the ILD diagnostic algorithms [1].
- Air leak after TBLC is usually transient and resolves after tube thoracostomy.

CONSENT FOR PUBLICATION

Not applicable.

CONFLICT OF INTEREST

The authors declare no conflict of interest, financial or otherwise.

ACKNOWLEDGEMENTS

The author acknowledges the support received from Dr. Noriah Othman, Department of Pathology, Serdang Hospital, Selangor, Malaysia.

REFERENCE

[1] Lauren KT, Christopher G, Tamera JC, *et al.* Diagnostic accuracy of transbronchial lung cryobiopsy for interstitial lung disease diagnosis (COLDICE): a prospective, comparative study. Lancet Respir Med 2020; 8(2): 171-81. [http://dx.doi.org/10.1016/S2213-2600(19)30342-X] [PMID: 31578168]

Case 25

Transbronchial Lung Cryobiopsy to Diagnose Eosinophilic Pneumonia

Wong Soo Fen[1], **Mona Zaria Nasaruddin**[1] and **Jamalul Azizi Abdul Rahaman**[1,*]

[1] *Department of Pulmonology, Serdang Hospital, Selangor, Malaysia*

Keywords: Transbronchial lung cryobiopsy (TBLC), Eosinophilic pneumonia, Ground glass opacity, Organizing pneumonia, Interstitial fibrosis.

Presentation

A 48-year-old lady presented with chronic cough for three years and worsening effort tolerance. She worked in the timber, electronics and camphor factories before.

Comorbidities

Diabetes Mellitus, allergic rhinitis.

Chest Imaging

HRCT thorax showed bilateral asymmetrical (right > left) upper lobe predominant ground glass opacity with associated cystic airspaces giving rise to reticular pattern and traction bronchiectasis. Peribronchovascular ground glass opacity with perilobular density at the lingular segment of left upper lobe suggestive of organizing pneumonia pattern (Fig. **1**).

Intervention

EBUS TBNA and TBLC *via* rigid bronchoscopy. EBUS TBNA of stations 4R and 7 lymph nodes followed by TBLC of RB2 with 2.4mm ERBE flexible cryoprobe.

***Corresponding author Jamalul Azizi Abdul Rahaman:** Department of Pulmonology, Serdang Hospital, Selangor, Malaysia; E-mail: jamalulazizi@gmail.com

Jamalul Azizi Abdul Rahaman & Tinku Joseph (Eds.)

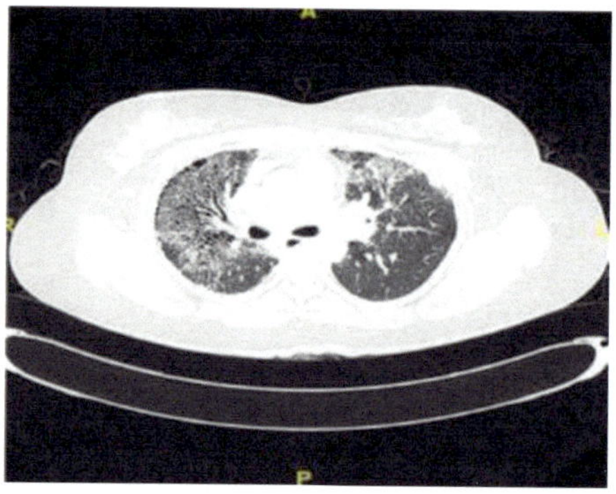

Fig. (1). Axial HRCT thorax showed right upper lobe predominant ground glass opacity with associated cystic airspaces giving rise to reticular pattern and traction bronchiectasis. Left lung: Lingular peribronchovascular ground glass opacity with perilobular density.

Complications

Nil. Patient was discharged well on the following day.

Post-Intervention

EBUS TBNA showed reactive lymph nodes. HPE of TBLC showed interstitial fibrosis and chronic inflammation with the presence of eosinophils in the alveoli, suggestive of eosinophilic pneumonia (Figs. **2a** and **b**). She was treated with oral prednisolone with symptomatic improvement and there was no worsening of the CXR.

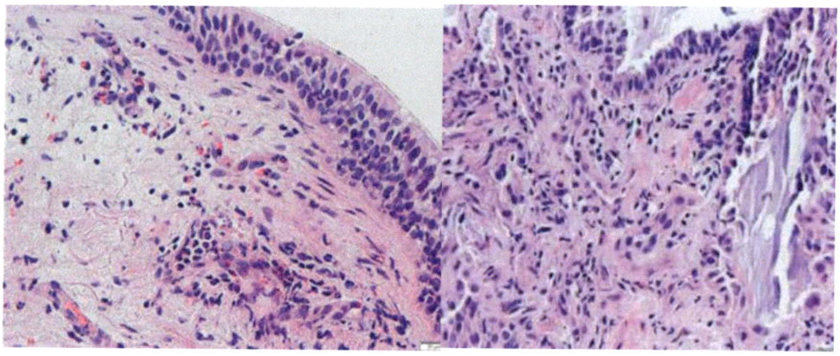

Fig. (2). **(a)** (Left) Bronchial tissue lined by pseudostratified columnar epithelium with stroma infiltrated by eosinophils, neutrophils and lymphocytes (H & E x400). (**b**) (Right) Chronic inflammatory infiltrates consisting of lymphocytes and eosinophils. Alveolar macrophages admixed with eosinophils are noted within the alveolar lumen (H & E x400).

Learning Points

- TBLC is a useful diagnostic tool in ILD diagnostic algorithm and can obviate the need for surgical lung biopsy in some cases. The COLDICE study showed high levels of agreement between TBLC and surgical lung biopsy for both histopathological interpretation and multidisciplinary discussion diagnoses [1].
- TBLC aids in the diagnosis of ILD in the appropriately selected patients and is an acceptable alternative to surgical lung biopsy with fewer complications [2].

Video

TBLC of the posterior segment of the right upper lobe with an endobronchial blocker to control bleeding.

CONSENT FOR PUBLICATION

Not applicable.

CONFLICT OF INTEREST

The authors declare no conflict of interest, financial or otherwise.

ACKNOWLEDGEMENTS

The authors acknowledge the support received from Dr. Noriah Othman, Department of Pathology, Serdang Hospital, Selangor, Malaysia.

REFERENCES

[1] Lauren KT, Christopher G, Tamera JC, *et al.* Diagnostic accuracy of transbronchial lung cryobiopsy for interstitial lung disease diagnosis (COLDICE): a prospective, comparative study. Lancet Respir Med 2020; 8(2): 171-81.

[2] Anne MO, Louise B, Alberto C, *et al.* Transbronchial lung cryobiopsy (TBLC) in the diagnosis of interstitial lung disease: experience of first 100 cases performed under conscious sedation with flexible bronchoscope. Ir J Med Sci 2021; 190(4): 1509-17.
[http://dx.doi.org/10.1016/S2213-2600(19)30342-X] [PMID: 31578168]

Case 26

A Case of Unilateral Interstitial Lung Disease – Transbronchial Lung Cryobiopsy Solved the Mystery

Tinku Joseph[1,*] and **Meghana Subash**[1]

[1] *Division of Interventional Pulmonology, Amrita Institute of Medical Sciences, Kochi, India*

Keywords: Lung cryobiopsy, Lipoid pneumonia, Unilateral ILD, Rigid Bronchoscopy, Cryoprobe.

Presentation

A 61-year-old gentleman, cardamom plantation worker with a history of exposure to pesticides presented with complaints of progressive breathlessness, productive cough, low grade fever on and off and bilateral lower limb edema for 3 months. He was previously treated for community acquired pneumonia. On examination, the patient was pale. Chest examination revealed bilateral fine crepitations and rhonchi. Pulmonary function test showed a mixed obstructive and restrictive ventilatory defect. 6MWT showed no desaturation and distance covered was around 48 meters. Sputum studies were negative for infection (Fig. **1**). ANA screening showed speckled 1+ and Rheumatoid factor was negative.

Comorbidities

Type 2 Diabetes mellitus, systemic hypertension, coronary artery disease (status post PTCA) and dyslipidemia.

Chest Imaging

CXR showed bilateral non-homogenous opacities in bilateral lung fields. CT chest showed interlobular and intralobular septal thickening with ground glass opacities in right middle and lower lobes along with crazy paving pattern likely to be interstitial pneumonia or lymphangitis carcinomatosa (Fig. **2**).

*__Corresponding author Tinku Joseph:__ Division of Interventional Pulmonology, Amrita Institute of Medical Sciences, Kochi, India; E-mail: tinkujoseph2010@gmail.com

Jamalul Azizi Abdul Rahaman & Tinku Joseph (Eds.)

Intervention

In view of inconclusive diagnosis, after a multi-disciplinary ILD board meeting, decision was made to do transbronchial lung cryobiopsy (TBLC) for obtaining a tissue diagnosis. BAL was performed prior to TBLC (Fig. **3**). The site for TBLC was localised based on HRCT findings and rigid bronchoscopy-guided multiple transbronchial lung cryobiopsies were obtained from right lower lobe (RB7, RB9 segments) and right middle lobe (RB5 segment) using 1.9mm flexible cryoprobe under real time fluoroscopy (Fig. **4**). Adequate haemostasis was achieved using 5F Fogarty balloon and local adrenaline instillation.

Complications

No immediate or delayed post procedure complications.

Post-Intervention

BAL showed lymphocyte predominant inflammation and was negative for mycobacterial, fungal and bacterial infections. Histopathological examination of lung biopsy specimens showed alveolar septal (interstitial) cellular infiltrate with ill-formed granuloma at many places. No definitive giant cells were seen. The alveolar lumina showed focally fibrinous exudate along with foamy macrophages (Fig. **5**). Alveolar lining at places showed prominence to type II pneumocytes. No DAD change, fibrosis or fibroblastic foci identified. The case was discussed in the ILD multi-disciplinary team and a diagnosis of right lower lobe lipoid pneumonia was made on the basis of TBLC histopathology and clinico-radiological correlation.

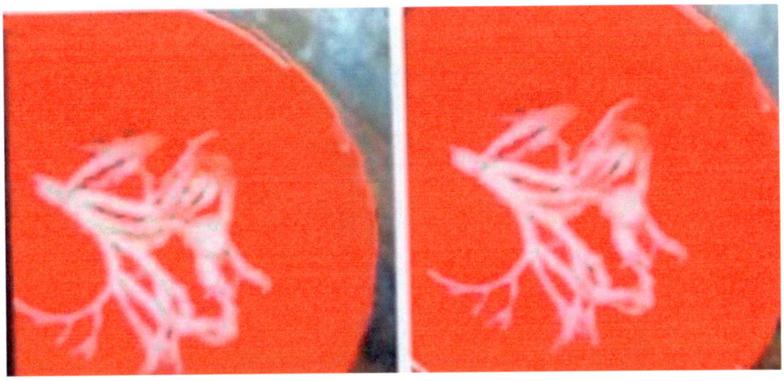

Fig. (1). Sputum sample of patient showing bronchial casts.

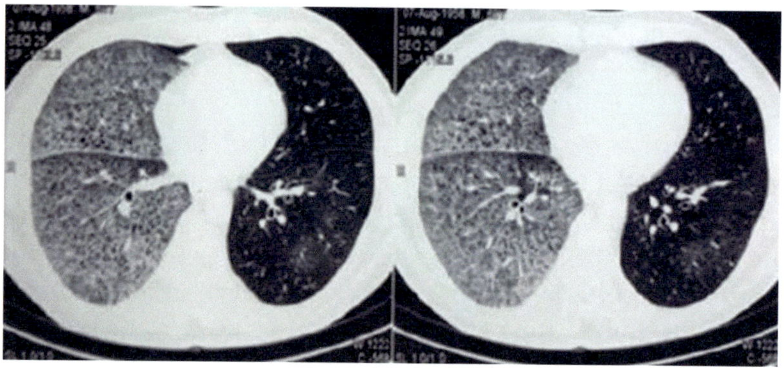

Fig. (2). CT chest showing right lower lobe GGOs with microcystic pattern.

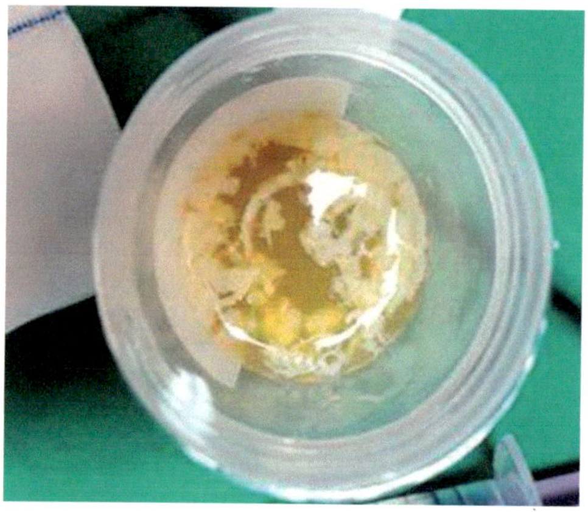

Fig. (3). BAL sample showing thick yellow aspirate with multiple bronchial casts.

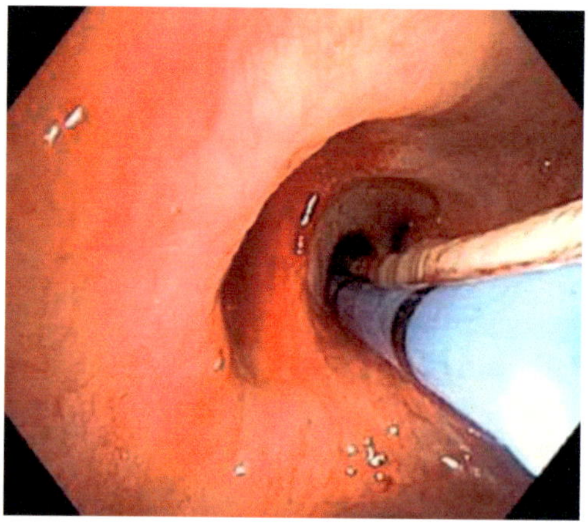

Fig. (4). Bronchoscopic image showing flexible cryoprobe (blue colour) and 5F Fogarty balloon (white colour).

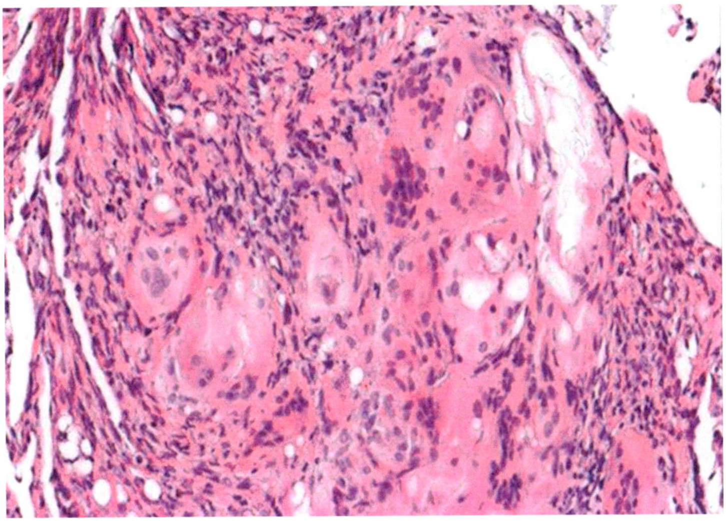

Fig. (5). Histopathology: The alveolar lumina shows focally fibrinous exudate along with foamy macrophages.

Learning Points

- TBLC is a novel technique for sampling lung tissue for diagnosis of idiopathic interstitial pneumonias.
- TBLC is less invasive than surgical lung biopsy in obtaining lung biopsy, with minimal complications [1].
- All cases of TBLC procedures should be discussed in ILD-MDT meetings prior to and after the procedure.

CONSENT FOR PUBLICATION

Not applicable.

CONFLICT OF INTEREST

The authors declare no conflict of interest, financial or otherwise.

ACKNOWLEDGEMENT

Declared none.

REFERENCE

[1] Simmons A, Rouf E, Whittle J. Not Your Typical Pneumonia: A Case of Exogenous Lipoid Pneumonia. J Gen Intern Med 2007; 22(11): 1613-16.
[https://doi.org/10.1007/s11606-007-0280-7]

Section B

Therapeutic Interventional Pulmonology

Case 1

Benign Central Airway Obstruction

Central Airway Obstruction due to Cryptococcus Neoformans

Rosmadi Ismail[1,*]

[1] *Sunway Medical Centre, Selangor, Malaysia*

Keywords: Benign tracheal mass, Cryptococcus neoformans, Interventional bronchoscopy, Central airway obstruction, Mechanical debulking.

Presentation

A 47-year-old lady, presented with recurrent intermittent haemoptysis over 3 months. She denied weight loss or febrile episodes.

Comorbidities

None.

Chest Imaging

CT-thorax showed a lobulated lower tracheal mass on the right lateral wall, right upper lobe nodule and mediastinal lymphadenopathy (Figs. **1a** and **b**).

She had CT guided biopsy of the right upper lobe nodule and the histopathological examination was consistent with non-specific inflammatory process and negative for AFB.

Initial flexible bronchoscopy showed lower tracheal mass with increased vascularity.

Intervention

Rigid bronchoscopy showed an intraluminal broad-based mass arising from the lateral wall of the distal end of trachea extending 2.0cm inferiorly till the right upper

*Corresponding author **Rosmadi Ismail:** Sunway Medical Centre, Selangor, Malaysia; E-mail: rismacc@yahoo.com

Jamalul Azizi Abdul Rahaman & Tinku Joseph (Eds.)

lobe opening. (Fig. **2a**) The mass caused an estimated 70-80% obstruction of the tracheal lumen. Flexible bronchoscope with an external diameter of 6.7mm was able to pass through the mass with slight difficulty.

The mass was endoscopically debulked with a combination of electrosurgical snaring followed by piece meal removal with Erbe® cryoprobe. The mass was further trimmed off and haemostasis was secured with a combination of carbon dioxide laser and argon plasma coagulation (Figs. **2b-d**).

Complications

Nil.

Post-Intervention

Airways were more than 95% patent after the procedure (Fig. **3**). HPE revealed chronic granulomatous inflammation with micro-abscesses and fungal conidia suggestive of histoplasmosis (Fig. **4**). The tissue culture grew Cryptococcus neoformans.

The patient was treated with oral fluconazole and a repeat flexible bronchoscopy showed almost complete resolution of the tracheal lesion (Fig. **5**).

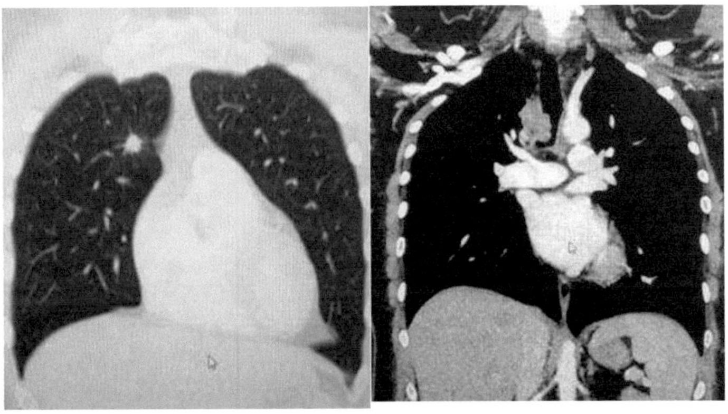

Fig. (1). (a) (Left) and **(b)** (Right) Coronal CT thorax showing a right upper lobe nodule and a lobulated lesion at lower trachea.

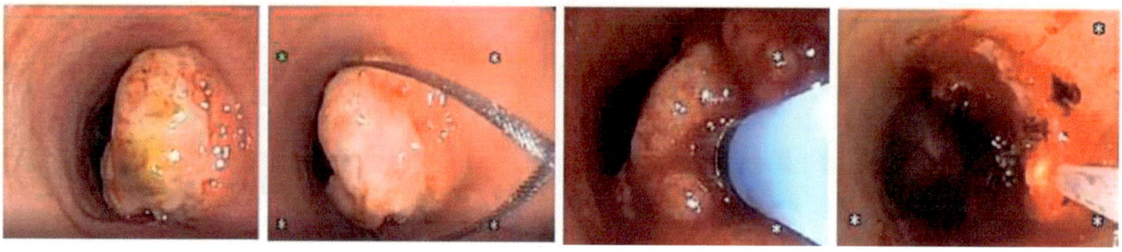

Fig. (2). (**a**) (1st image) Lower tracheal mass pre-procedure**.** **(b** and **c)** (2nd & 3rd images) Debulking with electrosurgical snaring and Erbe® cryoprobe. **(d)** (4th image) Further reduction of residual mass and securing haemostasis with CO_2 laser.

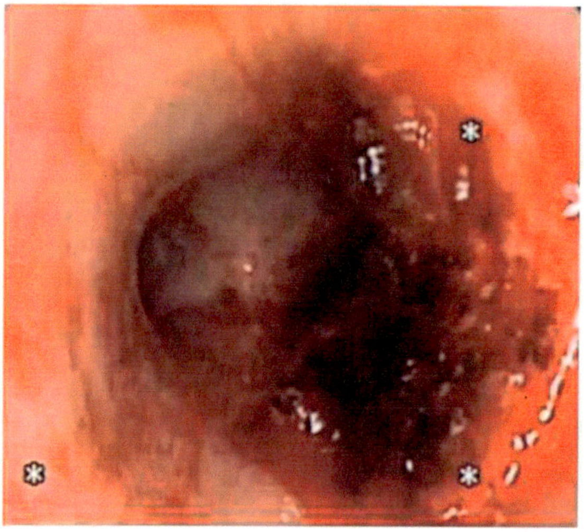

Fig. (3). Bronchoscopic view immediately post-procedure.

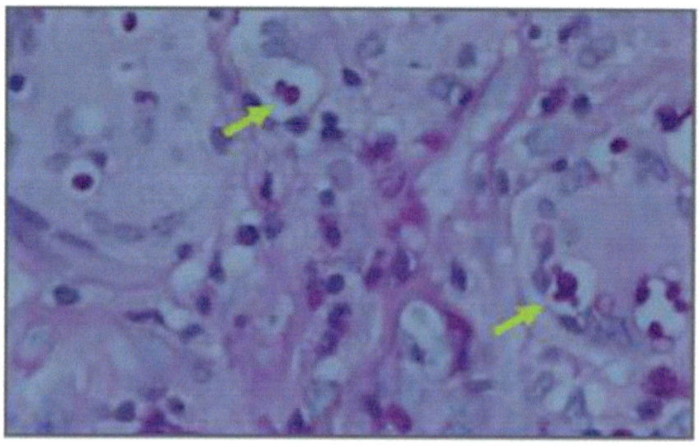

Fig. (4). PAS stain x400 showing the organism (arrow) in varying sizes.

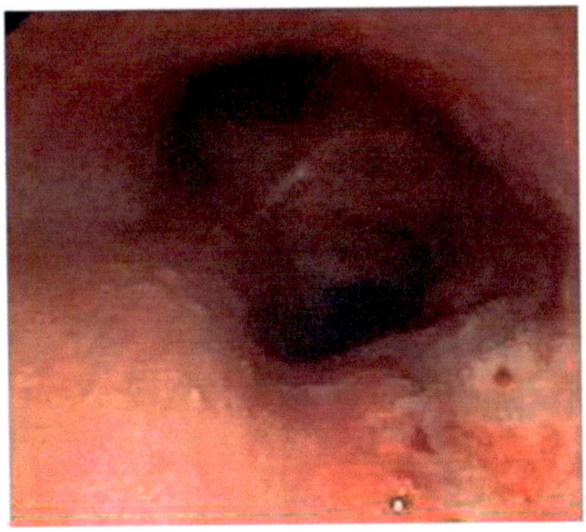

Fig. (5). After 2 months of treatment with oral fluconazole.

Learning Points

- Not all cancerous looking central airway lesions are malignant in nature. It is a good practice to send some of the recovered tissues for microbial studies.
- The recommended duration of antifungal therapy (fluconazole) in immunocompetent patient is between 3-6 months [1].

CONSENT FOR PUBLICATION

Not applicable.

CONFLICT OF INTEREST

The author declares no conflict of interest, financial or otherwise.

ACKNOWLEDGEMENTS

The author acknowledges the support received from Dr. Wan Muhaizan, Sunway Medical Centre, Malaysia.

REFERENCE

[1] Perfect JR, Dismukes WE, Dromer F, *et al*. Clinical practice guidelines for the management of cryptococcal disease: 2010 update by the infectious diseases society of America. Clin Infect Dis 2010; 50(3): 291-322.
[http://dx.doi.org/10.1086/649858] [PMID: 20047480]

Case 2

Micro Laryngeal Tube (MLT/MLS) Guided Debulking of Tracheo-Bronchial Lesions – An Alternative Option to Rigid Bronchoscopy

Tinku Joseph[1,*], **Sathish C. Reddy**[1], **Sreeraj Nair**[1] and **Tushara Madathil**[2]

[1] *Interventional Pulmonology Unit, Amrita Institute of Medical Sciences, Kochi, India*

[2] *Department of Cardiac Anaesthesia, Amrita Institute of Medical Sciences, Kochi, India*

Keywords: MLS tube, Microlaryngeal tube debulking, Benign central airway lesions, Rhinosporidiosis, Rigid bronchoscopy.

Presentation

A 62-year-old gentleman, a known case of severe COPD presented with progressive shortness of breath, cough with scanty mucoid expectoration associated with multiple episodes of haemoptysis and change in voice quality in the last 1 month.

Comorbidities

Recurrent rhinosporidiosis.

Chest Imaging

CECT thorax showed multiple irregular hyper dense heterogeneously enhancing soft tissue attenuating lesions within the tracheal lumen and left main bronchus (Fig. **1**).

Intervention

Initial flexible bronchoscopy showed multiple broad-based lesions involving mid trachea, carina and near total occlusion of left main bronchus (Figs **2a** and **b**). Bronchoscopic biopsy of the lesions confirmed the etiology as rhinosporidiosis. The patient was scheduled initially to undergo rigid bronchoscopy guided resection

*Corresponding author Tinku Joseph: Interventional Pulmonology Unit, Amrita Institute of Medical Sciences, Kochi, India; E-mail: tinkujoseph2010@gmail.com

of tracheo-bronchial lesions. However, in view of inadequate ventilation and high risk of aspiration of blood during debulking, the procedure was done with the assistance of an extra-long, soft small sized microlaryn geal tube (MLT) (Figs. **3a** and **b**). It provided adequate ventilation for the patient and once the distal cuff of MLT was inflated, it prevented aspiration of blood associated with debulking. Also, since the tube size was small (5mm internal diameter), it provided adequate working space inside the tracheal lumen to pass a standard adult flexible bronchoscope and various flexible electro-surgical equipments when we performed this procedure. Entire tracheobronchial rhinosporidiosis lesions were debulked.

Complications

No major/minor intra/post-procedure complications were noted.

Post-Intervention

The patient was extubated on the table and discharged the next day in a symptom free state.

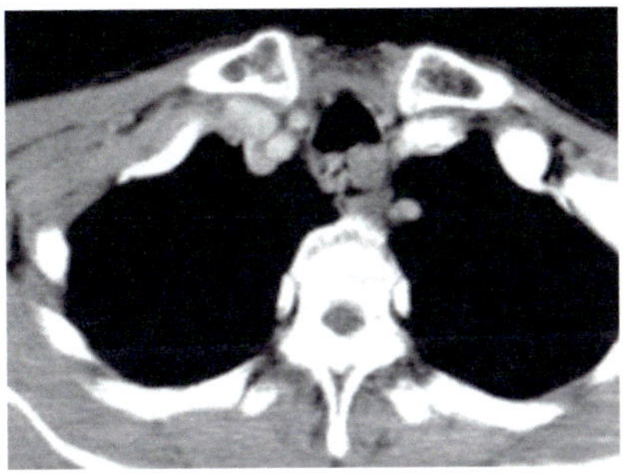

Fig. (1). Axial CT thorax showing polypoidal lesions within the tracheal lumen.

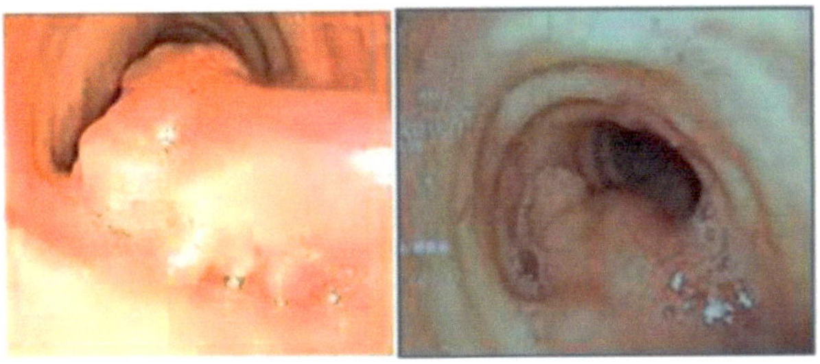

Fig. (2). (a) (Left) **(b)** (Right). Flexible bronchoscopy images showing rhinosporidiosis lesions within the tracheal lumen.

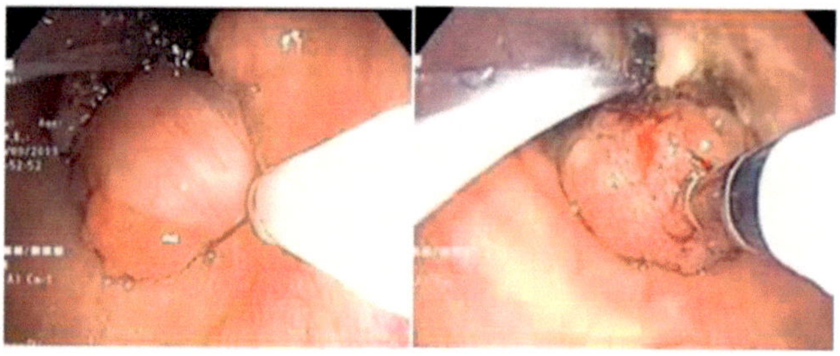

Fig. (3). (a) (Left) **(b)** (Right). MLT/MLS tube guided debulking of rhinosporidiosis tracheal lesions using snare electrocautery and cryoprobe.

Learning Points

- Extra-long, soft, small sized microlaryngeal tracheal tube (MLT/MLS) can be used as a possible alternative to rigid bronchoscope guided debulking of vascular lesions/ tumours [1].
- Tracheo-bronchial rhinosporidiosis is a difficult to treat condition, which may require frequent bronchoscopic procedures for symptom relief.
- Ablation of the base of the lesion is important to reduce the chances of recurrence.

Advantages of MLT/MLS Tube

- Prevents aspiration of blood into the airway during debulking procedure. Helps to maintain adequate ventilation when you debulk vascular central airway lesions.
- Increases the confidence level of the bronchoscopist and anaesthetist.

Disadvantages of Using an MLT/MLS Tube

- Reduces the working space when you perform the central airway debulking procedure.
- Possibility of damage to the upper airway structures due to the frequent passage of bronchoscope and electrodes around the narrowed airway due to the presence of MLT/MLS tube.

Video

The video shows MLT/MLS tube guided debulking of rhinosporidiosis tracheal lesions using snare electrocautery and cryoprobe.

CONSENT FOR PUBLICATION

Not applicable.

CONFLICT OF INTEREST

The author declares no conflict of interest, financial or otherwise.

ACKNOWLEDGEMENT

Declared none.

REFERENCE

[1] Kumar V, Garg R, Mishra R, Gupta N. Anesthetic concerns for rigid bronchoscopic debulking of tracheal growth in postpneumonectomy patient. J Anaesthesiol Clin Pharmacol 2018; 34(4): 563-64.
[https://doi.org/10.4103/joacp.JOACP_391_16]

Case 3

Multidimensional Approach for Tracheobronchial Papillomatosis Lesions

Tinku Joseph[1,*], **Sathish C. Reddy**[1] and **Gopan**[2]

[1] *Interventional Pulmonology Unit, Amrita Institute of Medical Sciences, Kochi, India*

[2] *Department of Cardiac Anaesthesia, Amrita Institute of Medical Sciences, Kochi, India*

Keywords: Airway benign lesions, Endobronchial electrocautery, Interventional Pulmonology, Tracheal papillomatosis, Rigid bronchoscopy.

Presentation

A 43-year-old male, presented with cough with scanty mucoid expectoration, dyspnoea on exertion of 5 months duration.

Comorbidities

Recurrent laryngeal papillomatosis, cerebrovascular disease, systemic hypertension, Type 2 diabetes mellitus.

Chest Imaging

CXR showed collapse consolidation of the left lower lobe (Fig. **1**).

CECT thorax showed lobar consolidation involving all the segments of left lower lobe and left lower lobe bronchus appeared occluded. No obvious focal intrapulmonary lesions.

Intervention

Initial flexible bronchoscopy done showed multiple papillomatous growth in the right vocal cord, mid trachea and left lower lobe basal segments (Fig. **2**). Subsequently, the patient underwent rigid bronchoscopy guided debulking of these lesions. The patient was intubated with a 13-14mm sized rigid bronchoscope. Using snare electrocautery, blunt probe electrocautery and flexible cryoprobe, the tracheal

*Corresponding author Tinku Joseph:** Interventional Pulmonology Unit, Amrita Institute of Medical Sciences, Kochi, India; E-mail: tinkujoseph2010@gmail.com and left lower lobe lobar bronchial lesions were debulked. The residual endotracheal sheet-like lesions were cored with the barrel of the rigid bronchoscope. The base of the lesions was subsequently ablated using cryoprobe and electrocautery (blunt probe). Later, the papillomatous lesions present over the vocal cord and nasopharynx were debulked using a coblator.

Complications

No immediate major post procedure complications were noted.

Post-Intervention

The upper and central airway lumen was recanalized post-procedure and the patient was extubated on table (Fig. **3**). HPE of the debulked tissue was suggestive of diffuse papillomatosis.

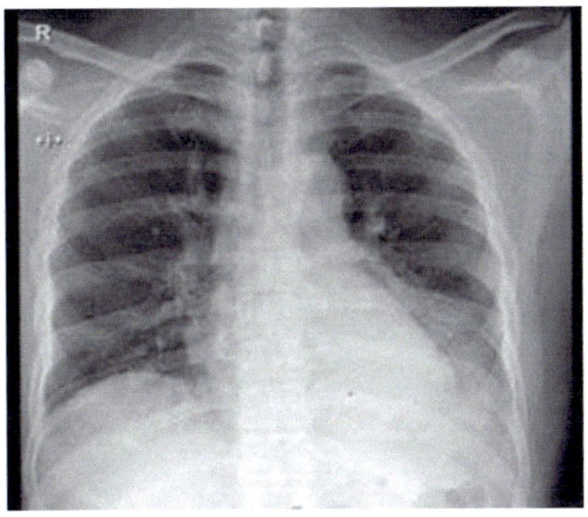

Fig. (1). CXR showing collapse consolidation of left lower lobe.

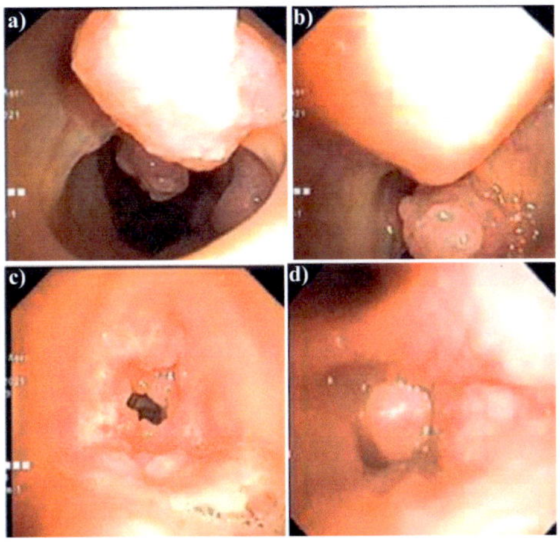

Fig. (2). Flexible bronchoscopy findings: Multiple broad-based sheet-like papillomatosis lesions involving the **a)** vocal cords **b)** subglottic space **c)** tracheal lumen **d)** left lower lobe bronchus.

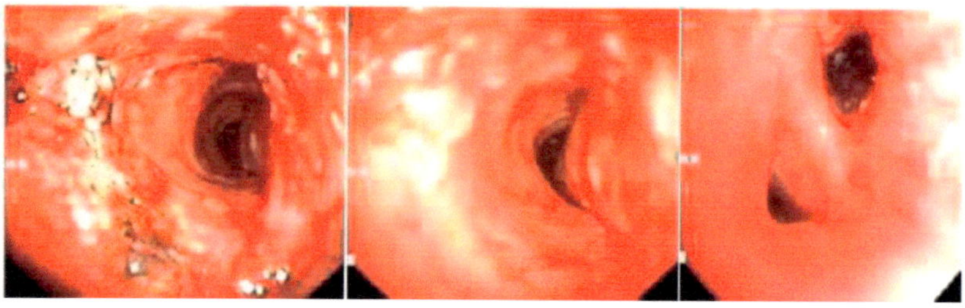

Fig. (3). Bronchoscopic images of recanalized subglottic space, tracheal lumen and left lower lobe bronchus.

Learning Points

- Tracheo-bronchial papillomatosis is a slow growing condition, treatment is ineffective with high recurrence rates (more than 90%) [1].
- Overall, it carries a poor prognosis. The disease gradually progresses leading to respiratory failure.
- Bronchoscopic ablative techniques/surgical excision is considered as a palliative measure to relieve the obstructive symptoms.

CONSENT FOR PUBLICATION

Not applicable.

CONFLICT OF INTEREST

The author declares no conflict of interest, financial or otherwise.

ACKNOWLEDGEMENT

Declared none.

REFERENCE

[1] Kalanjeri S, Hoffman S, Farver C, Almeida FA. Diffuse Tracheal Papillomatosis. Am J Respir Crit Care Med 2017; 195(1): 134-35.
[http://dx.doi.org/10.1164/rccm.201606-1242IM] [PMID: 27676185]

Case 4

Endoscopic Treatment for Inflammatory Myofibroblastic Tumor of the Trachea

Tang Jeat Thong[1], **Mona Zaria Nasaruddin**[1] and **Jamalul Azizi Abdul Rahaman**[1,*]

[1] *Department of Pulmonology, Serdang Hospital, Selangor, Malaysia*

Keywords: Debulking, Endoscopic treatment, Intraluminal mass, Inflammatory myofibroblastic tumor, Tracheal mass.

Presentation

26-year-old male, intermittent hemoptysis for 2 years.

Comorbidities

None.

Chest Imaging

CT angiography and CECT thorax revealed a well-defined heterogeneously enhancing broad-based lobulated intraluminal soft tissue lesion within the trachea arising from the right anterolateral wall of the trachea 4.5cm above the main carina (Fig. **1**). It measured 1.3 x 1.4 x 1.7cm. There was no calcification or fat component within the lesion. There was no extraluminal extension of the lesion.

Flexible bronchoscopy revealed a polypoidal mass at the distal trachea causing 90% occlusion of the trachea (Fig. **2**).

Intervention

Nd: YAP laser coagulation followed by snare electrocautery and cryoextraction of the tumor *via* rigid bronchoscopy. After the debulking, the base of the tumor was carbonized with Nd: YAP laser.

[*]**Corresponding author Jamalul Azizi Abdul Rahaman:** Department of Pulmonology, Serdang Hospital, Selangor, Malaysia; E-mail: jamalulazizi@gmail.com

Complications

Mild bleeding (<50ml).

Post-Intervention

Successfully achieved airway patency with symptom improvement (Fig. **3**). HPE revealed inflammatory myofibroblastic tumor (Fig. **4**).

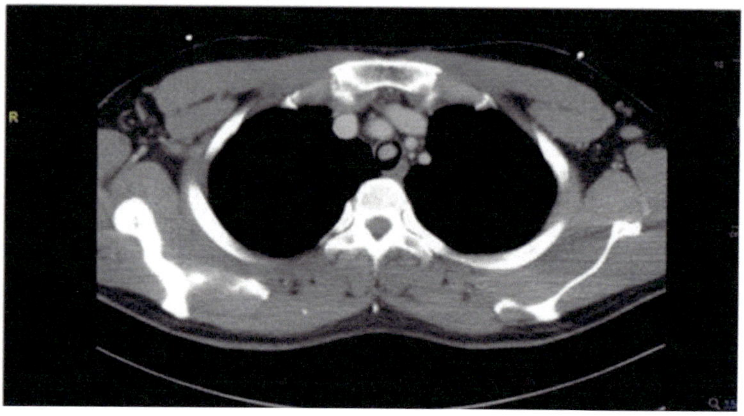

Fig. (1). Axial CECT thorax shows a well-defined broad-based lobulated intra-luminal lesion arising from the right anterolateral wall of the trachea.

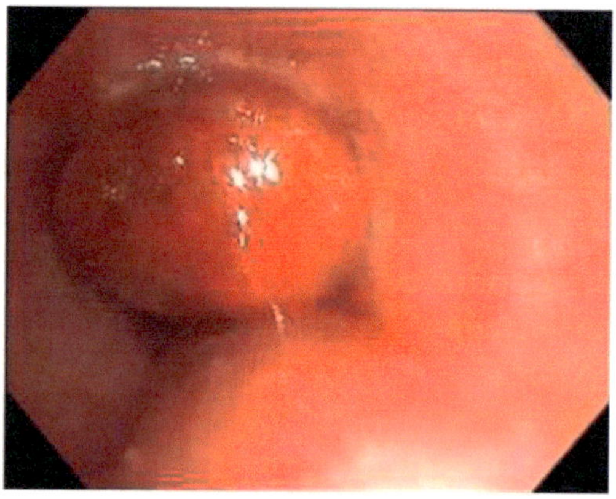

Fig. (2). Pre-debulking.

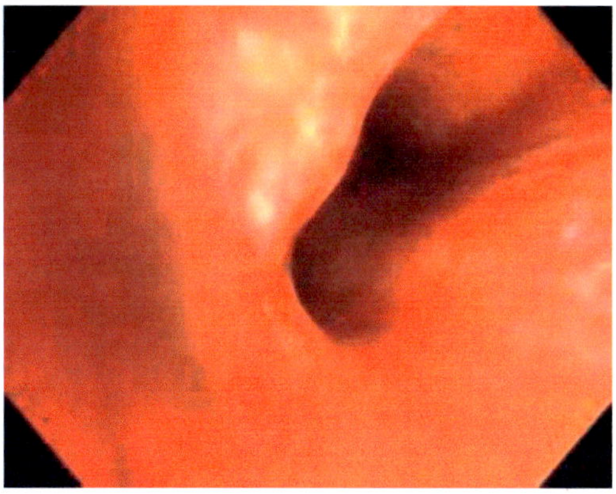

Fig. (3). Post-debulking.

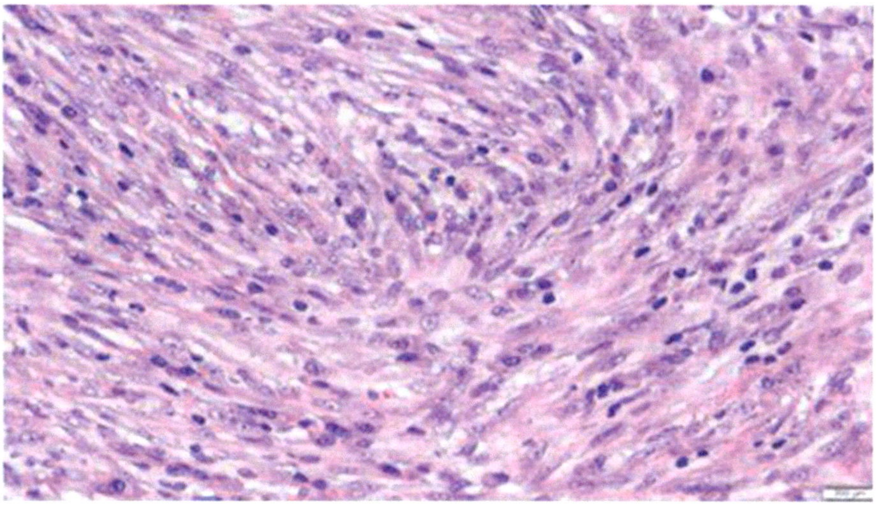

Fig. (4). Lesional tissue is composed of proliferation of spindle cells arranged in fascicular and vague storiform patterns set in collagenous to loose background. These spindle cells exhibit uniform fusiform to oval nuclei, pinpoint nucleoli and eosinophilic cytoplasm. Numerous plasma cells and lymphocytes intermingle within the lesion.

Learning Points

- This procedure was performed to relieve the immediate central airway obstruction (CAO) and was not intended to be the definitive treatment. The patient was advised for tracheal resection but he wanted to discuss with his family first and eventually was lost to follow-up. This is a benign neoplasm affecting young patients with local invasion, distant metastasis and local recurrence and therefore, a complete resection is the treatment of choice [1].

- Endoscopic treatment can be offered at the initial presentation to relieve CAO prior to surgical resection [2].

Video

Endoscopic resection of the tracheal tumour using Nd: YAP laser, snare electrocautery and cryoextraction.

CONSENT FOR PUBLICATION

Not applicable.

CONFLICT OF INTEREST

The author declares no conflict of interest, financial or otherwise.

ACKNOWLEDGEMENTS

The authors acknowledge the support received from Dr. Norhafizah Mohtarrudin, Department of Pathology, Faculty of Medicine and Health Sciences, Universiti Putra Malaysia, 43400 Serdang, Selangor, Malaysia.

REFERENCES

[1] Fabre D, Fadel E, Singhal S, *et al.* Complete resection of pulmonary inflammatory pseudotumors has excellent long-term prognosis. J Thorac Cardiovasc Surg 2009; 137(2): 435. [http://dx.doi.org/10.1016/j.jtcvs.2008.07.009] [PMID: 19185166]

[2] Yang F, Zhang W, Han C, *et al.* A case of pulmonary inflammatory myofibroblastic tumor treated with bronchoscopic therapy plus lobectomy. J Cardiothoracic Surg 2021; 16: 144. [http://dx.doi.org/10.1186/s13019-021-01528-5] [PMID: 34039398]

Case 5

Endoscopic Treatment of Pulmonary Mucormycosis in an Immunocompetent Patient

Khai Lip Ng[1,*], **Mona Zaria Nasaruddin**[1] and **Jamalul Azizi Abdul Rahaman**[1]

[1] *Department of Pulmonology, Serdang Hospital, Selangor, Malaysia*

Keywords: Endobronchial tumour, Immunocompetent, Mucormycosis, Multimodality, Pregnant.

Presentation

A 31-year-old pregnant lady with chronic cough, weight loss and on and off haemoptysis for 1 month. Retroviral screening was negative.

Comorbidities

None.

Chest Imaging

CXR showed a left 'lung mass' with pleural effusion. CT thorax showed a left hilar mass with infiltration of the left main bronchus and mediastinal lymphadenopathy and presence of consolidation with tree-in-bud and satellite nodules (Fig. **1**). Flexible bronchoscopy revealed a whitish endobronchial mass totally occluding the left main bronchus 2cm from the main carina (Fig. **2**).

Intervention

Debulking *via* rigid bronchoscopy. A bronchial rigid tube (EFER-DUMON bronchoscope, BT-2101, tube diameter 12.00mm/11.00mm, length 36cm, colour coded black) was advanced into the ostium of the left main bronchus. Snare electrocautery was done. After removing the endobronchial mass, copious secretions were seen coming from the left upper and lower lobes. The airway mucosa was unhealthy and multiple nodules were seen along the left main bronchus. Cryobiopsy of the nodules was performed (Fig. **3**). Argon plasma

*Corresponding author Khai Lip Ng: Department of Pulmonology, Serdang Hospital, Selangor, Malaysia; E-mail: khailip08@yahoo.com

Jamalul Azizi Abdul Rahaman & Tinku Joseph (Eds.)

coagulation (APC) was applied on the unhealthy mucosa. The left main bronchus was patent after the procedure. Provisional diagnosis was lung malignancy.

Complications

None.

Post-Intervention

Cough and haemoptysis improved after the procedure. HPE showed inflamed tissue with fungal organism (Fig. **4**). There was no granuloma or malignancy seen. Its morphology favoured mucormycosis/zygomycosis. Fungal PCR showed Rhizopus microsporus. The patient was treated with 2 weeks of intravenous Amphotericin B. A repeat CXR after 2 weeks showed complete resolution of the hilar mass (Fig. **5a** and **b**).

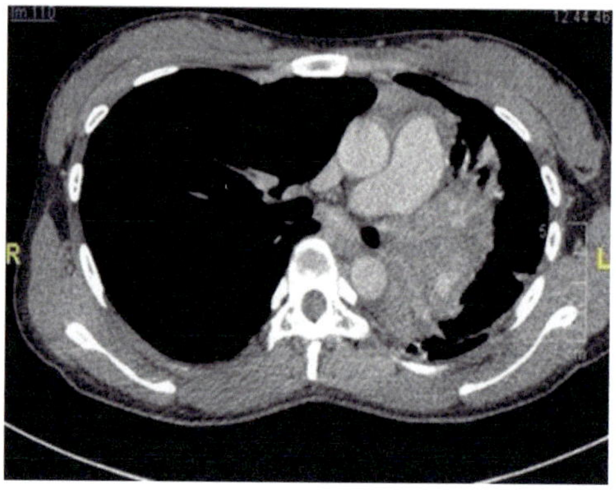

Fig. (1). CT thorax shows the left hilar mass with infiltration into the left main bronchus.

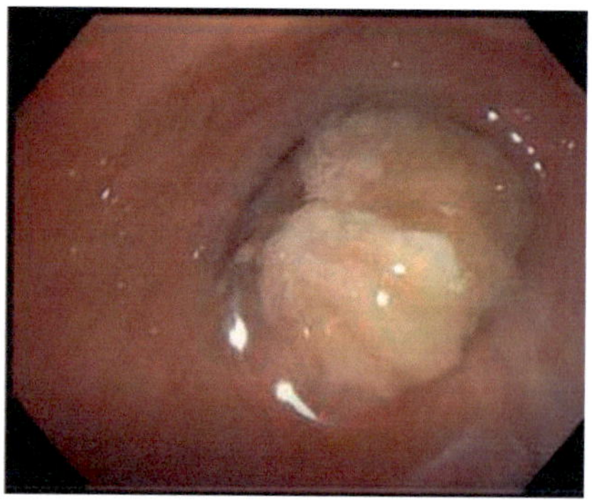

Fig. (2). Endoluminal mass in the left main bronchus.

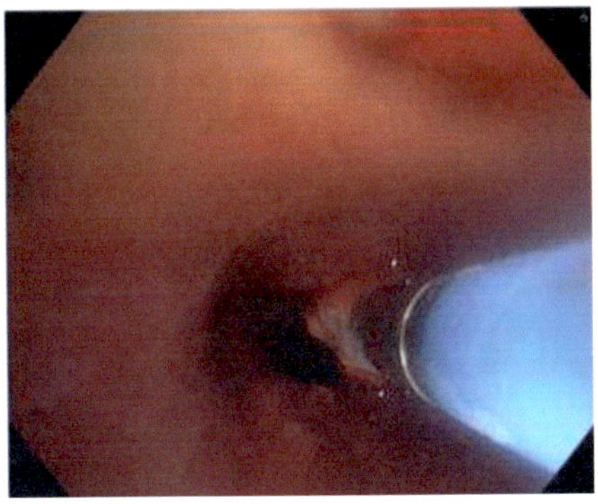

Fig. (3). Endoluminal mass removed *via* snare electrocautery, exposing the unhealthy mucosa and nodules beyond it. Cryoprobe was used to obtain large biopsy samples.

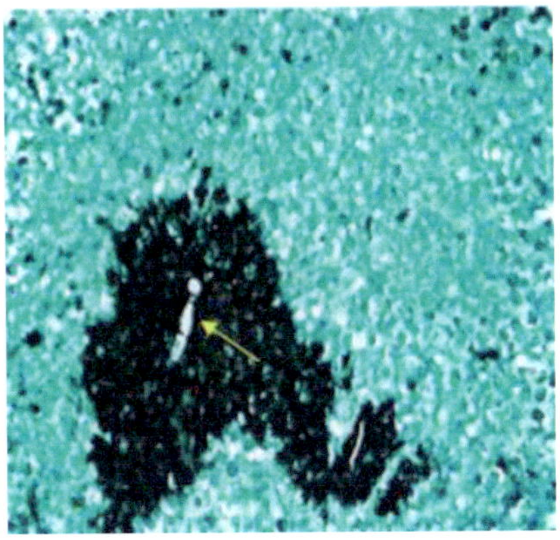

Fig. (4). HPE revealed fungal body (yellow arrow) under Giemsa Stain.

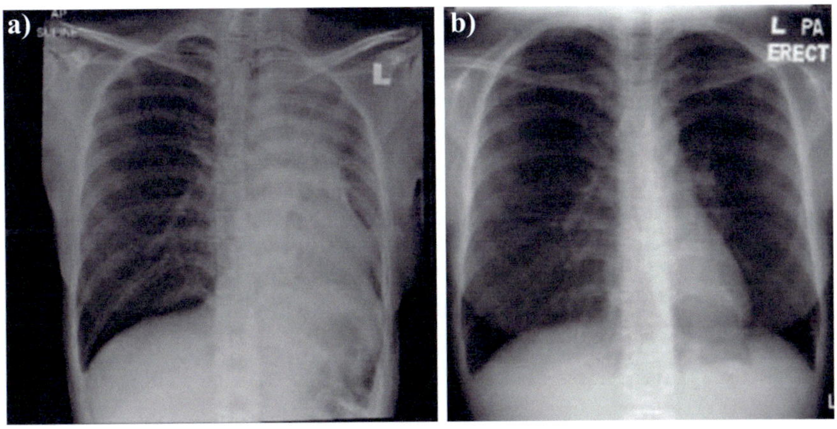

Fig. (5). (a) CXR before debulking showing a left 'lung mass'. **(b)** CXR after Amphotericin B.

Learning Points

- Although rare, mucormycosis has been reported in immunocompetent patients. A proactive approach to obtain tissue diagnosis is important as it is potentially curable if treated early. Endoscopic intervention followed by medical treatment can give the best outcome [1].

Video

Debulking of the endobronchial mass in the left main bronchus using snare electrocautery, cryoprobe and APC.

CONSENT FOR PUBLICATION

Not applicable.

CONFLICT OF INTEREST

The author declares no conflict of interest, financial or otherwise.

ACKNOWLEDGEMENTS

The authors acknowledge the support received from Dr. Noriah Othman, Department of Pathology, Serdang Hospital, 43000 Serdang, Selangor, Malaysia.

REFERENCE

[1] Ng KL, Huan N-C, Zaria M, *et al.* Pulmonary mucormycosis masquerading as endobronchial tumour in an immunocompetent pregnant young lady. Respirol Case Rep 2021; 9(2): e00704. [http://dx.doi.org/10.1002/rcr2.704] [PMID: 33364028]

Case 6

Emergent Endoscopic Treatment for TB-Associated Tracheal Stenosis Mimicking Asthma in a Young Adult

Nai-Chien Huan[1,*], **Mona Zaria Nasaruddin**[1] and **Jamalul Azizi Abdul Rahaman**[1]

[1] *Department of Pulmonology, Serdang Hospital, Selangor, Malaysia*

Keywords: Asthma mimicker, Balloon dilatation, Smear positive pulmonary TB, Tracheal stenosis, Topical mitomycin C.

Presentation

A 32-year-old lady with smear positive pulmonary TB who was still on treatment presented with recurrent episodes of shortness of breath (Modified Borg Dyspnoea Scale 6 at rest: severe) and orthopnoea. She was treated as adult-onset asthma and was empirically commenced on inhaled corticosteroids and short acting beta2-agonist without improvement.

Comorbidities

Nil.

Chest Imaging

CT thorax showed a significant luminal narrowing of the upper one third of the trachea (Fig. **1**). Flexible bronchoscopy revealed a complex tracheal stenosis (length > 1.0cm, about 3.0cm below the vocal cords) with an opening diameter of approximately 2.0mm (Myers-Cotton grade 3). Unable to pass the flexible bronchoscope through the stenotic segment.

*Corresponding author **Nai-Chien Huan:** Department of Pulmonology, Serdang Hospital, Selangor, Malaysia; E-mail: naichien_1@yahoo.com

Jamalul Azizi Abdul Rahaman & Tinku Joseph (Eds.)

Intervention

Emergent balloon dilatation of the stenotic segment followed by application of topical mitomycin C. The intervention was performed *via* rigid bronchoscopy (Figs. **2a-c**).

Complications

None. She was discharged 2 days later.

Post-Intervention

The patient reported improvement in symptoms (Modified Borg Dyspnoea Scale 4 at rest: moderate) with significant improvement in her quality of life. Flexible bronchoscopy 6 weeks later showed no evidence of recurrence (Fig. **2d**).

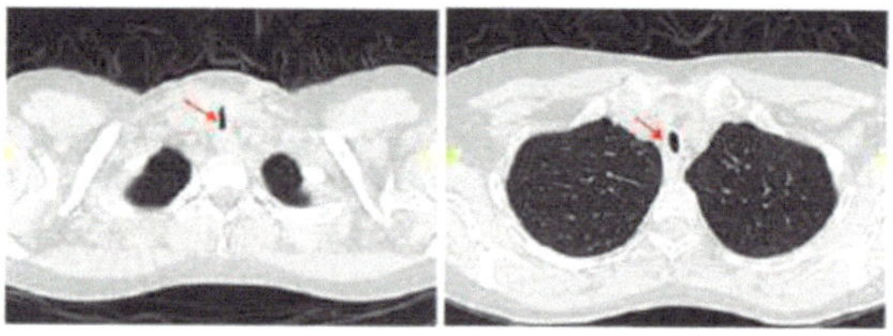

Fig. (1). CT images demonstrating critical stenosis at the upper one third of the trachea (red arrows).

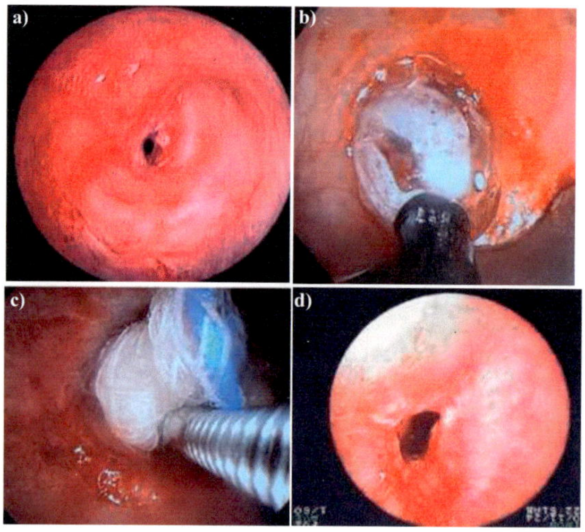

Fig. (2). (a) Severe tracheal stenosis with an opening of approximately 2.0mm. **(b)** Balloon dilatation of stenotic segment *via* rigid bronchoscopy (bevel of rigid bronchoscope marked with yellow circle). **(c)** Application of mitomycin C post-dilatation. **(d)** 6 weeks post-intervention – able to pass flexible bronchoscope beyond the stenotic segment.

Learning Points

- Tracheobronchial stenosis secondary to endobronchial tuberculosis (TSTB) is a debilitating complication usually seen in young females and sometimes misdiagnosed as asthma. It can happen while the patient is still on anti-TB medication [1]. When the stenosis affects the trachea, it can be life threatening. Immediate airway intervention is necessary to relieve the central airway obstruction as airway surgery is risky when the stenosis is complex, and the patient has not completed anti-TB medication. Flexible bronchoscopy should be performed to rule out TSTB in high risk patients with 'asthma-like' symptoms while on anti-TB medication. Topical mitomycin C is a useful adjunct in endoscopic treatment for TSTB to prevent or delay recurrence [1].

Video

Balloon bronchoplasty and topical mitomycin C to treat the tracheal stenosis.

CONSENT FOR PUBLICATION

Not applicable.

CONFLICT OF INTEREST

The author declares no conflict of interest, financial or otherwise.

ACKNOWLEDGEMENT

Declared none.

REFERENCE

[1] Huan C, Ng KL, Nasaruddin MZ, *et al.* Topical mitomycin-C as an adjuvant to multimodal endoscopic treatment for tracheobronchial stenosis secondary to endobronchial tuberculosis. Respirol Case Rep 2021; 9(3).
[https://doi.org/10.1002/rcr2.711] [PMID: 33532074]

Case 7

Mechanical 'Coring' as Part of Multimodality Treatment in Critical Post-TB Tracheal Stenosis

Nai-Chien Huan[1,*], **Mona Zaria Nasaruddin**[1] and **Jamalul Azizi Abdul Rahaman**[1]

[1] *Department of Pulmonology, Serdang Hospital, Selangor, Malaysia*

Keywords: Mechanical coring, Post-tuberculosis lung disease, Rigid bronchoscopy, Tuberculosis, Tracheal stenosis, Topical mitomycin C.

Presentation

A 57-year-old lady with a history of smear positive pulmonary TB 2 years ago. Recurrent episodes of shortness of breath and stridor for one year (Modified Borg Dyspnoea Scale 6 at rest: severe) due to tracheal stenosis. Prior to the current admission, she had undergone multiple endoscopic procedures (balloon dilatation and cauterisation) at another centre.

Comorbidities

Childhood asthma.

Chest Imaging

CT thorax demonstrated a significant luminal narrowing of the mid-trachea with a stenotic length of approximately 1.5cm (Fig. **1**). Flexible bronchoscopy showed a complex tracheal stenosis with an opening diameter of approximately 2.0mm (Myers-Cotton grade 3). Unable to pass the flexible bronchoscope through the stenotic segment.

Intervention

Rigid bronchoscopy followed by gradual balloon dilatation of the stenotic segment. Thereafter, mechan ical 'coring' of the stenotic segment was carefully performed with a rigid bronchial tube (outer diameter 10mm, length 36cm, colour coded red,

***Corresponding author Nai-Chien Huan:** Department of Pulmonology, Serdang Hospital, Selangor, Malaysia; E-mail: naichien_1@yahoo.com

Series 2 EFER-DUMON Bronchoscope, La Ciotat, France) before the application of topical mitomycin C (Figs. **2a-d**).

Complications

None. Discharged 2 days later.

Post-Intervention

Symptoms improved (Modified Borg Dyspnoea Scale 4 at rest: moderate) together with a resolution of orthopnoea. In view of the short segment stenosis with multiple recurrences despite endoscopic treatment, she was referred to a thoracic surgeon for tracheal resection and primary anastomosis.

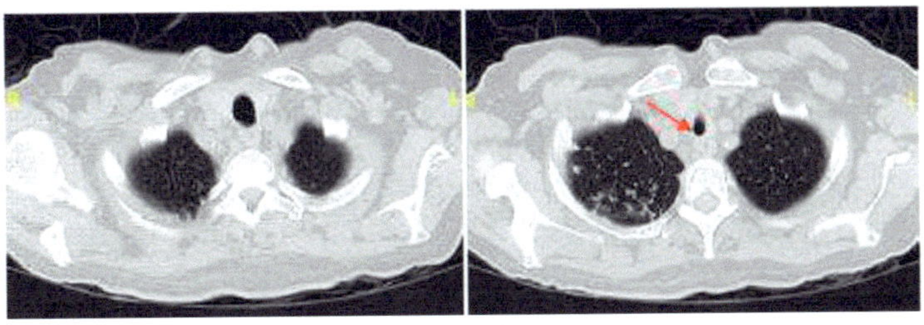

Fig. (1). Serial axial CT images (cranio-caudally) demonstrating critical stenosis at mid trachea (red arrow).

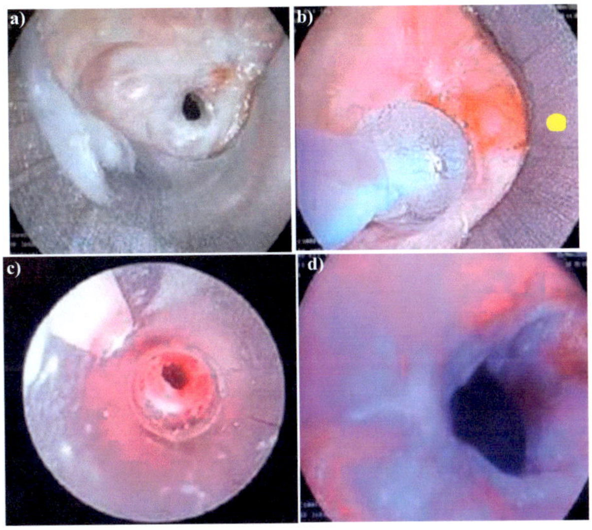

Fig. (2). (a) Severe tracheal stenosis with the opening of approximately 2.0mm. **(b)** Balloon dilatation of the stenotic segment via rigid bronchoscopy (bevel of rigid bronchoscope marked with yellow circle). **(c)** Mechanical 'coring' using a rigid bronchial tube. **(d)** Post-intervention - able to pass flexible bronchoscope beyond stenotic segment.

Learning Points

- Tracheobronchial stenosis is a serious complication of endobronchial TB and can develop several years post-TB treatment. It can be life-threatening when it affects the trachea. In this case, following balloon dilatation, we performed mechanical 'coring' of the stenotic segment followed by application of topical mitomycin C as a temporary measure to delay recurrence prior to definitive surgery [1]. Mechanical 'coring' must be done carefully after the initial balloon dilatation to avoid airway laceration or perforation.

Video

Balloon dilatation of the stenotic segment followed by mechanical 'coring' of the stenotic segment using a rigid bronchial tube (outer diameter 10mm, length 36cm, colour coded red, Series 2 EFER-DUMON Bronchoscope, La Ciotat, France).

CONSENT FOR PUBLICATION

Not applicable.

CONFLICT OF INTEREST

The author declares no conflict of interest, financial or otherwise.

ACKNOWLEDGEMENT

Declared none.

REFERENCE

[1] Huan C, Ng KL, Nasaruddin MZ, *et al.* Topical mitomycin-C as an adjuvant to multimodal endoscopic treatment for tracheobronchial stenosis secondary to endobronchial tuberculosis. Respirol Case Rep 2021; 9(3).
[http://dx.doi.org/10.1002/rcr2.711] [PMID: 33532074]

Case 8

Multimodal Endoscopic Management of Multi-Level Post-TB Tracheal Stenosis

Kho Sze Shyang[1,*], **Mona Zaria Nasaruddin**[1] and **Jamalul Azizi Abdul Rahaman**[1]

[1] *Department of Pulmonology, Serdang Hospital, Selangor, Malaysia*

Keywords: Airway stenosis, Balloon bronchoplasty, Mitomycin C, Rigid bronchoscopy, Tuberculosis.

Presentation

A 36-year-old lady with progressive worsening of exertional dyspnea associated with inspiratory stridor. She was diagnosed with smear and culture positive pulmonary TB four months earlier. Her initial constitutional symptoms improved after two months of intensive anti-TB therapy. However, her current symptoms gradually emerged and worsened during her maintenance therapy. Her modified medical research council (mMRC) scale was 3.

Comorbidities

None.

Chest Imaging

CT thorax showed right upper lobe consolidation with surrounding centrilobular nodules consistent with pulmonary TB. Three-dimensional (3D) airway reconstruction confirmed multilevel tracheal stenosis with the narrowest diameter measuring 4mm at two sites of mid trachea (Myers-Cotton grade 3) (Fig. **1**).

Intervention

Rigid bronchoscopy was performed under total intravenous anaesthesia with intravenous propofol and remi-fentanyl. She was intubated with 12mm rigid tracheoscope. Pre-intervention, patient's airway only allowed a slim flexible

*Corresponding author Kho Sze Shyang: Department of Pulmonology, Serdang Hospital, Selangor, Malaysia; E-mail: khosze@moh.gov.my

bronchoscope (outer diameter 3.8mm) to negotiate the stenotic segments (Figs. **2a** and **b**). Under direct vision, the stenotic tracheal segments were dilated gradually using controlled radial expansion balloon (CRE™, Boston Scientific, Marlborough, USA) from 7mm to 12mm with balloon occlusion time of two minutes for every millimeter of dilatation (Fig. **3a**). After dilatation to 12mm, the trachea allowed passage of a therapeutic flexible bronchoscope (outer diameter 6.2mm) with ease (Fig. **3b**). Topical mitomycin C (0.4mg/ml) soaked pledgets were applied directly on the tracheal mucosa using a rigid forceps (Figs. **4a** and **b**). A total of five topical applications were performed.

Complications

None. Patient was extubated post-procedure.

Post-Intervention

Immediate relief of breathlessness with improvement of mMRC scale from 3 to 1. Air entry was equal on chest auscultation and no stridor was heard. Surveillance bronchoscopy one month later showed a patent trachea and the patient was able to carry out daily activities with no recurrence of symptoms.

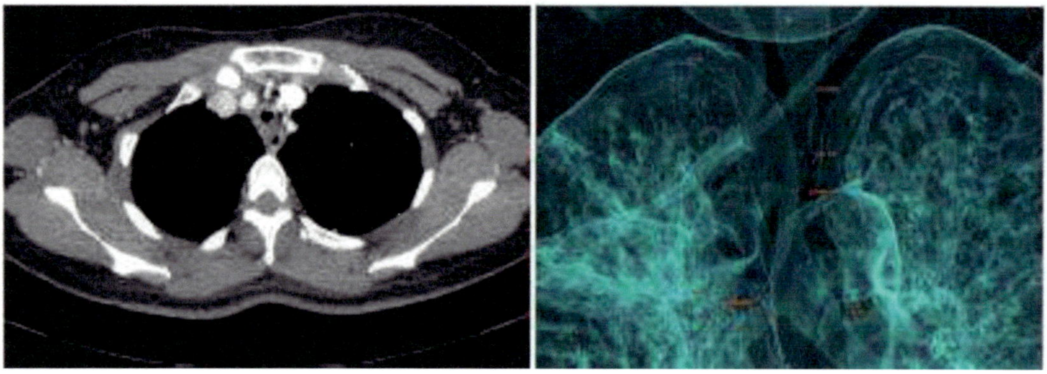

Fig. (1). Axial CT thorax with 3D airway reconstruction shows multilevel tracheal stenosis measuring around 4mm at two critical levels in mid trachea.

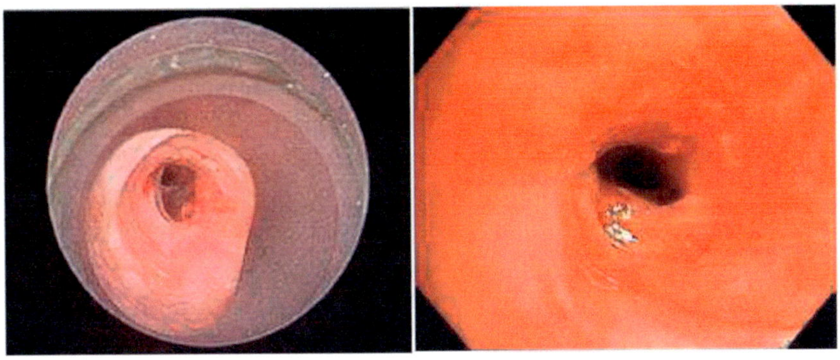

Fig. (2). (a) (Left) & **(b)** (Right). Critical tracheal stenosis pre-dilatation which only allows passage of 3.8mm flexible bronchoscope.

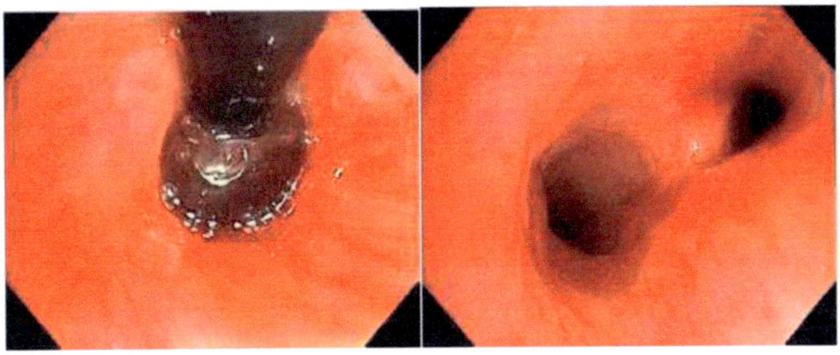

Fig. (3). (a) (Left) The stenotic segment was dilated gradually with CRE™ balloon from 7mm to 12mm sequentially. **(b)** (Right) Post-dilatation, therapeutic flexible bronchoscope (outer diameter 6.2mm) was able to negotiate the stenotic segment with ease.

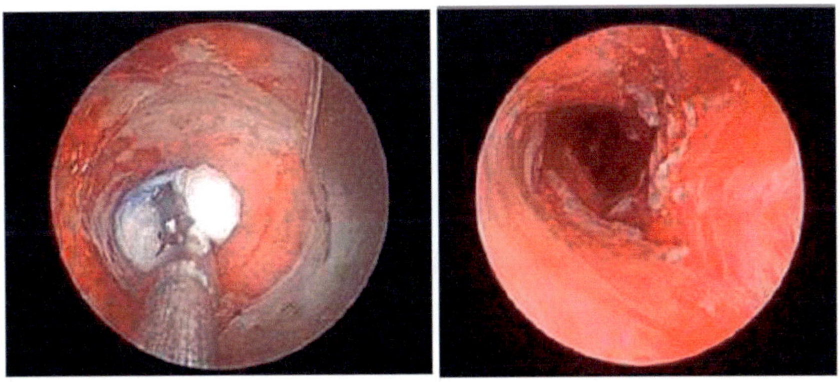

Fig. (4). (a) (Left) The stenotic segment was treated with topical mitomycin C (0.4mg/ml) by applying mitomycin C soaked pledgets directly on the tracheal mucosa using a rigid forceps. **(b)** (Right) Mucosal blanching was observed after mitomycin C application.

Learning Points

- Although open surgical repair remains the treatment of choice for post-TB central airway obstruction, very few patients are fit enough to undergo this high-risk procedure due to poor pulmonary reserve. Endoscopic interventions thus may remain the only option in these patients. Our early experience demonstrated that endoscopic interventions (balloon bronchoplasty combined with topical mitomycin C application *via* rigid bronchoscopy) can achieve good outcome in post-TB central airway obstruction, especially in patients with short segment stenosis without bronchomalacia or thick fibrous bands [1]. Interventional pulmonology remains an important option in the management of complicated, multilevel post-TB tracheal stenosis.

Video

Gradual balloon dilatation of the tracheal stenosis followed by topical mitomycin C application.

CONSENT FOR PUBLICATION

Not applicable.

CONFLICT OF INTEREST

The authors declare no conflict of interest, financial or otherwise.

ACKNOWLEDGEMENT

Declared none.

REFERENCE

[1] Huan C, Ng KL, Nasaruddin MZ, *et al.* Topical mitomycin-C as an adjuvant to multimodal endoscopic treatment for tracheobronchial stenosis secondary to endobronchial tuberculosis. Respirol Case Rep 2021; 9(3).
[http://dx.doi.org/10.1002/rcr2.711] [PMID: 33532074]

Case 9

Bronchoscopic Management of Post-Intubation Tracheal Stenosis (PITS) in a COVID-19 Treated Patient

Tinku Joseph[1,*] and **Sathish C. Reddy**[1]

[1] *Division of Interventional Pulmonology, Amrita Institute of Medical Sciences, Kochi, India*

Keywords: Electrocautery, Balloon bronchoplasty, Mitomycin C, Post-intubation tracheal stenosis, Rigid tracheoscope.

Presentation

A 51-year-old lady was initially treated for category C COVID-19 infection and was on prolonged mechanical ventilation support. A week after extubation, she developed worsening of breathlessness, orthopnoea and stridor. In view of these complaints, she was shifted to our hospital for further management.

Comorbidities

Post COVID status, right upper lobe bronchiectasis, Type II diabetes mellitus, systemic hypertension, old cerebrovascular accident, hypothyroidism.

Chest Imaging

CXR showed no obvious abnormality (Fig. **1**).

CT Neck and Chest revealed patchy air space opacities in the apical and basal segments of right lower lobe with subtle traction bronchiectasis and patchy air space opacities in basal segments of left lower lobe as well. There was reticular interstitial thickening in the basal segments of bilateral lower lobes in a predominant peripheral distribution and fibrotic bands in bilateral upper lobe. Narrowing of trachea was seen at C7-T1 level along a cranio-caudal length of 10mm, transverse diameter at the point of maximum narrowing was 6.5mm, and AP diameter was

*__Corresponding author Tinku Joseph:__ Division of Interventional Pulmonology, Amrita Institute of Medical Sciences, Kochi, India; E-mail: tinkujoseph2010@gmail.com

10.8mm. Irregularity of luminal contour was seen along the right lateral and posterior wall (Fig. **2**).

Intervention

Flexible bronchoscopy done immediately after hospital admission showed a web like (Type 1 PITS) pin hole stenosis 2.5cm below the level of vocal cords (Fig. **3**). In view of the significant stridor, the patient was shifted to the operation theatre immediately.

She was intubated using 11-12 mm rigid tracheoscope under IV sedation (propofol). Paralytics were avoided in view of critical airway compromise. The rigid tracheoscope was kept just below the vocal cords and airway was secured.

In order to get adequate tracheal luminal patency, initially the stenotic web was resected using electrocautery knife (Fig. **4**). The incisions were made at multiple ends. This was followed by serial CRE balloon dilatation using 12,13.5 and 15mm CRE balloon catheter (Fig. **5**). Post-procedure, 90 percent of the tracheal luminal patency was achieved and mitomycin C was applied locally to prevent restenosis (Figs. **6** and **7**). After the procedure, the patient was extubated on the table.

Complications

No immediate post-procedure complications were noted.

Post-Intervention

The patient was asymptomatic post-procedure and was discharged within 72 hours from the hospital. She was prescribed a 3-week course of tapering dose of oral corticosteroids in order to reduce the chances of re-stenosis and was advised surveillance bronchoscopy after 1 month.

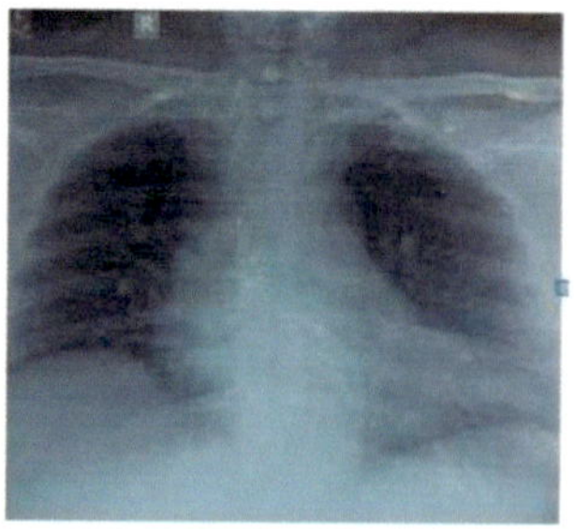

Fig. (1). Normal CXR.

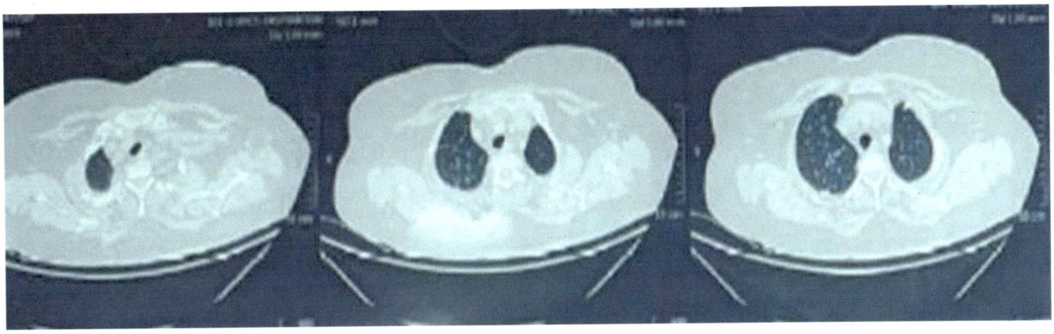

Fig. (2). CT chest: Narrowing of trachea with irregular luminal contour.

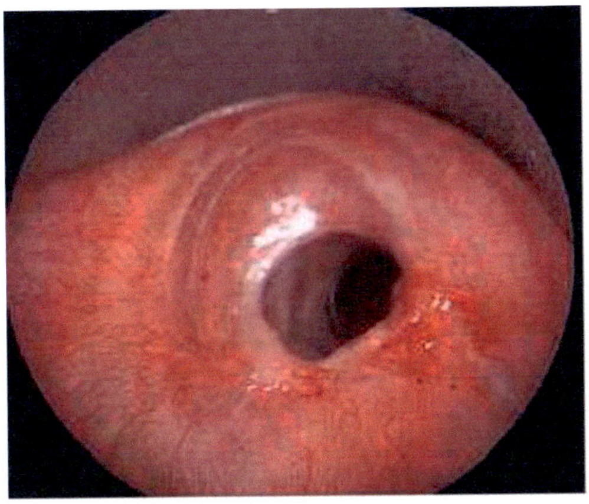

Fig. (3). Web-like stenosis 2.5cm below the level of vocal cords.

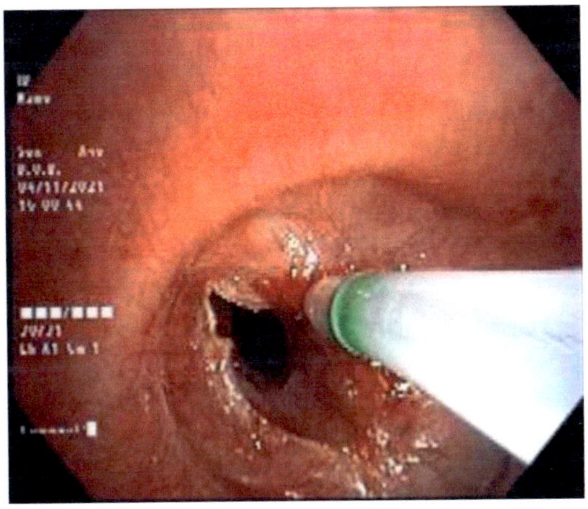

Fig. (4). Electrocautery knife incision of stenotic segment.

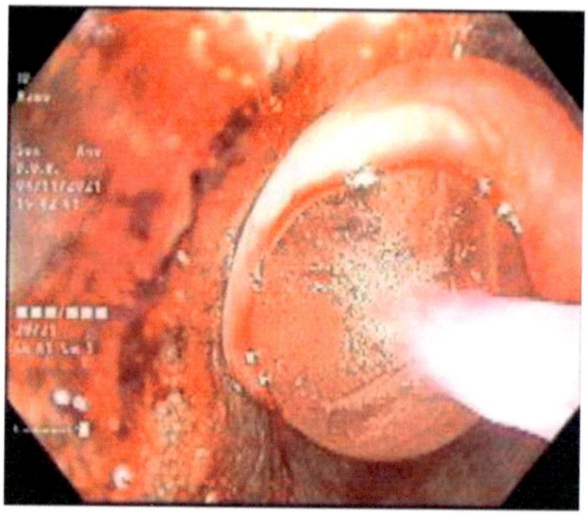

Fig. (5). Serial CRE balloon dilatation.

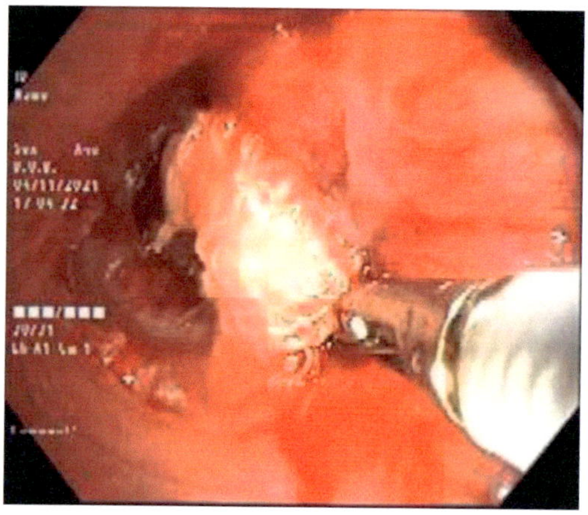

Fig. (6). Post-procedure mitomycin C application.

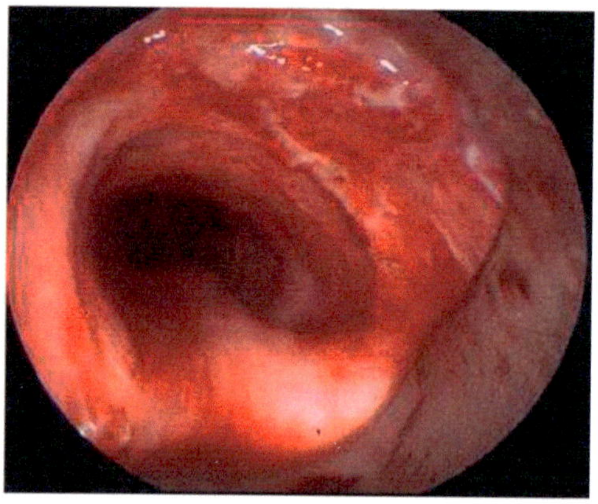

Fig. (7). Post-procedure: completely recanalized tracheal lumen.

Learning Points

- **Causes of Post Intubation (PITS) / Post Tracheostomy Tracheal Stenosis**

  - Prolonged intubation period.
  - Traumatic intubation.
  - Excessive cuff pressure of endotracheal tube.
  - Frequent suctioning through ET tube.
  - Due to abnormal wound healing with formation of excess granulation tissue around the tracheal stoma.
  - Fractured tracheal cartilage due to trauma or pressure necrosis.
  - High tracheostomy site.
  - History of previous intubation/tracheostomy.
  - Excessive use of corticosteroids.
  - Underlying disorders like autoimmune disorders, obstructive sleep apnoea, post radiation therapy for oropharyngeal and laryngeal malignancies, and gastroesophageal reflux disease.

- **Types of PITS**

  - Type 1: Simple (web-like) stenosis.
  - The length of stenosis is less than 1cm. No or minimal damage to tracheal cartilages.
  - Type 2: Complex stenosis.
  - Longer than 1 cm. Tracheal cartilages are damaged. Usually complicated with tracheomalacia.
  - Type 3: Pseudoglottic (A-shaped or tent-shaped) stenosis.
  - Subtype of the complex stenosis. Occurs due to dislocation or fracture of the tracheal cartilaginous rings with localized tracheomalacia.

- **Treatment Options**

  - Type 1: Bronchoscopic correction using electrocautery and balloon dilatation
  - Type 2: Bronchoscopic correction can be attempted along with stent placement (Chances of recurrence of stenosis are high).
  - Type 3: Surgical correction is the treatment of choice – Tracheal resection/ reconstruction and end-to-end anastomosis.
  - In many cases, a multidisciplinary approach combining bronchoscopic and surgical methods is used [1].

CONSENT FOR PUBLICATION

Not applicable.

CONFLICT OF INTEREST

The author declares no conflict of interest, financial or otherwise.

ACKNOWLEDGEMENT

Declared none.

REFERENCE

[1] Brichet C. Verkindre J. Dupont M, *et al.* Multidisciplinary approach to management of postintubation tracheal stenoses. Eur Respir J 1999; 13(4): 888-93. [http://dx.doi.org/10.1034/j.1399-3003.1999.13d32.x] [PMID: 10362058]

Case 10

Malignant Central Airway Obstruction

Endoscopic Treatment of Adenoid Cystic Carcinoma of the Trachea

Khai Lip Ng[1,*], **Mona Zaria Nasaruddin**[1] and **Jamalul Azizi Abdul Rahaman**[1]

[1] *Department of Pulmonology, Serdang Hospital, Selangor, Malaysia*

Keywords: Adenoid cystic carcinoma, Central airway obstruction, Debulking, Tracheal tumour, Radiotherapy.

Presentation

A 31-year-old man had cough and shortness of breath for 3 days, subsequently intubated for respirator distress. He was treated with antibiotics but showed no improvement in symptoms and CXR. Sputum direct smear for AFB was negative as was TB culture. Prior to the onset of the acute symptoms, he had been empirically treated as smear negative PTB for 5 months.

Comorbidities

Smoker of 15 pack years. Diagnosed as 'bronchial asthma' 2 years ago.

Chest Imaging

CXR showed narrowing of the mid trachea (Fig. **1**). CT thorax showed bilateral lower lobe pneumonia with seg mental consolidation and matted mediastinal lymphadenopathy.

In view of no response to anti-TB treatment, a repeat CT thorax was performed which showed a lobulated lesion in the lower paratracheal and precarinal regions encasing the trachea (Fig. **2**). The trachea was 50 percent narrowed.

Flexible bronchoscopy showed an intraluminal mass arising from 2 to 4 o'clock at mid trachea. Unable to get the flexible bronchoscope past the narrowed segment of the trachea.

*Corresponding author Khai Lip Ng: Department of Pulmonology, Serdang Hospital, Selangor, Malaysia; E-mail: khailip08@yahoo.com

Jamalul Azizi Abdul Rahaman & Tinku Joseph (Eds.)

Intervention

Emergent endoscopic treatment *via* rigid bronchoscopy. Electrocautery snare resection of the mass followed by cryobiopsy. The tumour was trimmed with semi-rigid long scissors. Haemostasis was secured with Nd: YAP laser and argon plasma coagulation.

Complications

None.

Post-Intervention

Airways were more than 95% patent after the procedure. HPE revealed adenoid cystic carcinoma (Fig. **3**). He was referred for radical radiotherapy.

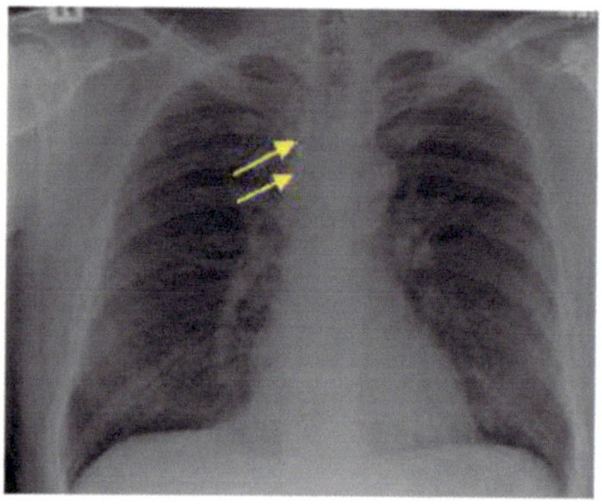

Fig. (1). CXR shows narrowing of the trachea (yellow arrows).

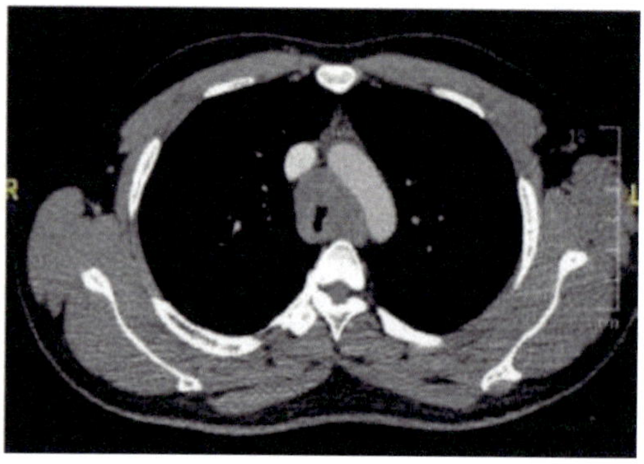

Fig. (2). Axial CT thorax shows a lobulated lesion at the paratracheal region causing narrowing of the trachea.

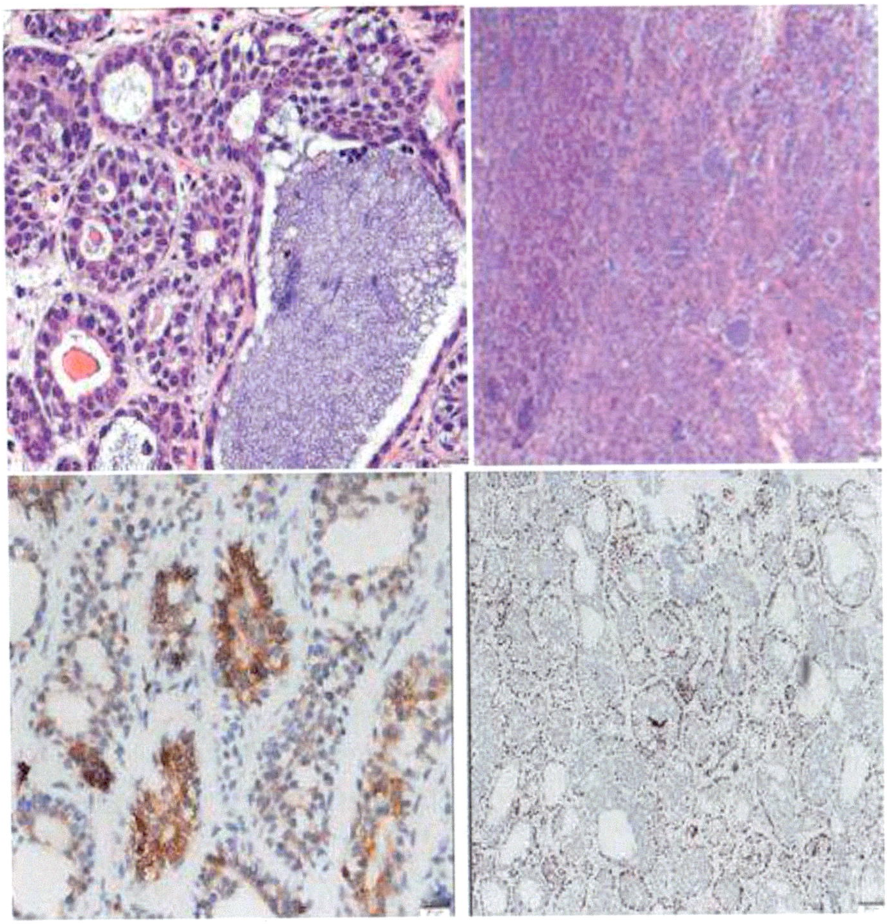

Fig. (3). Tumor arranged in cribriform structures and tubules, containing basophilic myxoid substance and eosinophilic hyalinised cores. The luminal cells are highlighted by CD117. The peripheral cells are highlighted by p63.

Learning Points

- This case highlights the importance of looking carefully at the CXR beyond the lung parenchyma since the narrowed segment of the trachea could be missed. Failure to respond to anti-TB treatment should prompt the treating physician to search for an alternative diagnosis such as malignancy. Adenoid cystic carcinoma can present with symptoms of central airway obstruction. Endoscopic management is necessary for rapid symptom relief prior to radical radiotherapy [1].

Video

Endoscopic resection of the mass using electrocautery snare and semi-rigid long scissors. Haemostasis was secured with Nd: YAP laser and argon plasma coagulation.

CONSENT FOR PUBLICATION

Not applicable.

CONFLICT OF INTEREST

The author declares no conflict of interest, financial or otherwise.

ACKNOWLEDGEMENTS

The authors acknowledge the support received from Dr. Suhashini Ganapaty, Department of Pathology, Serdang Hospital, 43000 Serdang, Selangor, Malaysia.

REFERENCE

[1] Lay G, Amichetti G, Dessiet M, *et al.* Adenoid cystic carcinoma (ACC) of the tracheo-bronchial tree treated with laser therapy and irradiation: report of two cases. Open Lung Can J 2009; 2: 31-4.
[http://dx.doi.org/10.2174/1876819900902010031]

Case 11

Recurrent Mucoepidermoid Carcinoma of the Bronchus

Khai Lip Ng[1,*], **Mona Zaria Nasaruddin**[1] and **Jamalul Azizi Abdul Rahaman**[1]

[1] *Department of Pulmonology, Serdang Hospital, Selangor, Malaysia*

Keywords: External beam radiotherapy, Laser, Mucoepidermoid carcinoma, Polypoidal mass, Recurrence.

Presentation

A 45-year-old gentleman with recurrent episodes of central airway obstruction was first seen in 2012 for prolonged cough. History of right middle and lower lobectomy 7 years earlier for 'atypical carcinoid tumour'. CT angiography showed a polypoidal lesion in the left main bronchus (LMB) and hence he was referred for endoscopic resection as he was deemed not suitable for surgical resection.

Comorbidities

None.

Chest Imaging

CT angiography showed a pedunculated polypoidal endobronchial lesion in the LMB 1.1 x 1. 4cm (First presentation in 2012) (Fig. **1**). Flexible bronchoscopy in 2012 revealed an oscillating polypoidal lesion with a stalk in the LMB 2.0cm from the main carina. The initial suspicion was recurrent carcinoid tumour.

Intervention

The first intervention in 2012 was a simple snare electrocautery of the LMB polypoidal lesion *via* rigid bronchoscopy (Fig. **2**). HPE was consistent with mucoepidermoid carcinoma (MEC). Subsequently, he underwent multiple tumour debulking procedures either under conscious sedation or *via* rigid bronchoscopy

*Corresponding author Khai Lip Ng: Department of Pulmonology, Serdang Hospital, Selangor, Malaysia; E-mail: khailip08@yahoo.com

Jamalul Azizi Abdul Rahaman & Tinku Joseph (Eds.)

(depending on the severity) due to the recurrent nature of the disease in the LMB over the next 8 years. In 2020, he had Nd: YAP laser-assisted tumour debulking followed by external beam radiotherapy.

Complications

None in any of these debulking procedures over 8 years.

Post-Intervention

Successful recanalization of LMB after each intervention but there were recurrences over the course of 8 years. The patient had 6-12 monthly surveillance bronchoscopy to look for tumour recurrence. There was a good response to radiotherapy in 2020 (Fig. **3**).

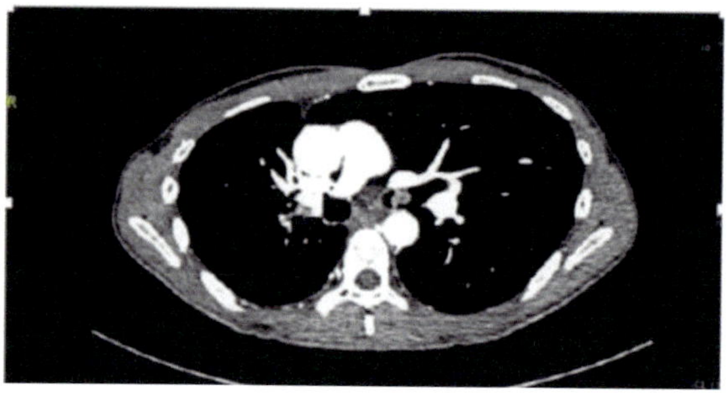

Fig. (1). CT angiography - Polypoidal mass in the left main bronchus.

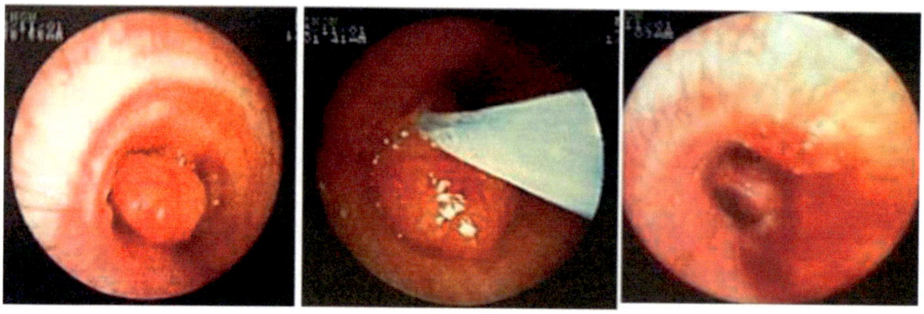

Fig. (2). First intervention in 2012. Left: Polypoidal tumour with a stalk causing obstruction of the left main bronchus; Middle: Snare electrocautery of the tumour; Right: Successful airway recanalization following snare electrocautery.

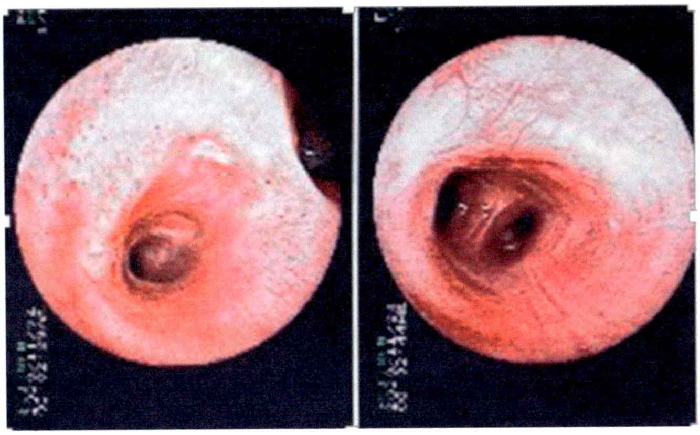

Fig. (3). Bronchoscopic appearance of the left main bronchus 2 months post-radiotherapy in 2020.

Learning Points

- What was thought to be a recurrent carcinoid tumour in the left main bronchus was confirmed to be an MEC. MEC usually arises from salivary glands such as parotid and submandibular glands. MEC with primary origin from the airways is rare, usually affecting young adults. In this case, surgical resection was not feasible due to its recurrent nature and repeat endoscopic approach was the best option for immediate relief of symptoms of central airway obstruction [1].

Videos

Snare electrocautery of the polypoidal tumour in the left main bronchus (first intervention in 2012).

Video 1(first intervention in 2012):

Nd: YAP laser-assisted debulking of the extensive tumour in the left main bronchus (most recent intervention in 2020).

Video 2 (most recent intervention in 2020):

CONSENT FOR PUBLICATION

Not applicable.

CONFLICT OF INTEREST

The author declares no conflict of interest, financial or otherwise.

ACKNOWLEDGEMENT

Declared none.

REFERENCE

[1] Khan AH, Faisal M, Ali RM, *et al*. Resolution of asthmatic symptoms following successful endoscopic resection of tracheal mucoepidermoid carcinoma. BMJ Case Rep 2019; 12: e226202.
[http://dx.doi.org/10.1136/bcr-2018-226202] [PMID: 30659001]

Case 12

Typical Low-Grade Carcinoid Tumour Causing Central Airway Obstruction

Khai Lip Ng[1,*], **Mona Zaria Nasaruddin**[1] and **Jamalul Azizi Abdul Rahaman**[1]

[1]*Department of Pulmonology, Serdang Hospital, Selangor, Malaysia*

Keywords: Haemoptysis, Carcinoid tumour, Central airway obstruction, Debulking, Surgical resection.

Presentation

A 40-year-old lady presented with haemoptysis and reduced effort tolerance for 5 months. She had multiple admissions treated for pneumonia.

Comorbidities

Nil.

Chest Imaging

CT thorax showed an intraluminal mass in the left main bronchus measuring 9mm x 11mm x 11mm (Fig. **1**). Flexible bronchoscopy revealed a polypoidal lesion in the left main bronchus 2.0cm from the main carina. The bronchoscopist was able to advance the scope beyond the lesion showing patent distal airways. Right main bronchus was patent.

Intervention

Endoscopic resection *via* rigid bronchoscopy. Nd: YAP laser photocoagulation was performed to devas cularize the mass. Snare electrocautery and flexible cryoprobe were used to obtain samples for histopathological examination. Rigid forceps was used to clear the tumour margin. Haemostasis was secured with Nd: YAP laser. The left main bronchus was 90 percent patent post-procedure (Figs. **2a-d**).

*Corresponding author Khai Lip Ng:** Department of Pulmonology, Serdang Hospital, Selangor, Malaysia; E-mail: khailip08@yahoo.com

Jamalul Azizi Abdul Rahaman & Tinku Joseph (Eds.)

Complications

Nil.

Post-Intervention

The patient was successfully extubated after the procedure. HPE showed typical low-grade carcinoid. 68-Gallium DOTATATE PET CT showed a residual GaTate avid endobronchial nodule in the left main bronchus with no metastasis or nodal involvement. The patient was referred to the cardiothoracic surgeon for sleeve resection and primary anastomosis.

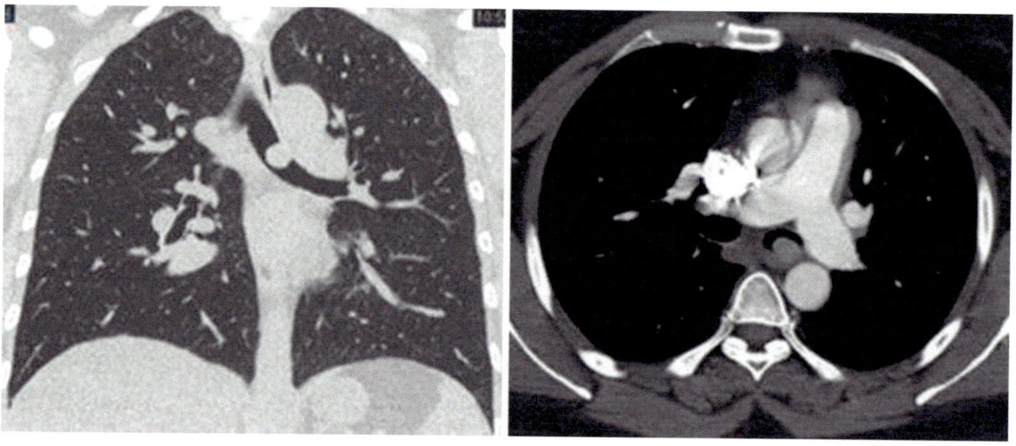

Fig. (1). Coronal and axial CT images show a pedunculated mass in the left main bronchus.

a) **b)**

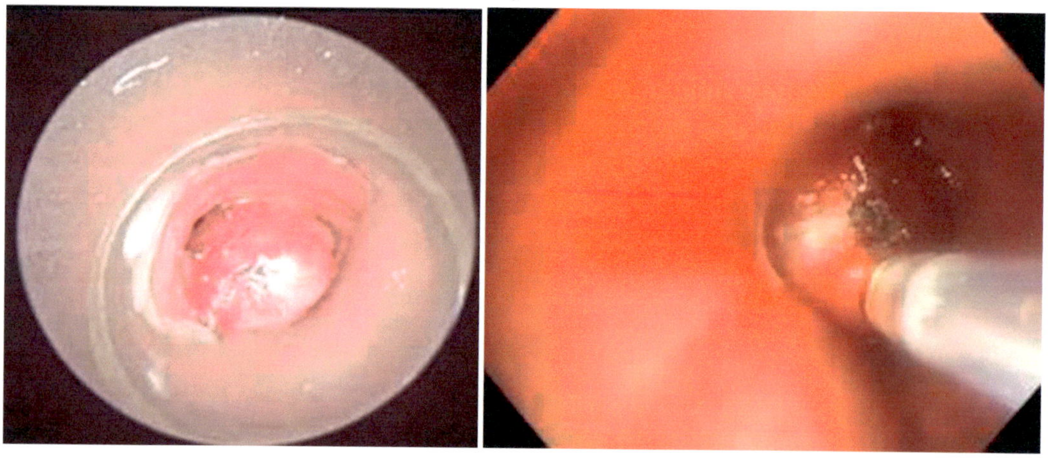

(Fig. 2) contd.....

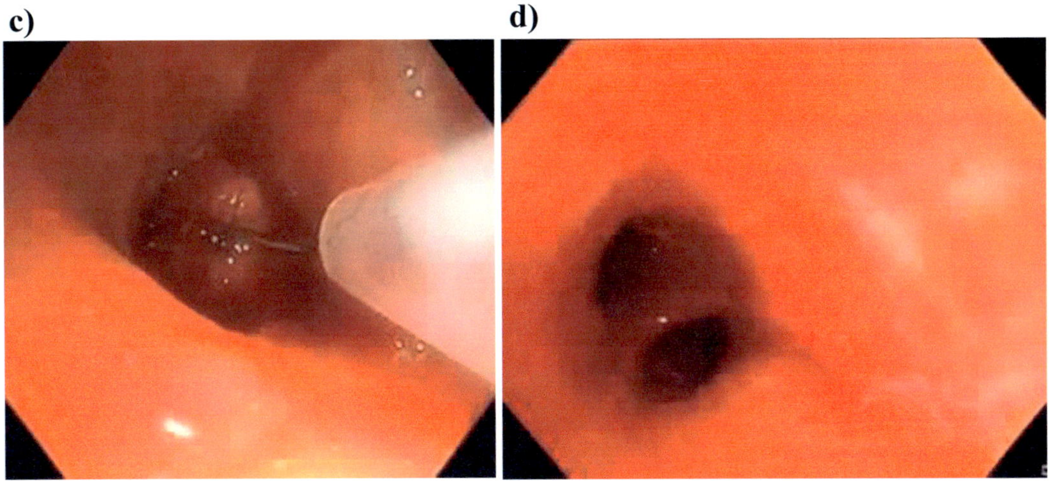

Fig. (2). (a) Pre-debulking. **(b)** The tumour was de-vascularized using Nd: YAP laser, **(c)** Debulked. using snare electrocautery and flexible cryoprobe. **(d)** Left main bronchus was patent post-debulking.

Learning Points

- Flexible bronchoscopy should be offered as part of the assessment of a patient with recurrent pneumonia to exclude an endobronchial lesion in the central airways. Although surgery is the gold standard of lung carcinoid treatment, endoscopic treatment including Nd: YAP laser may be offered as a safe stand-alone procedure in the treatment of typical carcinoid tumour in the central airways [1].

Video

Endoscopic resection of the carcinoid tumour using Nd: YAP laser, snare electrocautery, flexible cryoprobe and rigid forceps.

CONSENT FOR PUBLICATION

Not applicable.

CONFLICT OF INTEREST

The author declares no conflict of interest, financial or otherwise.

ACKNOWLEDGEMENT

Declared none.

REFERENCE

[1] Neyman K, Sundset A, Naalsund A, *et al.* Endoscopic treatment of bronchial carcinoids in comparison to surgical resection: a retrospective study. J Bronchol Interv Pulmonol 2012; 19(1): 29-34.
[http://dx.doi.org/10.1097/LBR.0b013e3182446b52] [PMID: 23207260]

Case 13

Debulking of Tumour (Muco-Epidermoid Carcinoma) Involving Right Main Bronchus Causing Complete Collapse of Right Middle and Lower Lobes

Tinku Joseph[1,*]

[1]*Division of Interventional Pulmonology, Amrita Institute of Medical Sciences, Kochi, India*

Keywords: Central airway tumour, Interventional pulmonology, Mucoepidermoid carcinoma, Rigid bronchoscopy, Tumour debulking.

Presentation

A 33-year-old gentleman visited our department with complaints of progressive breathlessness, cough and occasional haemoptysis.

Comorbidities

Nil.

Chest Imaging

CXR showed complete collapse of his right middle and lower lobes.

CECT chest revealed complete collapse of the right middle and lower lobes with right main bronchus cut off and enlarged subcarinal, left lower paratracheal, right upper and lower paratracheal lymphadenopathy.

Intervention

Bronchoscopic evaluation showed a fleshy growth involving right bronchus intermedius distal to upper lobe bronchus with a pin hole opening (Fig. **1**). He

[*]**Corresponding author Tinku Joseph:** Division of Interventional Pulmonology, Amrita Institute of Medical Sciences, Kochi, India; E-mail: tinkujoseph2010@gmail.com

Jamalul Azizi Abdul Rahaman & Tinku Joseph (Eds.)

underwent EBUS-TBNA initially which showed the presence of reactive lymphadenopathy and bronchoscopic biopsy from the mass lesion showed evidence of mild grade mucoepidermoid carcinoma. Various treatment options including VATS guided right middle lobe and lower lobe lobectomy were discussed with the patient, but he refused to undergo surgery. For symptom palliation, the patient underwent rigid bronchoscopy guided debulking of the tumour. He was intubated with 12-13mm size rigid bronchoscope. Once the airway was secured, the tumour was ablated at multiple points for 20 to 30 seconds using a 2.4mm flexible cryoprobe to reduce the vascularity of the lesion (Fig. **2**). Subsequently, the lesion was debulked using snare electrocautery (Fig. **3**). The debulked tissue was retrieved using a flexible cryoprobe (Fig. **4**). Haemostasis was achieved using 5F Fogarty balloon and local instillation of cold saline and adrenaline. The base of the lesion was later ablated using cryoprobe. Post-procedure, the right bronchus intermedius was completely recanalized and the patient was extubated on the table (Fig. **5**).

Complications

No immediate or delayed post-procedure complications were noted.

Post-Intervention

His follow up CXR showed completely expanded right middle and lower lobes. During his review visit after one month, the patient was asymptomatic and flexible bronchoscopy showed patent, clear broncho-pulmonary segments.

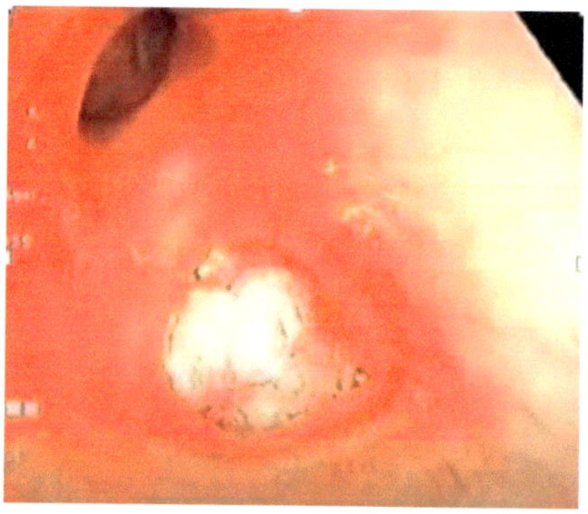

Fig. (1). Bronchoscopic view: Tumourous growth occluding right bronchus intermedius.

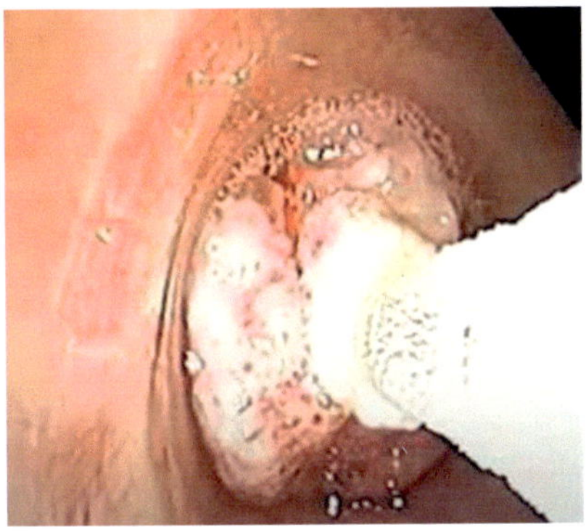

Fig. (2). Cryoablation of the tumour.

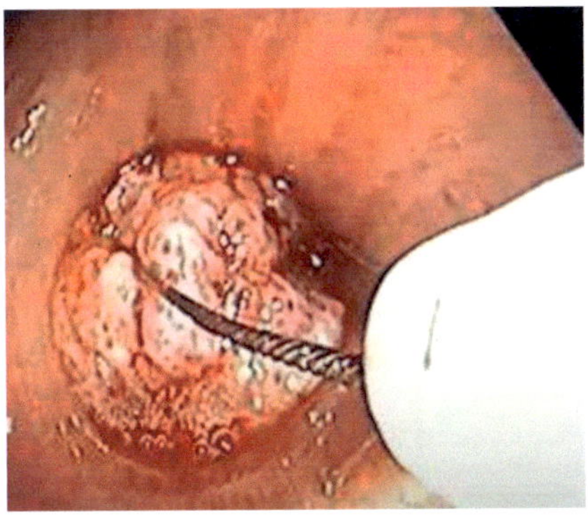

Fig. (3). Debulking using snare electrocautery.

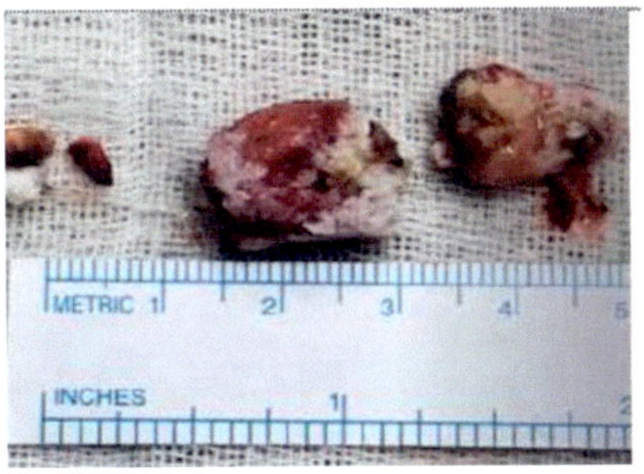

Fig. (4). The debulked tissue.

Learning Points

- Cryoablation of tumour prior to debulking helps to reduce the bleeding associated with the procedure [1]. This is an extremely useful technique especially when dealing with extremely vascular airway tumours.

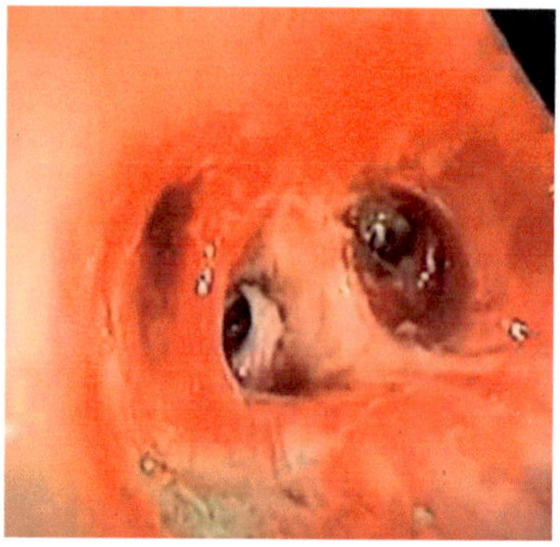

Fig. (5). Completely recanalized right bronchus intermedius.

Video

Cryo-assisted tumour debulking using snare electrocautery.

CONSENT FOR PUBLICATION

Not applicable.

CONFLICT OF INTEREST

The author declares no conflict of interest, financial or otherwise.

ACKNOWLEDGEMENT

Declared none.

REFERENCE

[1] Inoue M, Nakatsuka S, Jinzaki M. Cryoablation of early-stage primary lung cancer. Biomed Res Int 2014; 521691.

Case 14

Massive Haemoptysis Secondary to a Bleeding Pseudo-Aneurysm

Nai-Chien Huan[1,*], **Mona Zaria Nasaruddin**[1] and **Jamalul Azizi Abdul Rahaman**[1]

[1] *Department of Pulmonology, Serdang Hospital, Selangor, Malaysia*

Keywords: Massive hemoptysis, Respiratory emergency, Rigid bronchoscopy, Pseudo-aneurysm, Bronchial artery embolisation.

Presentation

A 70-year-old lady with recurrent haemoptysis. Diagnostic flexible bronchoscopy revealed what looked like a bleeding 'tumour' in the right main bronchus. The patient quickly desaturated and flexible bronchoscopy had to be abandoned. She was immediately intubated and required mechanical ventilation for acute respiratory failure.

Comorbidities

Hypertension, active smoker of 40 pack years.

Chest Imaging

CT thorax showed pulmonary infiltrates over the right upper lobe.

Intervention

Emergency rigid bronchoscopy. Extensive blood clots were seen in the right main bronchus, left main bronchus, right middle lobe and both lower lobes. A 2.4mm ERBE flexible cryoprobe was used to remove blood clots piecemeal to facilitate mechanical ventilation (Fig. **1**). After the removal of blood clots, airway examination showed no tumour in the airways. The source of the bleeding appeared to arise from the right upper lobe and hence the residual blood clots in the right

[*]**Corresponding author Nai-Chien Huan:** Department of Pulmonology, Serdang Hospital, Selangor, Malaysia; E-mail: naichien_1@yahoo.com

upper lobe were not removed for fear of re-bleeding. Thereafter, the patient underwent CT pulmonary angiography followed by bronchial artery embolization (BAE) (Figs. **2** and **3**). Findings were suggestive of a bleeding right bronchial artery pseudo-aneurysm.

Complications

The patient developed multiple episodes of desaturations due to blood clots in the endotracheal tube after intubation before she underwent rigid bronchoscopy. Rigid bronchoscopy and BAE were otherwise uneventful.

Post-Intervention

Successful haemostasis attained post BAE. Liberated from mechanical ventilation after 5 days and discharged 2 weeks later.

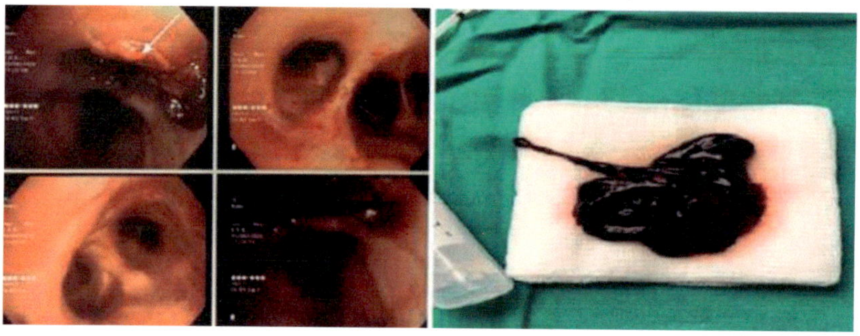

Fig. (1). Patent airways with residual blood clots in the right upper lobe (white arrow) post-rigid bronchos copy.

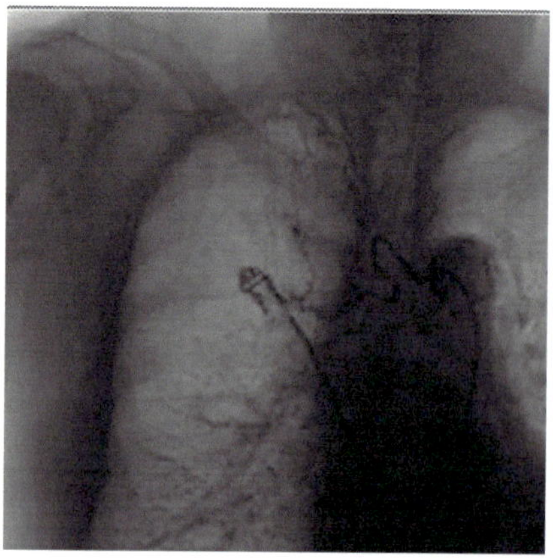

Fig. (2). Pseudo-aneurysm arising from a branch of right bronchial artery.

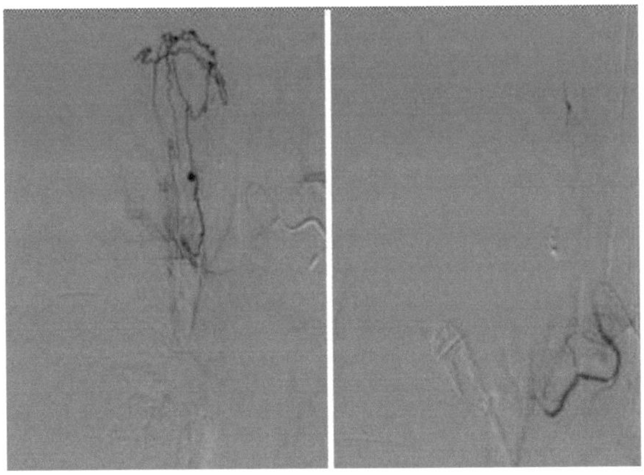

Fig. (3). Resolution of the pseudo-aneurysm before (left image) and after (right image) BAE.

Learning Points

- Rigid bronchoscopy is the gold standard in the management of massive life-threatening haemoptysis for successful removal of huge blood clots causing central airway obstruction prior to a more definitive treatment such as BAE. Multiple instruments (flexible cryoprobe, suction catheter, flexible forceps, en dobronchial blocker) can be passed down the rigid tube which acts as a conduit to manage massive airway bleeding effectively. BAE is an established treatment method for massive haemoptysis and should be available in any interventional pulmonary centres managing haemoptysis [1].

CONSENT FOR PUBLICATION

Not applicable.

CONFLICT OF INTEREST

The author declares no conflict of interest, financial or otherwise.

ACKNOWLEDGEMENT

Declared none.

REFERENCE

[1] Frood R, Karthik S, Mirsadraee S, *et al*. Bronchial artery embolisation for massive haemoptysis: immediate and long-term outcomes-a retrospective study. Pulmonary Ther 2020; 6: 107-17. [http://dx.doi.org/10.1007/s41030-020-00112-x] [PMID: 32185642]

Case 15

Haemorrhage Post Biopsy of a Bronchial Carcinoid: What can be Done when Airway Interventions are Unsuccessful?

Sangeta Vadivelu[1], **Kho Sze Shyang**[1], **Mona Zaria Nasaruddin**[1] and **Jamalul Azizi Abdul Rahaman**[1,*]

[1] *Department of Pulmonology, Serdang Hospital, Selangor, Malaysia*

Keywords: Angiography, Airway intervention, Bronchial carcinoid, Bleeding, Endobronchial biopsy.

Presentation

A 41-year-old female presented spontaneous left-sided pneumothorax requiring a chest tube insertion. There was a history of motor vehicle accident 1 month prior to the pneumothorax.

Comorbidities

None.

Chest Imaging

CT thorax (done as part of the assessment for pneumothorax) incidentally revealed a 'vascular lesion' in the right lower lobe. CT pulmonary angiography (CTPA) confirmed the lesion was a solitary pulmonary nodule in the right lower lobe measuring 2.4cm anteroposterior diameter, 2.6cm in width and 2.8cm in intercommissural diameter (CC) over the anterior segment of the right lower lobe (Fig. **1**). Flexible bronchoscopy revealed a smooth round tumour sitting at the ostium of the right lower lobe bronchus (Fig. **2**). Endobronchial biopsy was performed with a 2mm flexible forceps. The patient had recurrent bleeding post-bronchoscopy which could not be controlled with cold saline.

*__Corresponding author Jamalul Azizi Abdul Rahaman:__ Department of Pulmonology, Serdang Hospital, Selangor, Malaysia; E-mail: naichien_1@yahoo.com

Intervention

Emergency exploration *via* rigid bronchoscopy. Airway examination during rigid bronchoscopy revealed blood clots over the right main bronchus with active bleeding. Blood clots were extracted using a 2.4mm ERBE flexible cryoprobe. Multiple attempts to secure haemostasis using adrenaline (1:10000) flush, endobronchial Watanabe spigot and argon plasma coagulation failed. She was then reintubated with a 35F double lumen endotracheal tube to isolate the healthy left lung (Fig. **3**).

An urgent CPTA was performed to look for collaterals and for feasibility of embolisation; however, there were no collaterals visualised. She was then referred to the cardiothoracic surgeon for an emergency thoracotomy and lobectomy. Intraoperative findings - right lower lobe endoluminal tumour which was almost completely obstructing the lumen, right lower paratracheal (4R) and right interlobar (11R) lymph nodes (Fig. **4**). Post-operatively, she was transferred to the intensive care. She had a smooth post-operative recovery and was transferred back to the surgical ward 2 days later. The output from the chest tube was insignificant and minimal bubbling ceased gradually. CXR taken on her second post-operative day showed a well expanded right upper lobe and the chest tube was removed (Fig. **5**).

Complications

None.

Post-Intervention

The patient was discharged from the hospital in a stable condition. Resected specimens sent for urgent HPE showed a circumscribed, polypoid endobronchial tumour with neoplastic cells arranged in organoid nesting pattern and trabeculae. The cells had fine granular chromatin, inconspicuous nucleoli, moderate to abundant eosinophilic cytoplasm with mitosis seen at $7/2mm^2$. The stroma is vascularised composed of small, delicate blood vessels with areas of haemorrhage with no necrosis. The immunohistochemical stains were positive for Chromogranin A, Synaptophysin, Ki-67. The resected right lower paratracheal and interlobar lymph nodes were free from malignancy. The final diagnosis was typical carcinoid tumour; pathological staging pT2a pNo (Fig. **6**).

24-hour urinary excretion of 5-Hydroxyindoleacetic acid (5-HIAA) was only slightly elevated but serum Chromogranin A was significantly high. Other blood investigations were unremarkable.

Gallium-68 DOTATATE PET CT study showed a somatostatin receptor avid focus at the right temporofrontal region of the brain possibly due to meningioma. Otherwise, there was no Ga-68 DOTATATE avid local tumour recurrence in the lung or any abnormal uptake seen elsewhere throughout the body. The patient is currently undergoing regular oncology follow-up at the National Cancer Institute.

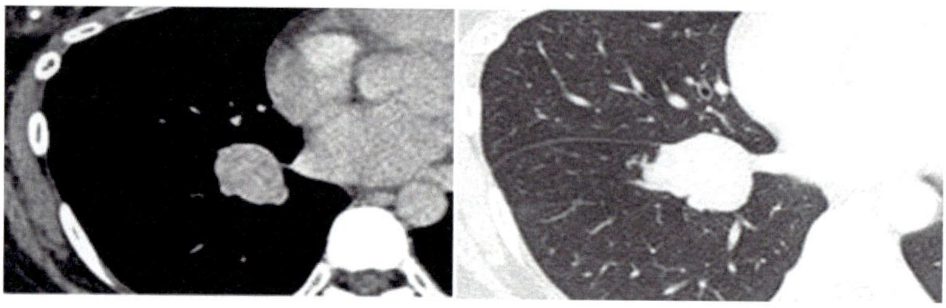

Fig. (1). Axial CTPA images show a nodule over the anterior segment of the right lower lobe.

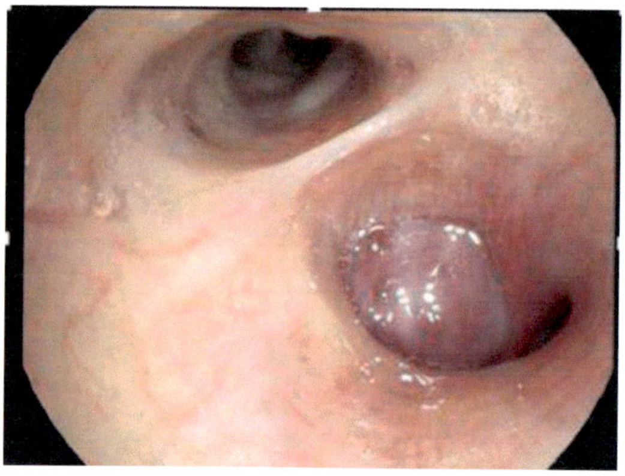

Fig. (2). Initial flexible bronchoscopy revealed a smooth round tumour at the ostium of the right lower lobe bronchus.

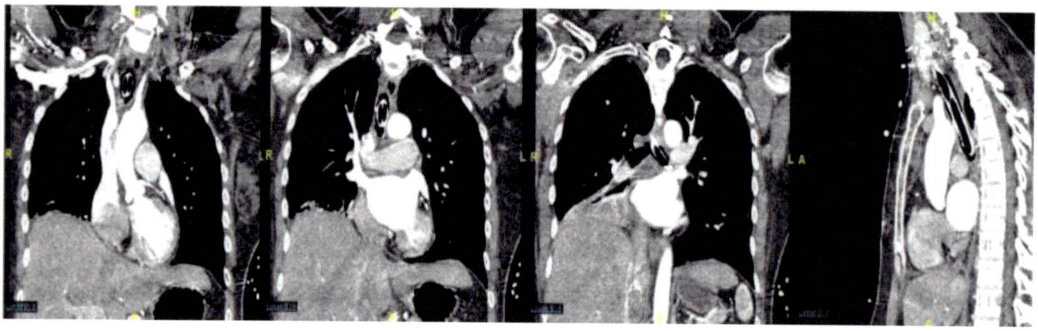

Fig. (3). Double lumen endotracheal tube (bronchial limb pushed into left main bronchus) to isolate the healthy left lung.

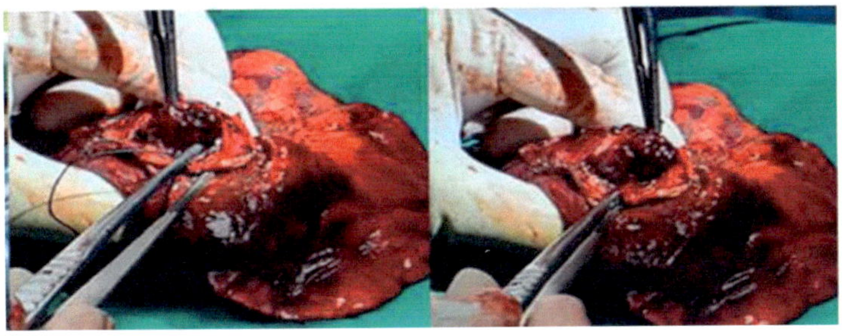

Fig. (4). Intraoperative images showing obstructive right lower lobe endobronchial tumour.

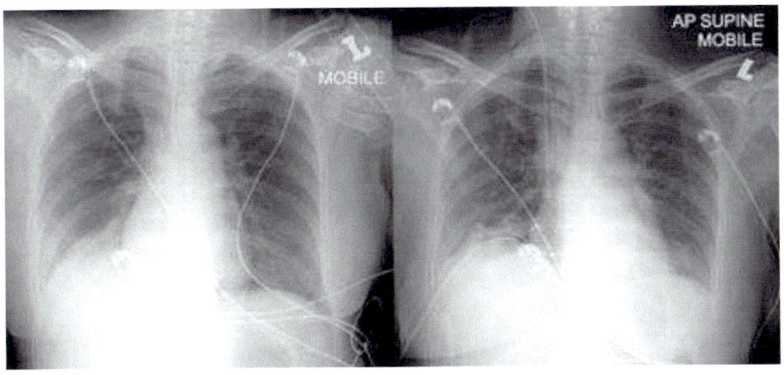

Fig. (5). CXR pre (right) and post (left) right lower lobectomy.

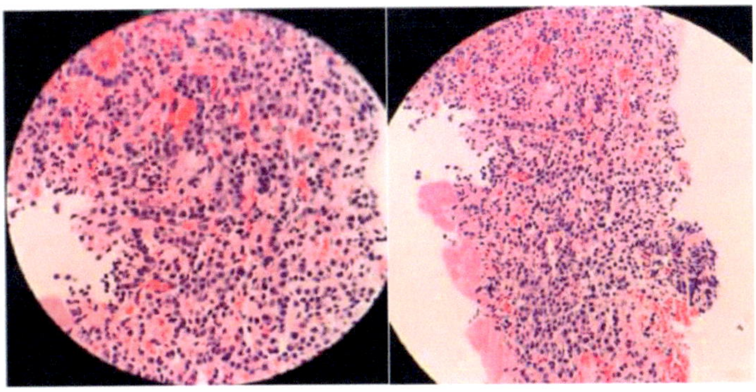

Fig. (6). Histological section showing neoplastic cells in organoid nesting pattern with fine granular chromatin and eosinophilic cytoplasm.

Learning Points

- Massive bleeding after endobronchial biopsy can occur and therefore the bronchoscopist should work closely with anaesthetists, interventional radiologists and cardiothoracic surgeons to handle this complication.

- Double lumen endotracheal lube can be useful in the management of massive airway bleeding when interventions *via* rigid bronchoscopy are unsuccessful to stabilise the patient prior to embolization or surgical resection.
- Tumour markers may obviate the need for biopsy in typical bronchial carcinoids to avoid massive bleeding after endobronchial biopsy [1, 2].

CONSENT FOR PUBLICATION

Not applicable.

CONFLICT OF INTEREST

The author declares no conflict of interest, financial or otherwise.

ACKNOWLEDGEMENTS

The authors acknowledge the support received from Dr. Suhashini Ganapaty, Department of Pathology, Serdang Hospital, 43000 Serdang, Selangor, Malaysia.

REFERENCES

[1] Lamberts SW, Hofland LJ, Nobels FR. Neuroendocrine tumor markers. Front Neuroendocrinol 2001; 22(4): 309-39. [http://dx.doi.org/10.1006/frne.2001.0218] [PMID: 11587555]

[2] Eriksson B, Öberg K, Stridsberg M. Tumor markers in neuroendocrine tumors. Digestion 2000; 62(Suppl. 1): 33-8. [http://dx.doi.org/10.1159/000051853] [PMID: 10940685]

Case 16

Airway Fistula

Watanabe Spigot for Persistent Pyopneumothorax with Bronchopleural Fistula

Chai Chan Sin[1] and **Tie Siew Teck**[1,*]

[1] *Division of Respiratory Medicine, Sarawak General Hospital, Kuching, Malaysia*

Keywords: Pyopneumothorax, Computer tomography of lung, Persistent air leak, Endobronchial Watanabe spigot.

Presentation

A middle-aged gentleman presented with one month of productive cough, haemoptysis, fever and right pleuritic chest pain. CXR revealed a right upper lobe (RUL) cavitating consolidation with right hydropneumothorax. Diagnostic thoracentesis drained pus, thus a chest drain was inserted. However, despite drainage and antimicrobial therapy, the right lung remained unexpanded with persistent air leak for more than one week. CT thorax demonstrated a bronchopleural fistula (BPF) at the RUL. Cardiothoracic team deemed the patient was a high surgical risk.

Comorbidities

COPD.

Chest Imaging

CXR during admission and after chest tube insertion showed right hydro-pneumothorax, right upper lobe cavity and right lung patchy consolidation (Figs.**1a** and **b**). CT thorax demonstrated BPF at RB3a (Posterior subsegment of RB3) (Fig. **2**).

Intervention

After discussing with the patient, we performed flexible bronchoscopy under conscious sedation. A 4F balloon catheter (B5-2C balloon catheter; Olympus,

***Corresponding author Tie Siew Teck:** Division of Respiratory Medicine, Sarawak General Hospital, Kuching, Malaysia; E-mail: tiest@moh.gov.my

Jamalul Azizi Abdul Rahaman & Tinku Joseph (Eds.)

Japan) was inflated and observed for 2-3 minutes to see any reduction in the air leak. The air leak stopped completely after occlusion of the right upper lobe bronchus but not when individual segmental bronchi were occluded.

Subsequently, under deep sedation and endotracheal intubation, three Endobronchial Watanabe Spigot (EWS) with different diameters were inserted *via* flexible bronchoscope-one each into RB1 (7 mm), RB2b (5 mm), and RB3a (5 mm). First, a nylon thread was attached to the EWS for the ease of retrieval if needed. The EWS was then grabbed with a flexible forceps and inserted under direct vision of the flexible bronchoscope (Fig. **3**). The air leak stopped immediately once all EWS were in place but unfortunately recurred 1 hour post procedure during spontaneous respiration. However, the right pneumothorax showed some reduction.

Hence, the procedure was repeated a week later, with the removal of sub-segmental RB2b and RB3a EWS, which were replaced with two segmental EWS, inserted into RB2 (6mm) and RB3 (7mm), respectively (Fig. **4**). The air leak resolved completely, the chest drain was removed the following day, and the patient was discharged the day after with antibiotic.

Complications

None.

Post-Intervention

During the subsequent follow-up, serial CXRs demonstrated significant improvement of the right pleu ral thickening (Fig. **5**). Symptoms resolved with good weight gain and return to work. CT thorax at two months showed all EWS were in place with no recurrence of pyopneumothorax. The EWS were removed *via* flexible bronchoscopy six months later. Minimal granulation tissue was noted at the RUL bronchus with minimal secretion upon EWS retrieval. Patient remained well and the right lung remained fully expanded.

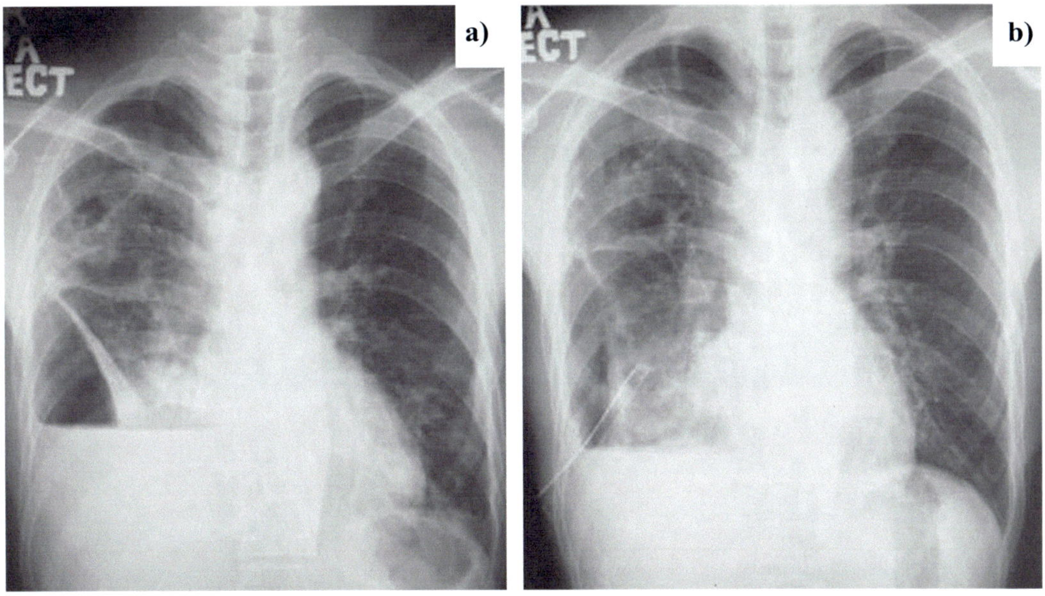

Fig. (1). (a) (Left) CXR during admission before chest tube insertion. **(b)** (Right) After chest tube insertion) showing right hydropneumothorax, right upper lobe cavity and right lung patchy consolidation.

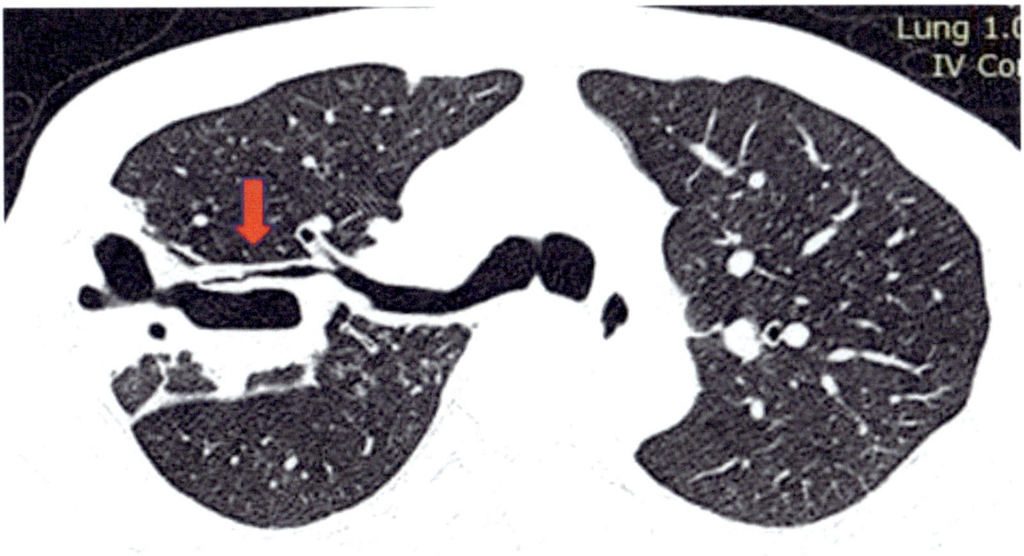

Fig. (2). CT thorax demonstrating bronchopleural fistula at RB3a (red arrow).

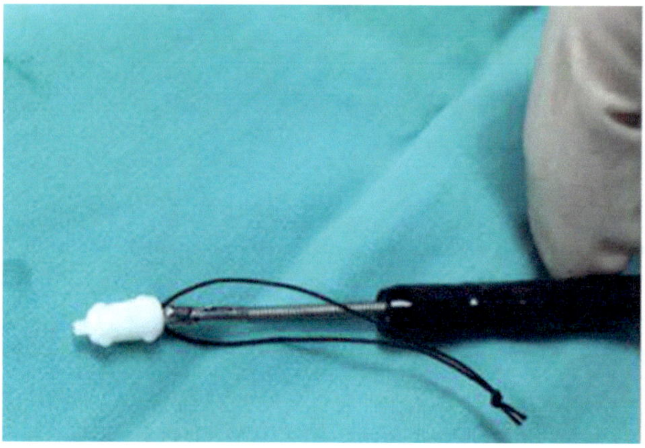

Fig. (3). EWS grasped with flexible forceps.

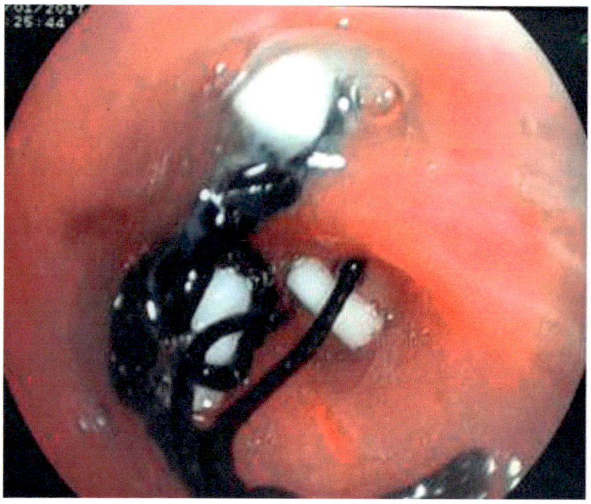

Fig. (4). EWS inserted at right upper lobe segmental bronchi.

Learning Points

- EWS can be used to treat persistent air leak due to BPF that is not suitable for surgical intervention [1]. EWS offers a simple and relatively inexpensive modality for endobronchial blockage.
- However, localization of airway responsible for the air leak can be difficult at times. This is because some of these fistulas are not demonstrable on CT thorax. Sometimes, there are multiple fistulas responsible for the air leak. The Chartis system (Pulmonx, USA) can be used for air leak identification if available.

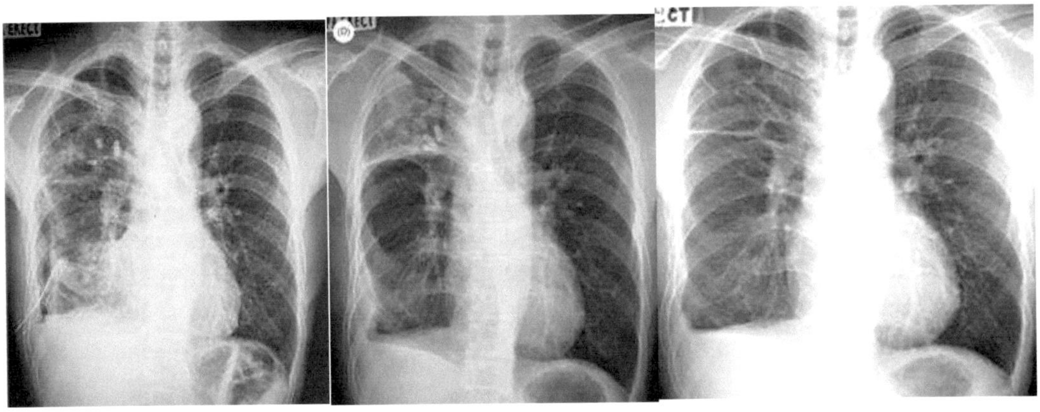

Fig. (5). Serial CXRs showing resolution of right pyopneumothorax. Left: Post first EWS insertion. Middle: Post second EWS insertion. Right: Post EWS removal six months after insertion.

- EWS may result in obstructive pneumonia due to its inability to let proper drainage of secretions. Hence, careful follow up of patient is needed, and if consolidation worsens, spigot removal is indicated.
- Endobronchial valve (EBV) is an alternative in persistent air leak if available.

CONSENT FOR PUBLICATION

Not applicable.

CONFLICT OF INTEREST

The author declares no conflict of interest, financial or otherwise.

ACKNOWLEDGEMENT

Declared none.

REFERENCE

[1] Chai CS, Chan SK, Kho SS, Yong MC, Tie ST. Successful treatment of pyopneumothorax with bronchopleural fistula using endobronchial Watanabe spigots. Respirol Case Rep 2020; 8(5): e00562.
[http://dx.doi.org/10.1002/rcr2.562] [PMID: 32313656]

Case 17

Airway Stent (Silicone)

Management of Iatrogenic Tracheal Tear with Silicone Y-Stent under V-V ECMO

Khai Lip Ng[1], **Mona Zaria Nasaruddin**[1,*] and **Jamalul Azizi Abdul Rahaman**[1]

[1] *Department of Pulmonology, Serdang Hospital, Selangor, Malaysia*

Keywords: ECMO, Iatrogenic, Tracheal tear, Subcutaneous emphysema, Y stent.

Presentation

A 23-year-old lady with palmar hyperhidrosis underwent bilateral video assisted thoracoscopy (VATS) and sympathectomy. She was intubated with a double lumen endotracheal tube after the second attempt. During the VATS procedure, there was desaturation and anterior chest wall subcutaneous emphysema was noted.

Comorbidities

None.

Chest Imaging

CXR showed gas around the pericardium (Fig. **1**). Flexible bronchoscopy on the table revealed a tracheal tear 1cm above the main carina and 4cm in length (Fig. **2**). No active bleeding was seen.

In an attempt to allow the tear to heal by itself, the patient was put on V-V ECMO for 1 week, but a repeat flexible bronchoscopy showed the tear had not healed.

Intervention

Insertion of a silicone Y-stent to cover the tear (Fig. **3**). As the patient was still on V-V ECMO, it was decided to do rigid bronchoscopy under V-V ECMO. Hence, the side-port of the rigid bronchoscope was not used for ventilation during the stent insertion.

***Corresponding author Mona Zaria Nasaruddin:** Department of Pulmonology, Serdang Hospital, Selangor, Malaysia; E-mail: mzaria78@yahoo.com

Jamalul Azizi Abdul Rahaman & Tinku Joseph (Eds.)

Measurements Prior to Y-Stent Insertion:

Main carina to proximal part of the tear: 5.5cm Main carina to right secondary carina: 1.5cm Main carina to left secondary carina: 4cm Silicone Y-stent: tracheal limb (6cm), right limb (1cm), left limb (2cm).

Complications

None.

Post-Intervention

Successful deployment of the Y-stent. The patient was kept intubated for 2 days while on V-VECMO. She was successfully extubated and discharged 3 days later. Surveillance bronchoscopy 1 month later showed the stent was *in situ*. CECT thorax 2 months after Y-stent insertion showed no pneumomediastinum or obvious tracheal wall defect. The Y-stent was removed, leaving granulation tissue at the tracheal tear site (Fig. **4**). The patient was discharged from follow-up subsequently.

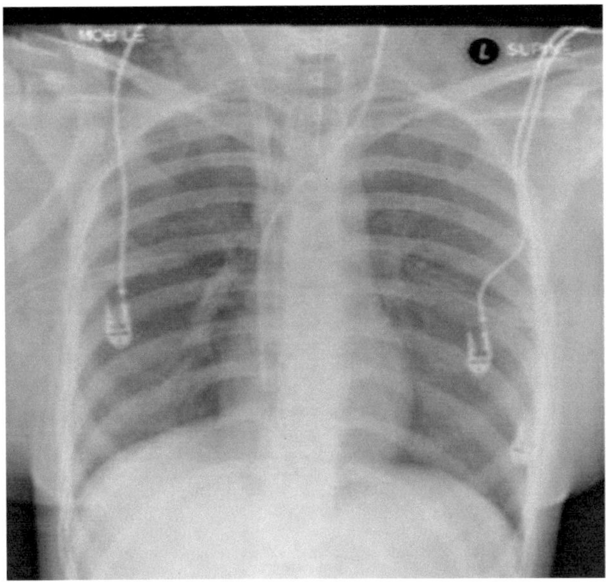

Fig. (1). CXR taken before stenting showing gas around the pericardium.

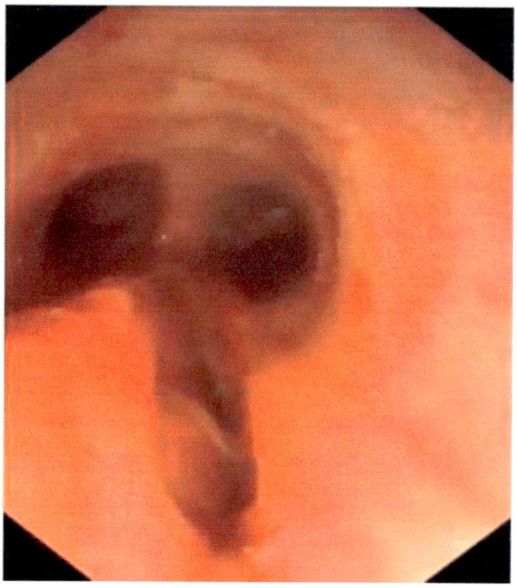

Fig. (2). Flexible bronchoscopy shows a 4cm tracheal tear at the posterior tracheal wall.

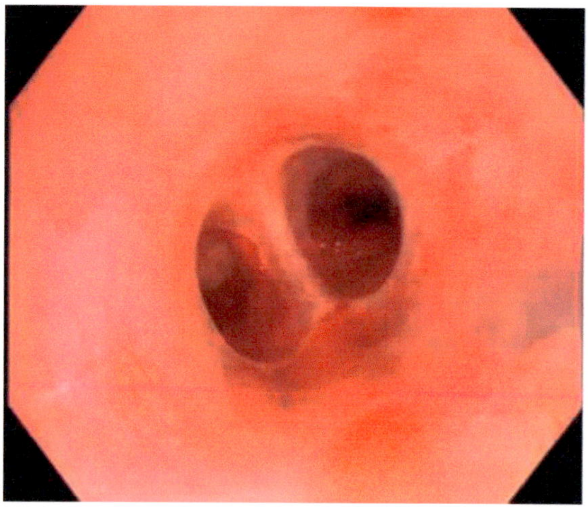

Fig. (3). Silicone Y-stent after deployment. The tracheal limb of the stent covered the whole length of the tracheal tear.

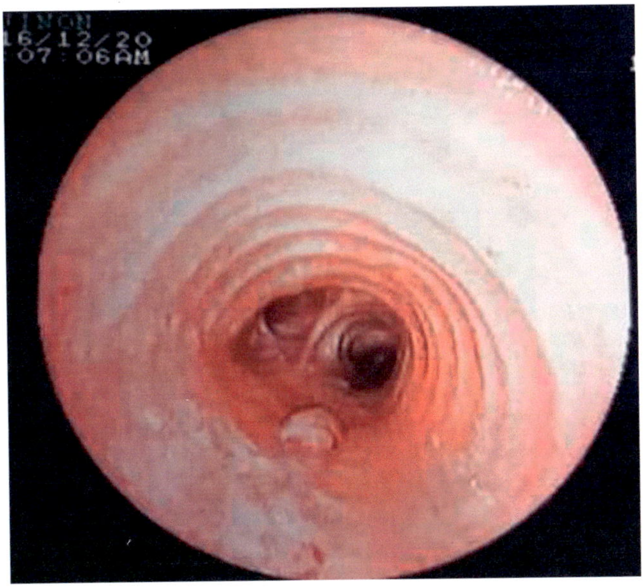

Fig. (4). Healed tracheal tear with granulation tissue after removal of silicone Y-stent.

Learning Points

- This was our first experience doing rigid bronchoscopy *via* ECMO. Tracheal laceration is a rare but potentially a serious complication of endotracheal intubation. Primary surgical repair is considered the preferred treatment. However, non-surgical management of tracheal tear has been described to avoid significant morbidity and mortality associated with surgical repair. Silicone Y-stent placement can be a suitable option in certain patients [1].

Video

Silicone Y-stent placement to cover the tracheal tear.

CONSENT FOR PUBLICATION

Not applicable.

CONFLICT OF INTEREST

The author declares no conflict of interest, financial or otherwise.

ACKNOWLEDGEMENT

Declared none.

REFERENCE

[1] Ghosh SB, Gupta A, Almeida FA, *et al.* Tracheal laceration successfully managed using silicone y-stent after failure of surgical repair. Chest 2010; 138(4_MeetingAbstracts): 59A. [http://dx.doi.org/10.1378/chest.10978]

Case 18

Silicone Y-Stent for Extrinsic Central Airway Obstruction due to Hodgkin's Lymphoma

Tie Siew Teck[1,*]

[1] *Division of Respiratory Medicine, Sarawak General Hospital, Kuching, Malaysia*

Keywords: Chemotherapy, Extrinsic central airway obstruction, Lymphoma, Rigid bronchoscopy, Silicone Y stent.

Presentation

A 23-year-old man presented with progressive dyspnoea for 1 month duration. He was previously well with no past medical or surgical history. There was also significant weight loss of 8kg and mild fever. On presentation, he was severely dyspnoeic at rest and arterial blood gases showed Type 2 respiratory failure. Lung auscultation revealed wheezing during both inspiratory and expiratory phases. Other physical examination was unremarkable. He was intubated and underwent USG guided trucut biopsy of the mediastinal mass, which confirmed Hodgkin's lymphoma.

Comorbidities

None.

Chest Imaging

CXR showed a large mediastinal mass (Fig. **1**). CT thorax showed a large heterogenous mass at the anterior mediastinum with severe compression of the distal trachea and both main bronchi (Fig. **2**).

Flexible bronchoscopy through the endotracheal tube showed a severe slit like pure extrinsic compression of the distal trachea and both main bronchi (Fig. **3**). Distal airways were patent.

*__Corresponding author Tie Siew Teck:__ Division of Respiratory Medicine, Sarawak General Hospital, Kuching, Malaysia; E-mail: tiest@moh.gov.my

Intervention

Rigid bronchoscopy under general anaesthesia. A silicone Y-stent was inserted using the pullback technique. The silicone stent remained partially compressed immediately post-stenting (Fig. **4**).

Complications

None.

Post-Intervention

The type 2 respiratory failure resolved after stenting and the patient was extubated after one day. He was able to lie flat and underwent chemotherapy subsequently. CT thorax and flexible bronchoscopy at two months post-stenting showed a well expanded stent with no significant granulation tissue (Figs. **5** and **6**). The stent was removed 2 months post-insertion with no complication.

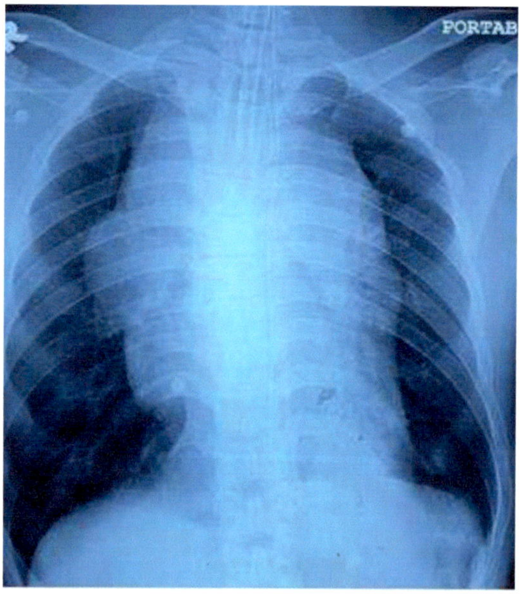

Fig. (1). CXR shows a large mediastinal mass.

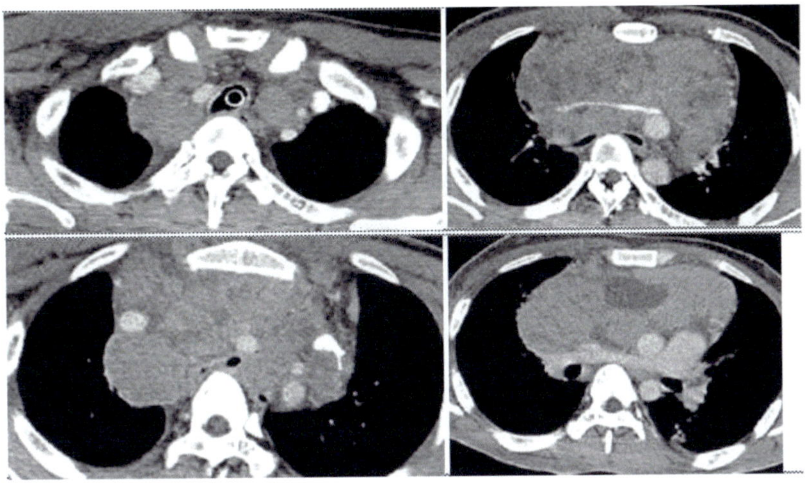

Fig. (2). CT thorax showing a large heterogenous mass at the anterior mediastinum with severe compression of the distal trachea and both main bronchi.

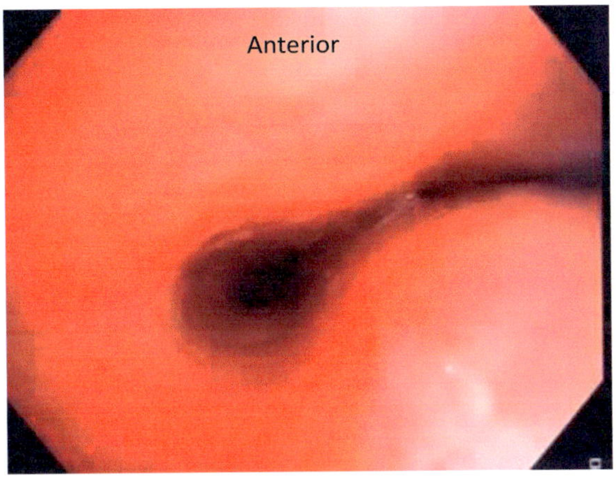

Fig. (3). Severe compression of the distal trachea and main bronchi.

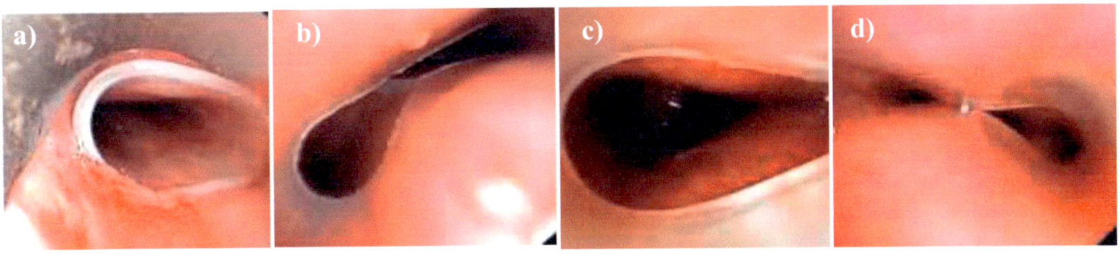

Fig. (4). Silicone Y-stent in position immediately post-stenting. **a)** Trachea. **b)** Main carina. **c)** Left main bronchus. **d)** Right main bronchus.

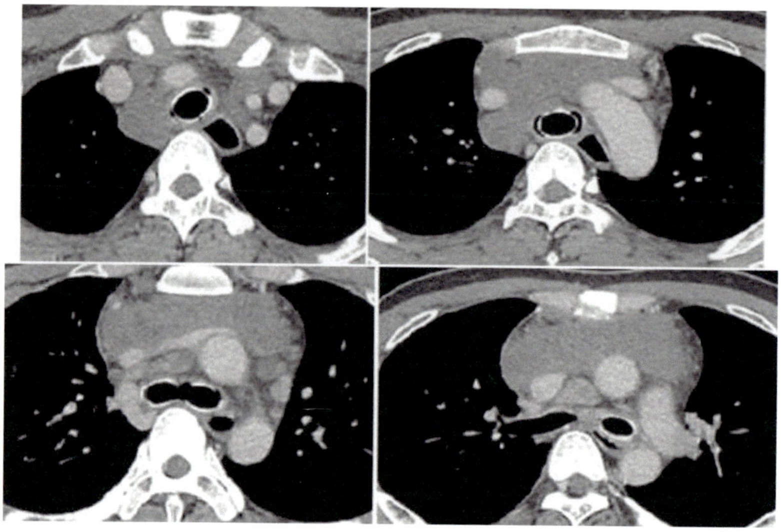

Fig. (5). CT thorax at two months post-stenting showing markedly smaller mediastinal mass and improved central airway compression.

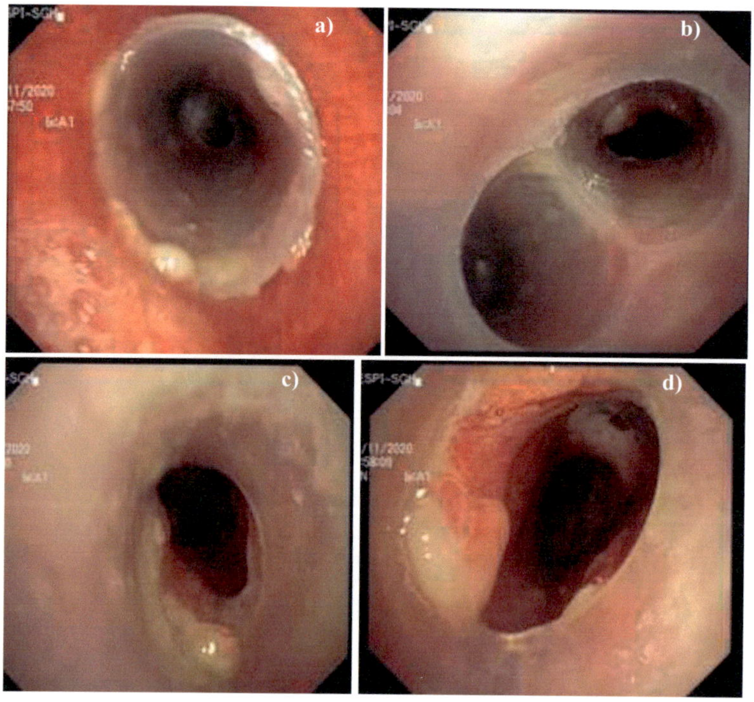

Fig. (6). Bronchoscopy at 2 months showing a well expanded stent with minimal granulation tissues at the proximal edges of the stent. **a)** Trachea. **b)** Main carina**. c)** Left main bronchus. **d)** Right main bronchus.

Learning Points

- Airway stenting is useful to relieve severe extrinsic central airway obstruction.
- Silicone stent is easier to remove compared to metallic stent. In this case, a silicone stent was used because stent removal was anticipated in the near future. Certain malignancies especially Hodgkin's lymphoma have good prognosis and prolonged survival. Hence the need for stent removal should be taken into consideration when selecting the type of stent.
- Silicone stent also has a greater ability to resist compression compared to some metallic stents and hence, better in relieving severe airway compression [1].
- Fully covered metallic stent can be used in similar conditions, however the operator must be experienced in removing it. Metallic stent removal can be difficult after a prolonged period of insertion, hence metallic stent should be removed as soon as possible or replaced with a silicone stent if prolonged stenting is needed.

CONSENT FOR PUBLICATION

Not applicable.

CONFLICT OF INTEREST

The author declares no conflict of interest, financial or otherwise.

ACKNOWLEDGEMENT

Declared none.

REFERENCE

[1] Freitag L. Airway stents. European Respiratory Monograph 2010. [http://dx.doi.org/10.1183/1025448x.00991409]

Case 19

Silicone Y-Stent for Extrinsic Central Airway Obstruction due to Mediastinal Lymphadenopathy

Tie Siew Teck[1,*]

[1] *Division of Respiratory Medicine, Sarawak General Hospital, Kuching, Malaysia*

Keywords: Extrinsic central airway obstruction, Lung cancer, Rigid bronchoscopy, Silicone Y stent, Radial EBUS cryobiopsy.

Presentation

A 70-year-old man presented with progressive dyspnoea of 3-month duration. On arrival, he was severely breathless at rest with Modified Medical Research Council (mMRC) Dyspnoea Scale of 4 and had to sit upright. Physical examination revealed bilateral noisy breath sounds.

Comorbidities

None.

Chest Imaging

CXR showed a right upper lobe lung mass (Fig. **1**) CT thorax showed a spiculated lung mass at the right upper lobe with severe extrinsic compression of the distal trachea by enlarged mediastinal lymphadenopathy (Fig. **2**). Flexible bronchoscopy showed a severe slit like pure extrinsic compression of the distal trachea (Fig. **3**). Distal airways were patent.

Intervention

Rigid bronchoscopy under general anaesthesia. The stenosis was dilated using CRE balloon and rigid bronchial tube. A silicone Y-stent was inserted using the pullback technique. The silicone stent remained partially compressed immediately post-stenting (Fig. **4**). A radial EBUS guided transbronchial cryobiopsy of the right upper lobe mass was performed at the same time and HPE showed lung adenocarcinoma (Fig. **5**).

[*]**Corresponding author Tie Siew Teck:** Division of Respiratory Medicine, Sarawak General Hospital, Kuching, Malaysia; E-mail: tiest@moh.gov.my

Jamalul Azizi Abdul Rahaman & Tinku Joseph (Eds.)

Complications

None.

Post-Intervention

The patient was extubated to room air after rigid bronchoscopy. He was able to lie flat and undergo radiotherapy and chemotherapy. His mMRC Dyspnoea Scale improved to 2 on discharge. CT thorax and flexible bronchoscopy at 2 months post-stenting showed a well expanded stent with some secretions in the stent (Figs. **6** and **7**).

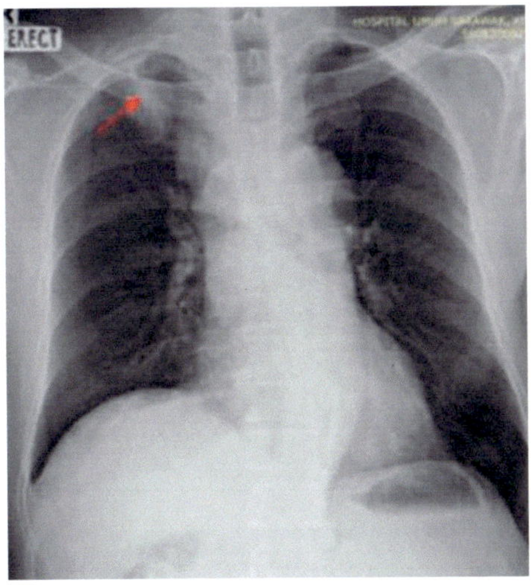

Fig. (1). CXR showing a lung mass at right upper lobe (red arrow).

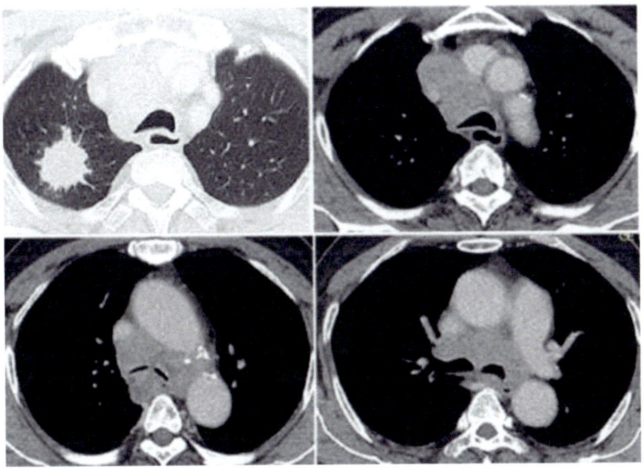

Fig. (2). Axial CT thorax shows a spiculated lung mass at right upper lobe with severe extrinsic compression of the distal trachea by enlarged mediastinal lymphadenopathy.

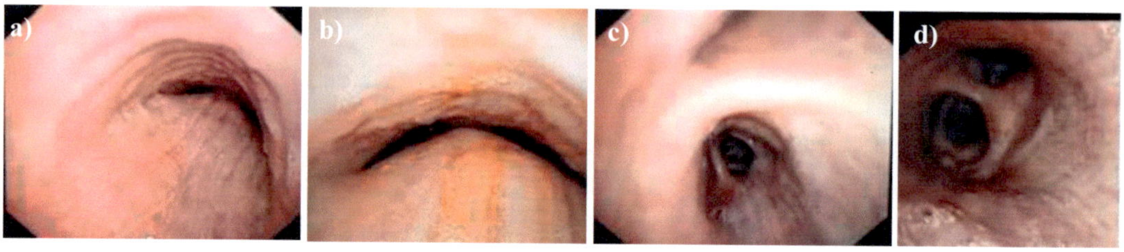

Fig. (3). Bronchoscopy images showing severe compression of the distal trachea and main bronchi. **a)** Proximal trachea. **b)** Distal trachea. **c)** Right main bronchus. **d)** Left main bronchus.

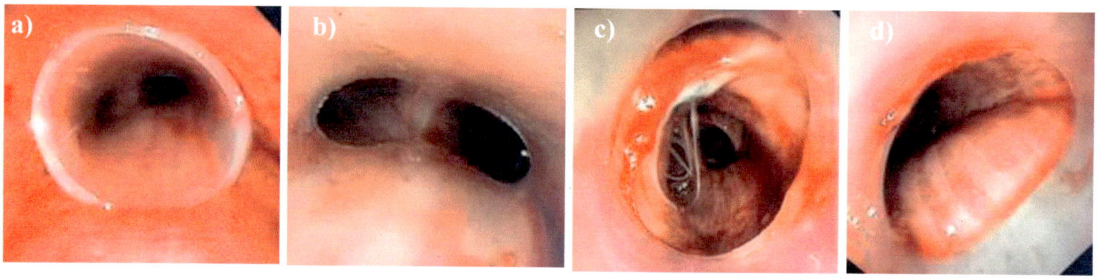

Fig. (4). Silicone Y-stent in position immediately post-stenting. **a)** Trachea. **b)** Main carina. **c)** Right main bronchus. **d)** Left main bronchus.

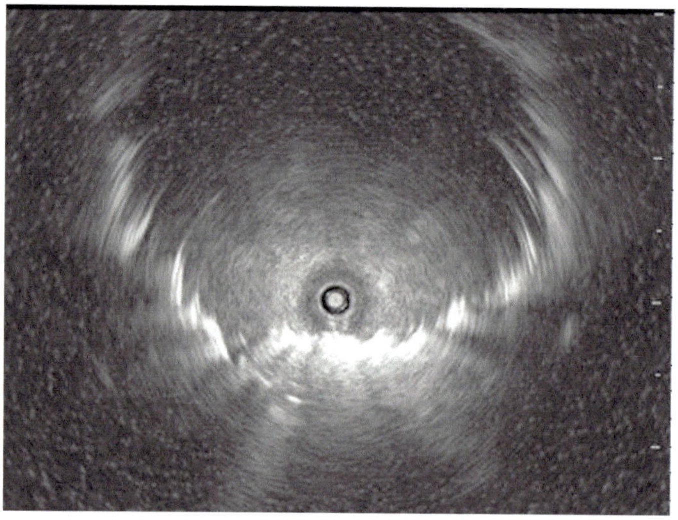

Fig. (5). Radial EBUS image of the right upper lobe lung mass.

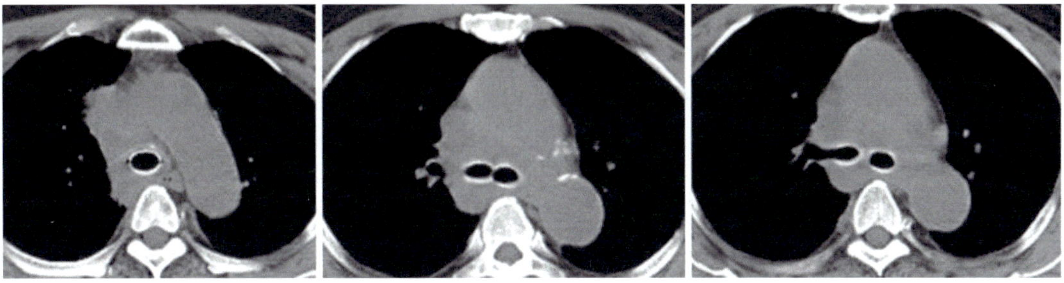

Fig. (6). CT thorax at two months post-stenting showing markedly smaller mediastinal mass and improved central airway compression.

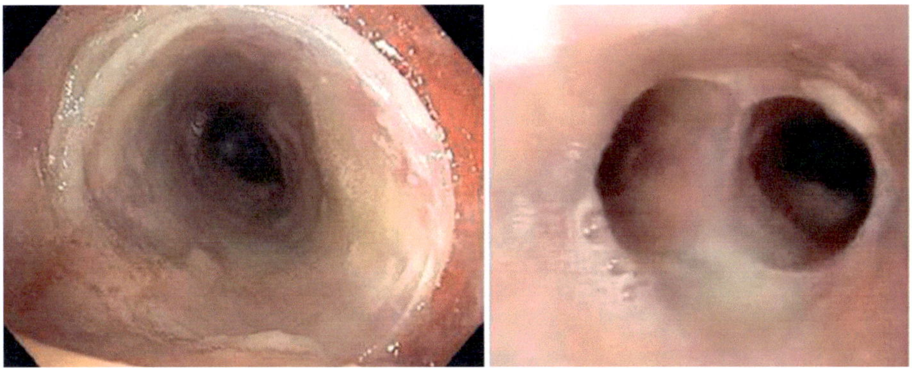

Fig. (7). Bronchoscopy at 2 months showing a well expanded stent with minimal granulation tissues at the proximal edge of the stent. (Left) Trachea. (Right) Main carina.

Learning Points

- Airway stenting is useful to relieve severe extrinsic central airway obstruction.
- Silicone stent has a better radial force compared to some metallic stents and hence is better in relieving severe airway compression [1]. It is also more durable compared to metallic stent with no risk of stent fracture. If stent removal is anticipated; silicone stent is the preferred choice due to the ease of removal.
- Silicone stent requires rigid bronchoscopy for insertion and removal.
- A disadvantage of silicone stenting is the difficulty of inserting the stent introducer distal to the stenotic site in some cases with severe stenosis. Metallic Y-stent is a good option in such cases due to its ease of insertion. Some operators also insert and remove metallic stent under conscious sedation without the need for rigid bronchoscopy.

CONSENT FOR PUBLICATION

Not applicable.

CONFLICT OF INTEREST

The author declares no conflict of interest, financial or otherwise.

ACKNOWLEDGEMENT

Declared none.

REFERENCE

[1] Freitag L. Airway stents. European Respiratory Monograph 2010. [http://dx.doi.org/10.1183/1025448x.00991409]

Case 20

Silicone Stent for Recurrent Post-Intubation Tracheal Stenosis

Khai Lip Ng[1], **Nai-Chien Huan**[1], **Rosmadi Ismail**[2], **Mona Zaria Nasaruddin**[1,*] and **Jamalul Azizi Abdul Rahaman**[1]

[1] *Department of Pulmonology, Serdang Hospital, Selangor, Malaysia*

[2] *Sunway Medical Centre, Selangor, Malaysia*

Keywords: Post-intubation tracheal stenosis, Stridor, Balloon dilatation, Recurrence, Silicone stent.

Presentation

A 31-year-old lady had worsening shortness of breath and stridor. Two weeks earlier, she had undergone rigid bronchoscopy with balloon dilatation and topical mitomycin C for tracheal stenosis. Recurrent tracheal stenosis was suspected.

Comorbidities

Diabetes mellitus, history of prolonged intubation (40 days) for severe diabetic ketoacidosis a year ago.

Chest Imaging

CXR demonstrated a significant luminal narrowing at mid-trachea (Fig. **1**).

Flexible bronchoscopy confirmed a complex mid-tracheal stenosis (length > 1cm) with an opening diameter of approximately 3.0mm (Myers-Cotton grade 3) (Fig. **2a**). Unable to pass the flexible bronchoscope through the stenotic segment.

Airway Intervention

Emergent rigid bronchoscopy with gradual balloon dilatation of the stenotic segment. In view of the rapid recurrence of symptoms after the previous balloon

*Corresponding author Mona Zaria Nasaruddin: Department of Pulmonology, Serdang Hospital, Selangor, Malaysia; E-mail: mzaria78@yahoo.com

Jamalul Azizi Abdul Rahaman & Tinku Joseph (Eds.)

dilatation, a silicone tracheal stent (15 millimetres in diameter, 50 millimetres in length; NOVATECH® GSS™ BD, Novatech, La Ciotat, France) was deployed after dilatation (Figs. **2b-d**). The tracheal lumen distal to the silicone stent was patent after stent deployment and adjustment (Fig. **3**).

Complications

No immediate procedure related complications were noted. The patient however developed fever post intervention and was given a week of intravenous antibiotics (piperacillin-tazobactam) for presumed hospital acquired pneumonia. She was discharged well.

Post-Intervention

Improvement in symptoms with the resolution of stridor.

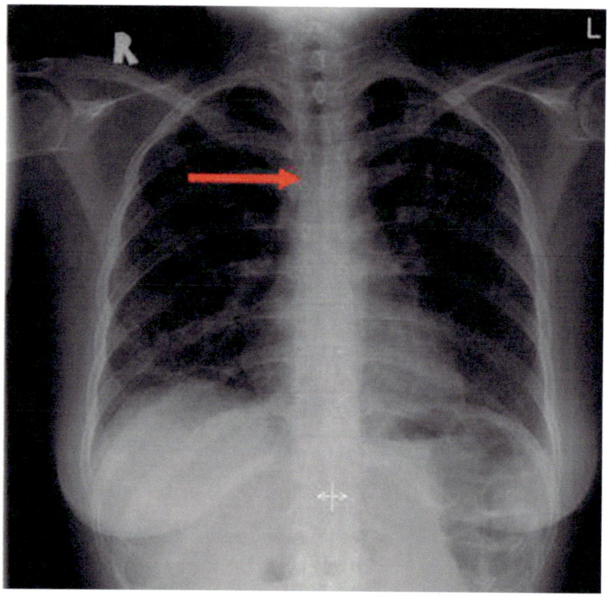

Fig. (1). CXR before dilatation and stenting showing significant narrowing at mid-trachea (red arrow).

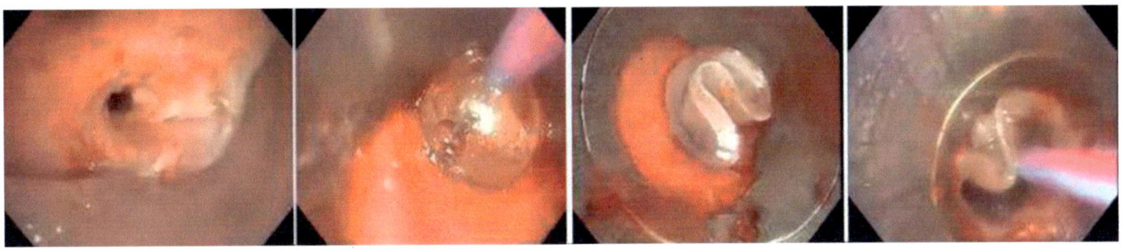

a) b) c) d)

Fig. (2). (a-d) Narrowing at mid-trachea of 3.0 mm diameter. Balloon dilatation was done followed by silicone stent insertion. Balloon catheter was inserted into the folded stent and inflated to unfold the stent.

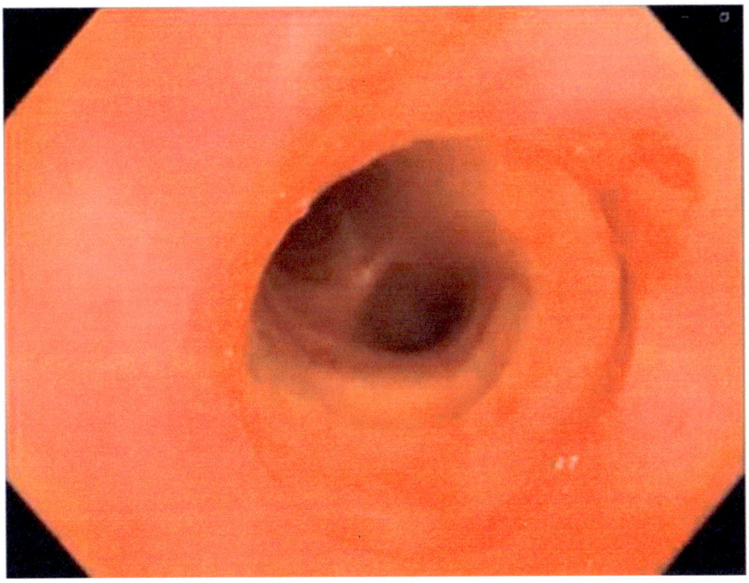

Fig. (3). Patent lower trachea after stenting.

Learning Points

- Post-intubation tracheal stenosis is potentially life-threatening. Endoscopic management in the form of balloon dilatation and mitomycin C application is an acceptable measure to provide symptomatic relief thereby improving the quality of life of patients. However, airway stenting might occasionally be required in the event of rapid recurrence of symptoms post-endoscopic intervention while waiting for a definitive treatment *i.e.*, airway reconstructive surgery [1].

Video

The placement of the silicone stent in the trachea after balloon dilatation.

CONSENT FOR PUBLICATION

Not applicable.

CONFLICT OF INTEREST

The author declares no conflict of interest, financial or otherwise.

ACKNOWLEDGEMENT

Declared none.

REFERENCE

[1] Kim, J-H, Jeong-Eun K, Kyung WK. The management of post-intubation/tracheostomy stenosis with silicone stent. Eur Respirat J 2011; 38: 612.

Case 21

Post Intubation Tracheal Stenosis: Hourglass Stent

Harikishan Gonuguntla[1,*] and **Belgundi Preeti Vidyasagar**[1]

[1] *Department of Interventional Pulmonology, Yashoda Hospital, Secunderabad, India*

Keywords: CT scan, Respiratory failure, Stenosis, Stridor, Vocal cords.

Presentation

A 34-year-old male patient presented to the emergency room with stridor. His past medical history suggests recent ICU admission for respiratory failure after organophosphate ingestion. He had a prolonged ICU stay on mechanical ventilatory support and was gradually weaned off. On his review consult, an ENT examination showed stenosis in the subglottic area, which was repaired by an ENT surgeon. He had recurrence of stenosis causing acute stridor necessitating an emergency room visit.

Comorbidities

None.

Chest Imaging

High resolution CT scan of the neck demonstrated narrowing of the trachea with the proximal stenotic part 2.5cm distal to the vocal cords. The location of the tracheal stenosis was confirmed prior to intervention (Fig. **1a**).

Intervention

Via a supraglottic device, under general anesthesia, using a flexible bronchoscope and electrosurgical knife (KD-31-C1, Olympus Medical systems, Tokyo, Japan) radial incisions were made to accommodate a CRE dilatation balloon (Fig. **1b**). Using the CRE dilatation balloon, the stenotic segment was dilated (Fig. **1c**). After an initial dilatation with flexible bronchoscope, the patient was intubated with a rigid tracheoscope (Outer diameter 12.00mm- Inner diameter 11.00mm EFER-DUMON SERIES 3 BT2201-3). CRE (controlled radial expansion balloons;

*Corresponding author **Harikishan Gonuguntla:** Department of Interventional Pulmonology, Yashoda Hospital, Secunderabad, India; E-mail: khailip08@yahoo.com

Jamalul Azizi Abdul Rahaman & Tinku Joseph (Eds.)

CRETM Pulmonary balloon dilatation catheter, 10mm/11mm/12mm, Bos ton scientific, Ireland) balloon dilation was done of the stenotic segment. The barrel of the rigid tube was negotiated through the stenotic segment further dilating it. A radiopaque silicone hourglass stent (SETX 14-12-14, STENING) was deployed through the rigid tracheoscope under fluoroscopy guidance (Fig. **1d**).

Complications

No complications were observed during the procedure.

Post-Intervention

The patient had complete resolution of stridor and was discharged after explaining the stent care in detail.

a) b)

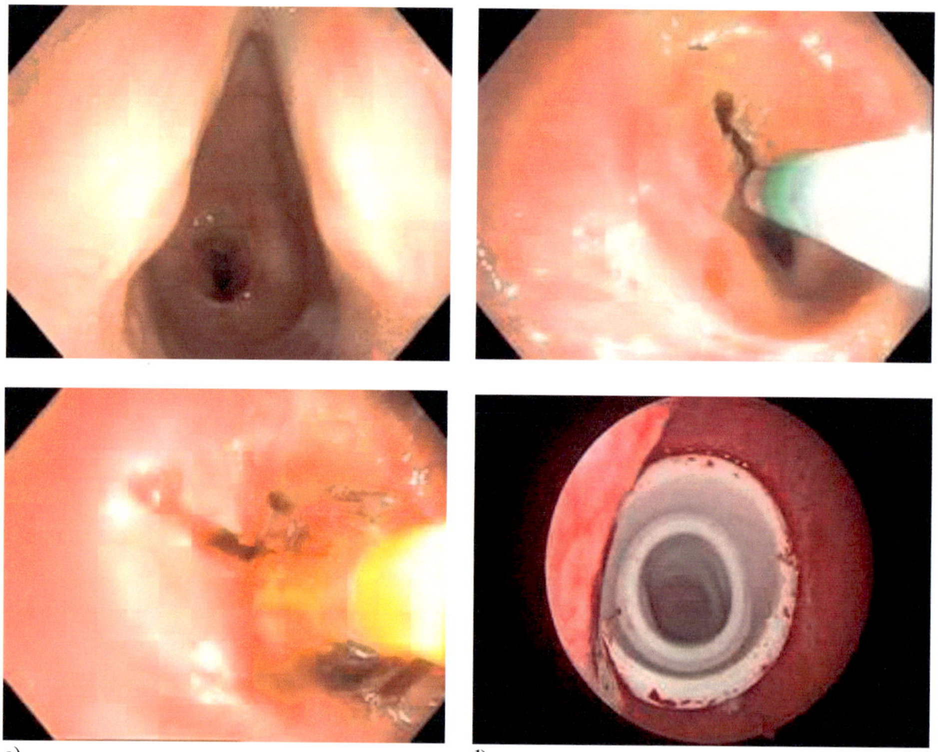

c) d)

Fig. (1). (a-d) Steps of bronchoscopic dilatation and stenting.

Learning Points

- Hourglass stents are useful in cases of post-intubation tracheal stenosis and have less chance of migration compared to the straight silicone stents [1].

Video

The placement of the silicone hourglass stent after dilatation of the sub-glottic stenosis with electrocautery knife and CRE balloon.

CONSENT FOR PUBLICATION

Not applicable.

CONFLICT OF INTEREST

The authors declare no conflict of interest, financial or otherwise.

ACKNOWLEDGEMENT

Declared none.

REFERENCE

[1] Sabath B, Casal RF. The (hour) glass half-full: modified silicone hourglass stents for the treatment of central airway obstruction. Cureus 2021; 13(6): e15501. [http://dx.doi.org/10.7759/cureus.15501] [PMID: 34268032] [PMCID: PMC8262651]

Case 22

Airway Stent (Metallic)

Tracheal Stenting for Malignant Central Airway Obstruction due to a large Thyroid Mass

Tinku Joseph[1,*] and **Sathish C. Reddy**[1]

[1] *Interventional Pulmonology Unit, Amrita Institute of Medical Sciences, Kochi, India*

Keywords: Central airway tumour, Interventional pulmonology, Rigid bronchoscopy, Self-expanding metallic stent (SEMS), Tracheal stenting.

Presentation

A 57-year-old lady presented with cough, worsening breathlessness of 6 months duration. She also had associated loss of appetite and loss of weight. She underwent partial thyroidectomy 4 months before at a tertiary care center and was diagnosed with Hashimoto thyroiditis. However, in spite of surgery, her general condition gradually deteriorated and developed significant stridor and orthopnoea and hence she was transferred to our hospital for further management.

Comorbidities

Post-COVID-19 lung fibrosis, COPD, Hashimoto thyroiditis, systemic hypertension and type 2 diabetes mellitus.

Chest Imaging

CXR showed no significant abnormality (Fig. **1**). CT thorax revealed a right thyroid lesion compressing the trachea with suspicious infiltration into the trachea (Fig. **2**).

CT neck with contrast showed a right thyroid lesion measuring 5.2cm x 5.2cm x 5cm causing significant compression of the trachea with intraluminal component and retrosternal extension (Fig. **3**). Larynx and pharynx appeared normal.

*Corresponding author Tinku Joseph: Interventional Pulmonology Unit, Amrita Institute of Medical Sciences, Kochi, India; E-mail: tinkujoseph2010@gmail.com

Jamalul Azizi Abdul Rahaman & Tinku Joseph (Eds.)

Intervention

Bronchoscopy showed critical narrowing of the tracheal lumen (lumen diameter 3mm and 1.5cm distal to vocal cords) with extrinsic compression and intraluminal growth, extending from subglottic space up to 2cm above the carina (Figs. **4** and **5**). Histopathological examination of the bronchoscopic biopsy specimen was suggestive of anaplastic carcinoma thyroid.

In view of significant stridor and poor prognosis of the disease after multi-disciplinary meeting, the plan was made to do palliative airway stenting to maintain luminal patency and subsequently radiate the patient. After obtaining a high risk procedure consent, the patient underwent a rigid bronchoscopy guided tracheal stenting. A 16mm diameter x 6cm length self-expanding covered metallic stent (SEMS) was used for the procedure. The size of the stent was measured during prior bronchoscopic evaluation of the airway and also on the basis of CT neck and chest findings. Both flexible bronchoscope and fluoroscopy were used for stent deployment as they helped in accurate positioning of the stent. Post-procedure, the entire tracheal lumen was recanalized and the patient was extubated on the table (Figs. **6** and **7**).

Complications

No immediate post-procedure complications noted.

Post-Intervention

The patient was comfortable after the procedure and she was symptom free. In order to prevent mucus retention inside the stent, she was given nebulized mucolytics and was discharged 48 hours post- procedure. Prior to discharge, a CXR was done to rule out stent migration. She was referred subsequently to radio therapy unit for palliative radiotherapy to reduce the size of the thyroid mass.

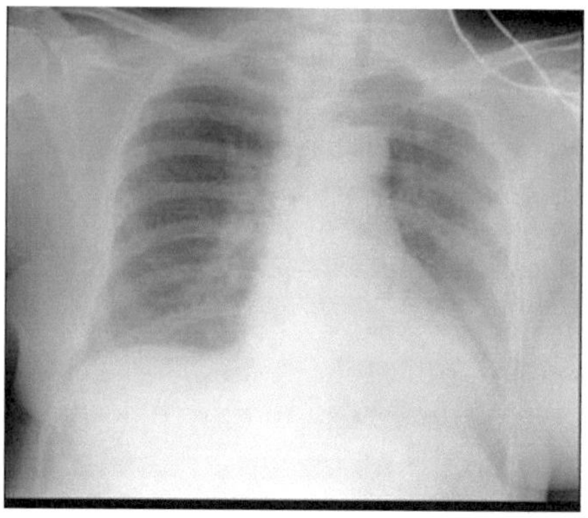

Fig. (1). Pre-procedure CXR.

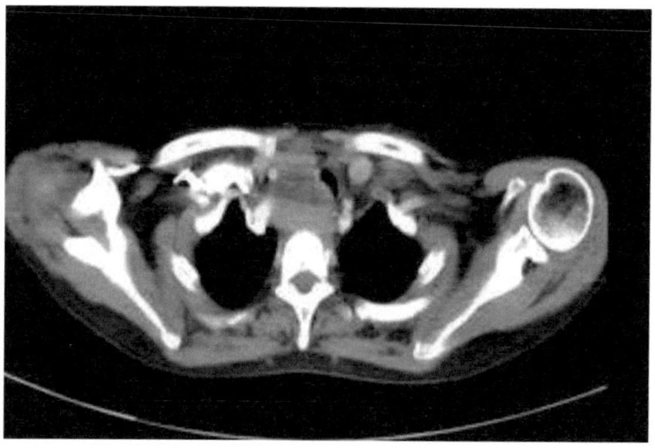

Fig. (2). CECT thorax: Right thyroid lesion compressing the trachea with suspicious infiltration into the trachea.

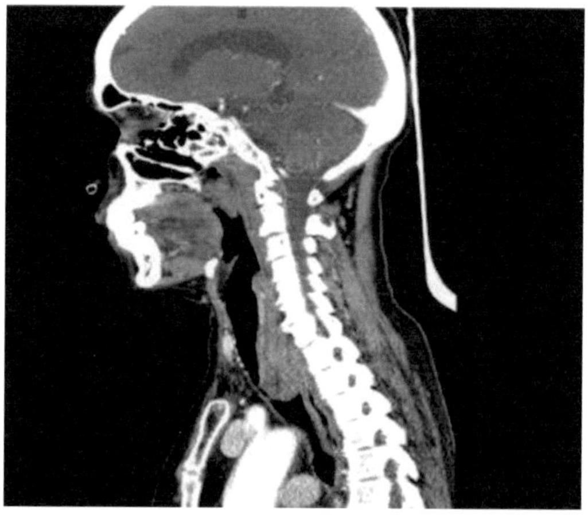

Fig. (3). CT neck: Compression of the trachea with intraluminal component.

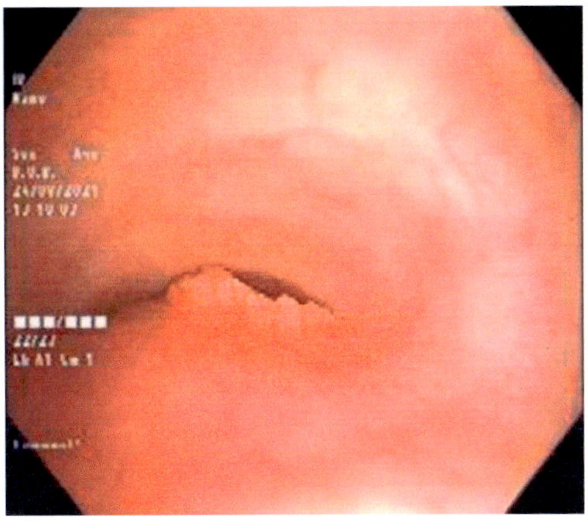

Fig. (4). Significantly narrowed tracheal lumen due to extrinsic and intrinsic compression.

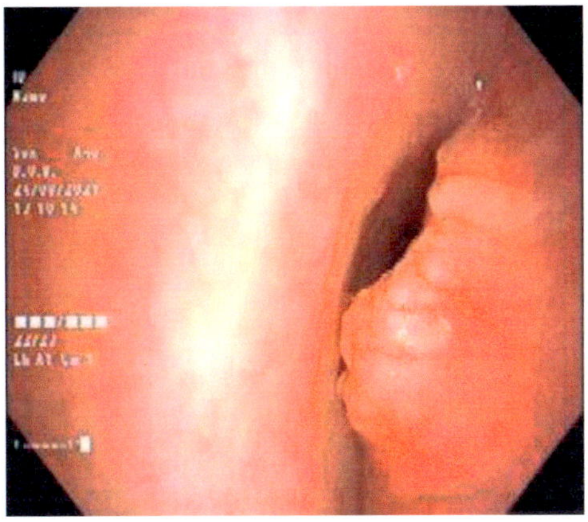

Fig. (5). Thyroid mass infiltrating into the tracheal lumen.

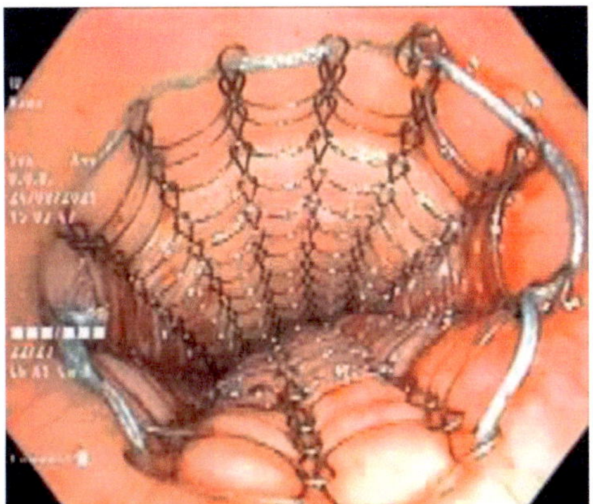

Fig. (6). Post-procedure: Proximal end of stent inside tracheal lumen.

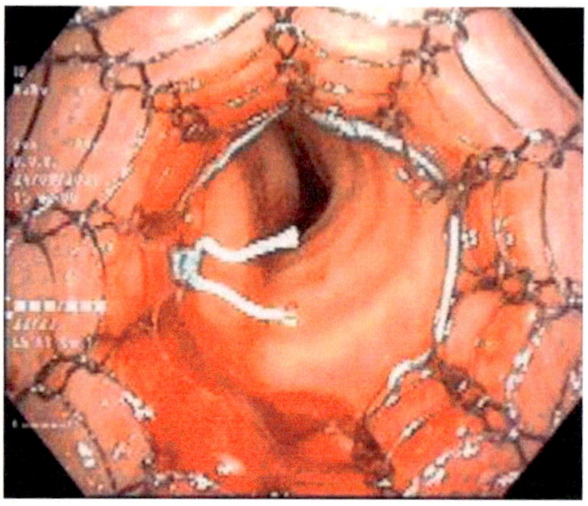

Fig. (7). Post-procedure: Distal end of stent showing completely recanalized tracheal lumen.

Learning Points

- Airway stenting has been well used in the treatment and palliation of patients with malignant stenosis and to a lesser extent in those with benign disease causing airway compromise.
- Stents are either constructed of silicone or metal, usually a nitinol, a nickel and titanium alloy.
- The different categories of stents have positive and negative attributes that play a role in choosing the proper stent.

Indications for Airway Stenting in Malignant Conditions

- Extrinsic compression [1].
- Endobronchial tumour with residual obstruction – post mechanical tumour debulking.
- Mixed intrinsic and extrinsic tumour.
- Tracheo-esophageal fistula.
- Loss of cartilage support due to tumour destruction.

Advantages of SEMS

- Fewer episodes of stent migration.
- Less airway obstruction due to improved secretion clearance.
- Ease of insertion using a flexible bronchoscope.
- Available sizes for larger airways.

Disadvantages of Using a SEMS

- Tumour in-growth.
- Difficulty in removing.
- Increased risk of stent fracture (500 to 1000 days).
- Should be avoided in benign conditions.

CONSENT FOR PUBLICATION

Not applicable.

CONFLICT OF INTEREST

The authors declare no conflict of interest, financial or otherwise.

ACKNOWLEDGEMENT

Declared none.

REFERENCE

[1] Pappalardo V, La Rosa S, Imperatori A, *et al*. Thyroid cancer with tracheal invasion: a pathological estimation. Gland Surg 2016; 5(5).

Case 23

Fully Covered Metallic Stent for Critical Tracheal Stenosis Secondary to Small Cell Lung Carcinoma

Nai-Chien Huan[1], **Mona Zaria Nasaruddin**[1,*], **Rosmadi Ismail**[2] and **Jamalul Azizi Abdul Rahaman**[1]

[1] *Department of Pulmonology, Serdang Hospital, Selangor, Malaysia*

[2] *Sunway Medical Centre, Selangor, Malaysia*

Keywords: Airway stenting, Central airway obstruction, Lung cancer, Respiratory emergency, Rigid bronchoscopy, Small cell lung cancer.

Presentation

A 67-year-old gentleman with a one-month history of progressively worsening shortness of breath (Modified Borg Dyspnoea Scale 9 at rest: almost maximal).

Comorbidities

COPD, chronic smoker of more than 20 pack years.

Chest Imaging

CT thorax demonstrated significant luminal narrowing of mid and lower trachea secondary to a massive mediastinal and right hilar mass with concurrent superior vena cava obstruction (Fig. **1a**).

Intervention

Rigid bronchoscopy, biopsy and debulking of the tracheal mass using a flexible cryoprobe (Fig. **1b**). Following that, a fully covered tracheal metallic stent (length 10cm, diameter 16mm, Niti-STM Tracheal Stent, Taewoong Medical, Gyeonggi-do, South Korea) was deployed at the site of the obstruction (Figs. **1c** and **d**).

Complications

No immediate complications.

[*] **Corresponding author Mona Zaria Nasaruddin:** Department of Pulmonology, Serdang Hospital, Selangor, Malaysia; E-mail: mzaria78@yahoo.com

Jamalul Azizi Abdul Rahaman & Tinku Joseph (Eds.)

Post-Intervention

Intervention was technically successful as it allowed re-canalization of the trachea facilitating mechanical ventilation. HPE revealed small cell lung carcinoma. Family members opted for conservative care. The patient eventually succumbed a month post-procedure due to disease progression and hospital acquired infection.

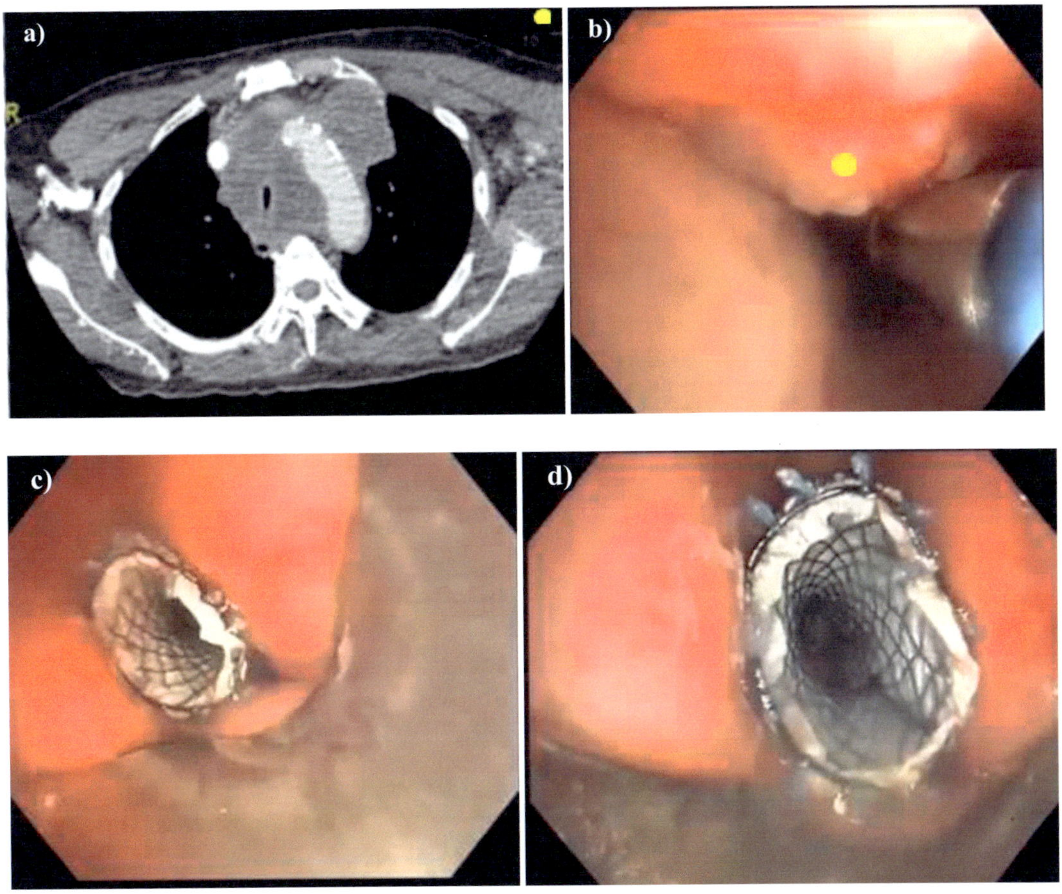

Fig. (1). CT thorax and bronchoscopy image. **a)** Axial CT thorax demonstrating narrowed main trachea due to the mass. **b)** Debulking of tracheal mass (yellow dot) with a flexible cryoprobe. **c)** Appearance of the stent immediately after deployment. **d)** Successful recanalization of the trachea after tumour debulking and stenting.

Learning Points

- Malignant central airway obstruction is a life-threatening medical emergency. Therapeutic bronchoscopy including airway stenting can facilitate mechanical ventilation and provide meaningful symptomatic relief. Nevertheless, technical success does not always translate into clinical benefits as seen in our case. The AQuIRE registry demonstrated an overall technical success rate of 93% [1]. Clinical factors associated with a higher rate of poorer outcome include American Society of Anaesthesiologists (ASA) score of greater than 3, renal failure, primary lung cancer, tracheoesophageal fistula and left mainstem disease [1]. Therefore, a careful risk and benefit assessment is required to ensure the best patient outcome.

Video

Placement of fully covered tracheal metallic stent (length 10cm, di ameter 16mm, Niti-STM Tracheal Stent, Taewoong Medical, Gyeonggi-do, South Korea).

CONSENT FOR PUBLICATION

Not applicable.

CONFLICT OF INTEREST

The authors declare no conflict of interest, financial or otherwise.

ACKNOWLEDGEMENT

Declared none.

REFERENCE

[1] Shafiq M, Lee H, Yarmus L, Feller-Kopman D. Recent advances in interventional pulmonology. Ann Am Thorac Soc 2019; 16(7): 786–796. [http://dx.doi.org/10.1513/AnnalsATS.201901-044CME] [PMID: 31145638]

Case 24

Palliative Stenting in Malignant Tracheal Narrowing

Muhammad Farid Fauad[1], **Muhammad Amin Ibrahim**[1], **Mona Zaria Nasaruddin**[2,*] and **Jamalul Azizi Abdul Rahaman**[2]

[1] *Respiratory Unit, Pusat Perubatan Pakar UiTM Sg Buloh, Malaysia*

[2] *Department of Pulmonology, Serdang Hospital, Selangor, Malaysia*

Keywords: Metastatic adenocarcinoma, Malignant tracheal narrowing, 3D reconstruction, Palliative, Partially covered stent.

Presentation

A 71-year-old lady presented with cough for one month and progressive shortness of breath for 2 weeks. CXR showed widened mediastinum and right-sided pleural effusion (Fig. **1**). Pleural fluid analysis showed metastatic adenocarcinoma likely lung primary. Immunohistochemical staining showed the malignant cells were strongly positive for TTF-1 and Napsin A but negative for thyroglobulin.

Comorbidities

Hypertension.

Chest Imaging

CT thorax showed a large soft tissue mass occupying the superior mediastinum measuring 8.2 x 10.0 x 9.5cm (APxWxCC) from the level of T1 vertebral body superiorly till T6 inferiorly. The mass was likely matted lymph nodes encasing the great vessels with local compression causing tracheal narrowing with preserved patency, right subclavianvein thrombosis, right brachiocephalic thrombosis with slit like vessel patency, left jugular vein thrombo sis and left brachiocephalic vein thrombosis (Figs. **2** and **3**). Numerous lung nodules and right pleural nodules with a large pleural effusion were observed. 3D reconstruction of the CT thorax showed significant anteroposterior compression at the mid-distal trachea (Fig. **4**).

*Corresponding author Mona Zaria Nasaruddin: Department of Pulmonology, Serdang Hospital, Selangor, Malaysia; E-mail: mzaria78@yahoo.com

Jamalul Azizi Abdul Rahaman & Tinku Joseph (Eds.)

Intervention

Rigid bronchoscopy was performed using the 10mm tracheal tube (EFER-DUMON) under general anaesthesia. Airway assessment showed mid to distal tracheal obstruction with predominantly extrinsic compression leading to significant anteroposterior compression at the distal trachea. Mucosal infiltration was seen at the lower left paratracheal wall. Endobronchial nodules with grossly abnormal mucosa were seen in both right and left main bronchi. Endobronchial biopsy was taken from the lower left paratracheal wall. Tracheal dilatation was performed with CRE balloon gradually up to 12mm. Boston Scientific Ultraflex (18 x 60mm) partially covered stent was inserted and deployed at the distal trachea. Post-stenting showed patent tracheal lumen (Fig. **5**).

Complications

None.

Post-Intervention

Intravenous dexamethasone and oral gefitinib were continued. In addition, palliative radiotherapy was planned for this lady. Intravenous heparin was given to address thrombosis in the great vessels. Endovenous recanalization with SVC stent placement could not be offered at this point as the patient was unable to lie in a supine position. The pleural fluid was further drained (Fig. **6**).

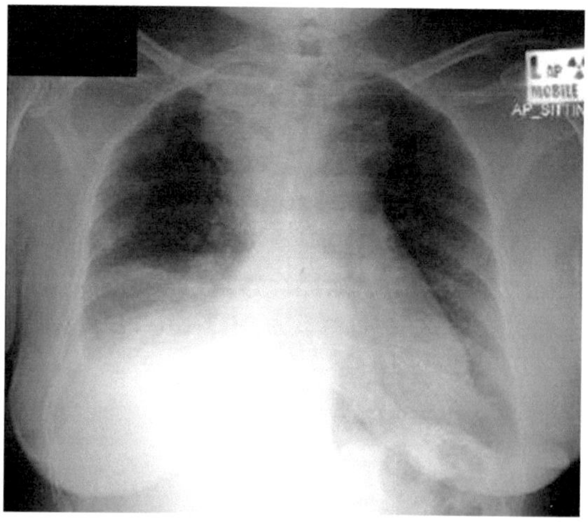

Fig. (1). CXR on presentation showed widened mediastinum and right pleural effusion.

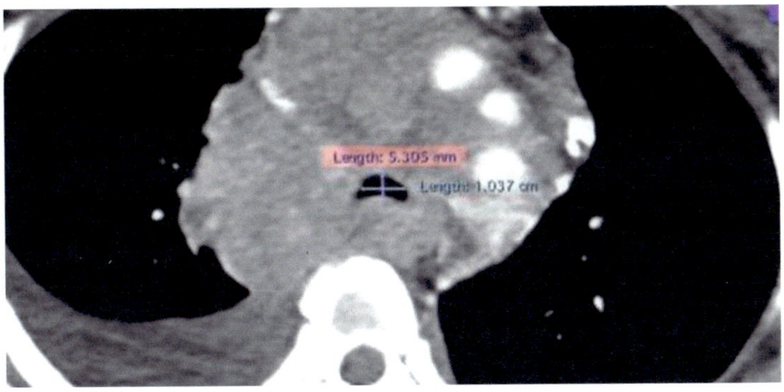

Fig. (2). Axial CT scan view showed narrowing of the distal trachea 5.3 x 10mm.

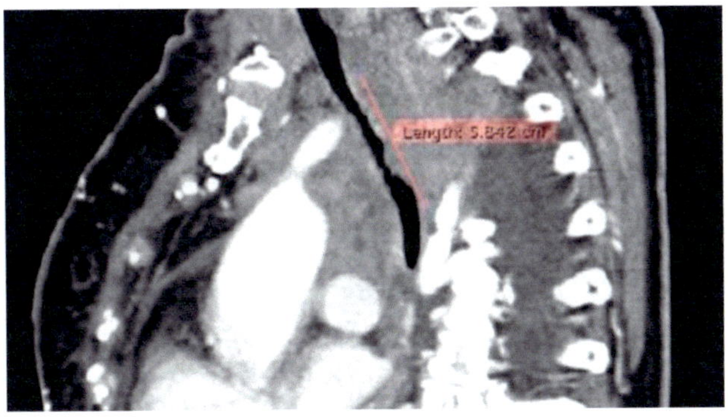

Fig. (3). Sagittal CT scan showing the tracheal narrowing length 58mm.

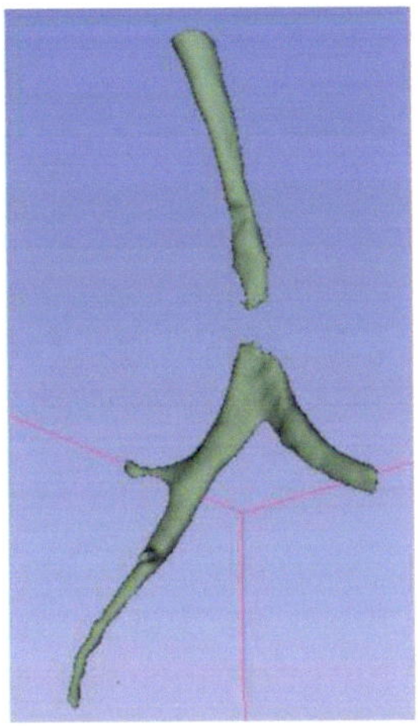

Fig. (4). 3D reconstruction of the CT thorax showed significant anteroposterior compression at the mid-distal trachea.

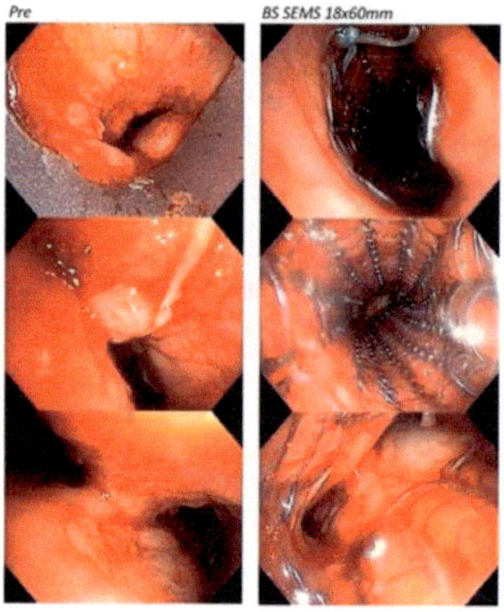

Fig. (5). Rigid bronchoscopy view showed mucosal infiltration at the lower left paratracheal wall and endobronchial nodules with grossly abnormal mucosa. Tracheal stent was successfully deployed at the distal trachea. The airway was patent after stenting.

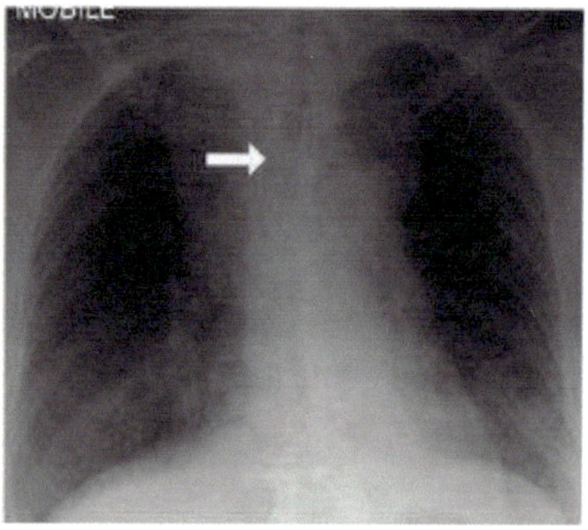

Fig. (6). CXR post-pleurul drainage and the tracheal stent (white arrow).

Learning Points

- Central airway obstruction in lung cancer often indicates advanced stage of the disease. The aim of intervention at this point is to alleviate the symptoms without curative intent [1]. Multimodality approaches to address the symptoms are required and among these interventions, tracheal stenting offers immediate relief of central airway obstruction [2]. This can lead to a significant clinical improvement and offer a better quality of life for the patient.

Video

Tracheal dilatation with CRE balloon followed by the deployment of Boston Scientific Ultraflex (18 x 60mm) partially covered stent at the distal trachea.

CONSENT FOR PUBLICATION

Not applicable.

CONFLICT OF INTEREST

The authors declare no conflict of interest, financial or otherwise.

ACKNOWLEDGEMENT

Declared none.

REFERENCES

[1] Simoff MJ, Lally B, Slade MG, *et al.* Symptom management in patients with lung cancer: Diagnosis and management of lung cancer, 3rd ed.; American College of Chest Physicians evidence-based clinical practice guidelines. Chest 2013; 143(5 Suppl): e455S-e497S. [http://dx.doi.org/10.1378/chest.12-2366] [PMID: 23649452]

[2] Boyd M, Rubio E. The utility of interventional pulmonary procedures in liberating patients with malignancy-associated central airway obstruction from mechanical ventilation. Lung. 2012; 190(5): 471-6. [http://dx.doi.org/10.1007/s00408-012-9394-8] [PMID: 22644069]

Case 25

Removal of Partially Covered Self-Expandable Metallic Tracheal Stent in a Stepwise Approach

Kho Sze Shyang[1,*], **Mona Zaria Nasaruddin**[1] and **Jamalul Azizi Abdul Rahaman**[1]

[1] *Department of Pulmonology, Serdang Hospital, Selangor, Malaysia*

Keywords: Airway stenting, Rigid bronchoscopy, Stent removal, Self-expandable metallic stent, Therapeutic bronchoscopy.

Presentation

A 36-year-old gentleman with constitutional symptoms and haemoptysis, admitted for decompensated respiratory failure requiring positive pressure ventilation. Urgent CT thorax showed a huge lung mass with mediastinal lymphadenopathy causing significant central airway obstruction (Fig. **1a**). Emergent rigid bronchoscopy with tumour debulking was performed followed by insertion of an 18 x 60mm partially covered self-expanding metallic stent (Ultraflex™, Boston Scientific, Marlborough, USA). The patient was extubated post-procedure. Endobronchial cryobiopsy established the diagnosis of diffuse large B cell lymphoma (DLBCL). The patient underwent four cycles of chemotherapy (cyclophosphamide, doxorubicin, vincristine, prednisolone) with good response showing reduction in the volume of mediastinal lymphadenopathy. However, two months post stent placement, the patient coughed out a short fragment of nitinol-stent wire. In view of good treatment response with evidence of stent fatigue, a decision for stent removal was made.

Comorbidities

Ex-smoker.

Chest Imaging

CT thorax showed a significant reduction of mediastinal lymphadenopathy (Fig. **1b**). A vertical air pocket was visualized between the stent and the right lateral wall of the trachea (Fig. **2**). Granulation tissue was also evident at both ends of the stent.

*Corresponding author Kho Sze Shyang: Department of Pulmonology, Serdang Hospital, Selangor, Malaysia; E-mail: khosze@moh.gov.my

Intervention

Rigid bronchoscopy was performed under total intravenous anaesthesia with cardiothoracic surgery backup. The patient was intubated with a 13mm rigid tracheoscope. Examination using a flexible bronchoscope confirmed granulation tissues at both uncovered ends of the stent. Disruption of the nitinol wire strand was noted at the mid-distal region of the stent lumen. A stepwise approach was used for the removal of the SEMS:

Step 1: Cryo-debridement was performed over the granulation tissues using a 2.4mm flexible cryoprobe (ERBE, Medizintechnik, Tübingen, Germany) at both uncovered ends of the stent (Fig. **3**). Cryo-activation was performed with direct visualization and limited to superficial granulation tissue removal to avoid incidental dislodgement of the stent. Debridement was performed until the whole circumference of the stent was visible distally and proximally.

Step 2: The tracheoscope was then advanced towards the stent. The proximal end of the stent was telescoped into the rigid tracheoscope lumen (Fig. **4a**). The rigid forceps was then inserted gently between the stent and tracheal wall, aiming to loosen the stent (Fig. **4b**).

Step 3: Next, the stent was grasped using the rigid forceps at its proximal end and gently twisted from 0 to 90 degree, observing for any resistance. The stent was then removed in a twisting motion and gently pulled into the lumen of the rigid tracheoscope (Fig. **5**). Gradually, the stent was freed from its distal granulation tissue and was removed in one piece through the rigid tracheoscope (Fig. **6**). Total duration of stent *in situ* was exactly 100 days.

Step 4: Residual granulation tissue and bleeding was coagulated with Nd: YAP laser (Fig. **7a**). All distal secretions were aspirated.

Complications

None. The patient was extubated post-procedure.

Post-Intervention

Airway was patent albeit it was still extrinsically compressed (Fig. **7b**).

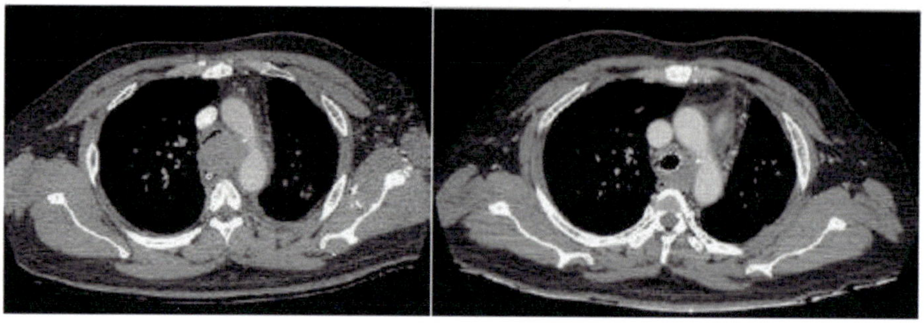

Fig. (1). (a) (Left) Axial CT thorax on presentation showing critical tracheal compression with only a slit like opening. **(b)** (Right) CT scan prior to the removal of the stent showing a patent airway with the stent *in situ*.

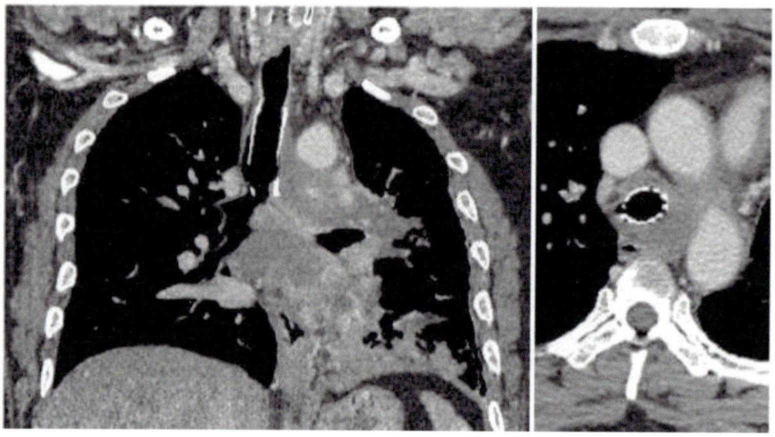

Fig. (2). Vertical air pocket was seen between the stent and right lateral wall of the trachea on coronal and axial CT thorax.

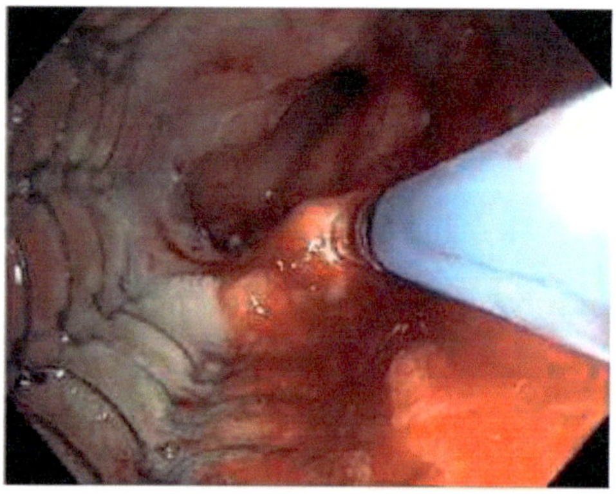

Fig. (3). Cryo-debridement performed over the granulation tissues at the distal end of the stent.

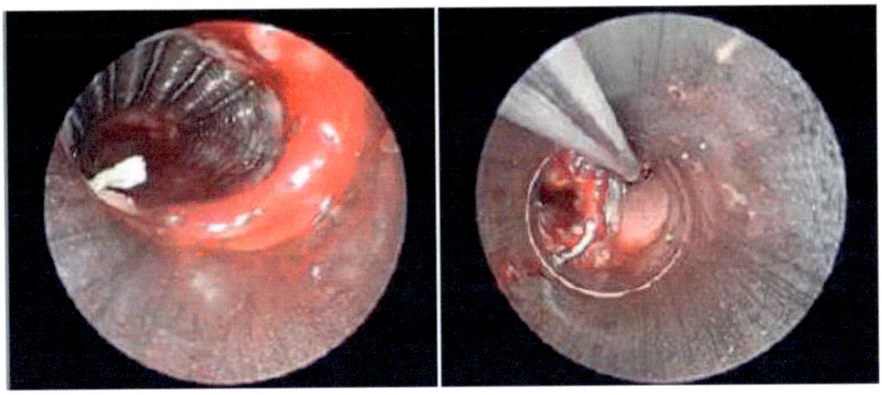

Fig. (4). (a) (Left) The proximal end of the stent was telescoped into the rigid tracheoscope. **(b)** (Right) The rigid forceps was then inserted gently between the stent and tracheal wall.

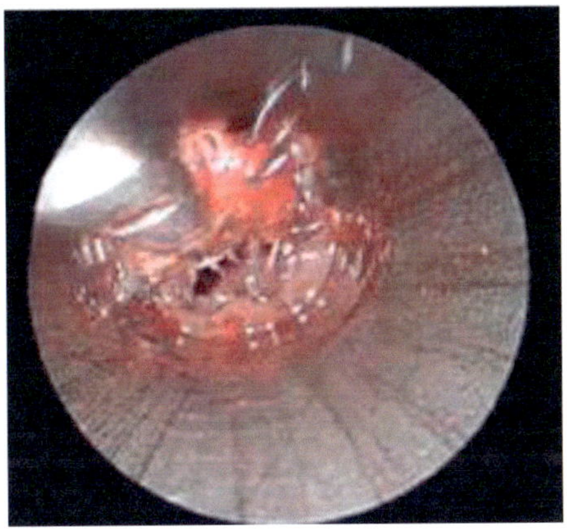

Fig. (5). The stent was grasped and removed through the rigid tracheoscope in a twisting motion.

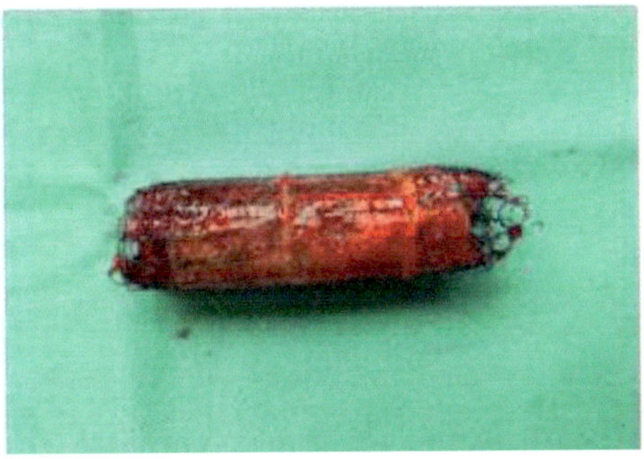

Fig. (6). The Ultraflex™ SEMS was removed in one piece with a total duration of 100 days *in situ*.

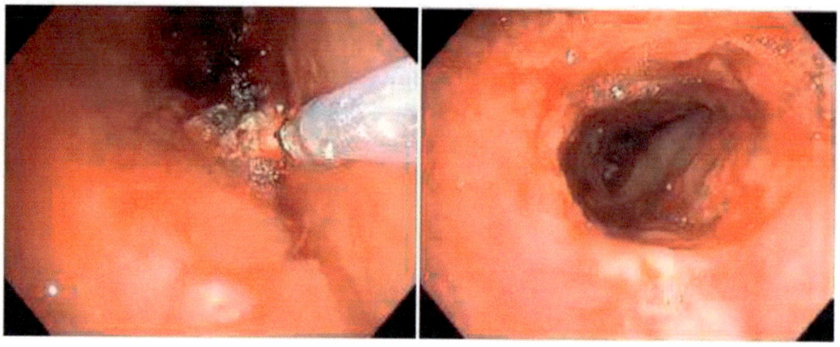

Fig. (7). (a) (Left) Residual granulation tissue and bleeding was coagulated with Nd: YAP laser. **(b)** (Right) Airway remained patent after stent removal.

Learning Points

- Airway stenting is frequently a life-saving procedure in patients with malignant central airway obstruction. The usage of self-expanding metallic airway stent (SEMS) has increased lately due to its user-friendly deployment system. However, long term SEMS usage is frequently associated with complications such as granulation tissue, stent migration and stent fracture. Hence, SEMS should be removed as soon as it is feasible. A previous study had demonstrated the safety and feasibility of SEMS removal with a median duration of 35 days (range, 2-595 days) [1]. As bronchoscopic technique has matured and advanced over the years, more advanced ancillary tools are now available to complement this complex procedure, including the use of cryo-technology [2]. Although the removal of SEMS is feasible, proper communication and collaborative planning with anesthesiology and thoracic surgery are of utmost importance to ensure safety to the patient.

Video

Removal of the self-expandable metallic stent *via* rigid bronchoscopy.

CONSENT FOR PUBLICATION

Not applicable.

CONFLICT OF INTEREST

The authors declare no conflict of interest, financial or otherwise.

ACKNOWLEDGEMENT

Declared none.

REFERENCES

[1] Shah SK, Jennings JH, Diaz-Mendoza JI, *et al.* Removal of self-expanding metallic stents. J Bronchology Interv Pulmonol 2016; 23(4): 279-82. [http://dx.doi.org/10.1097/LBR.0000000000000322] [PMID: 27764006]

[2] Majid A, Palkar A, Myers R, *et al.* Cryotechnology for staged removal of self-expandable metallic airway stents. Ann Thorac Surg 2013; 96: 336-38. [http://dx.doi.org/10.1016/j.athoracsur.2013.03.002] [PMID: 23816097]

Case 26

3D Printed Airway Stents

Patient Specific 3D Printed Silicone Stent for Treatment of Focal Bronchomalacia

Marcela Azevedo[1] and **Thomas R. Gildea**[1,*]

[1] *Department of Pulmonary, Allergy and Critical Care Medicine & Transplant Center, Respiratory Institute, Cleveland Clinic, Cleveland, Ohio, USA*

Keywords: 3D printing, Airway stenting, Bronchomalacia, Tracheal stenosis, Y-stent.

Presentation

A 45-year-old female undergoes evaluation for suspected excessive dynamic airway collapse due to or thopnea, persistent cough and recurrent pulmonary infections requiring multiple hospitalizations.

Comorbidities

Asthma, Systemic Lupus Erythematosis.

Chest Imaging

CT of the chest revealed near complete collapse of the bronchus intermedius on exhalation but less than 50 percent reduction in the anterior-posterior diameter of the trachea and left mainstem bronchus consistent with focal bronchomalacia (Fig. **1**).

Airway inspection with flexible bronchoscopy revealed complete obstruction of bronchus intermedius and approximately 75 percent obstruction of the right mainstem bronchus (RMSB) with tidal breathing (Fig. **2**).

Intervention

After failed conservative therapies, the patient underwent tubular silicone stent placement under rigid bronchoscopy of the right mainstem with a notch created at

[*]**Corresponding author Thomas R. Gildea:** Department of Pulmonary, Allergy and Critical Care Medicine & Transplant Center, Respiratory Insti tute, Cleveland Clinic, Cleveland, Ohio, USA; E-mail: gildeat@ccf.org

2cm for the right upper lobe (Fig. **3**). Over the following 10 years, her airway was managed with serial therapeutic bronchoscopies and stent revisions. Multiple stent revisions were required for stent exchange due to mucous plugging and frequent infections. Other stent length-based revisions were required due to bronchus intermedius malacia and right upper lobe obstruction. A variety of locations for notch placement for the right upper lobe were attempt ed with frequent obstruction but adequate drainage. Recurrent migration of the stent into the trachea (Fig. **4**) led to upsizing the diameter of the stent from 14mm to 16mm. While a 16mm tubular stent also migrated due to the small size, an 18mm stent was too large and could not be unfolded in the airway. After failed proper seating of tubular stents of various diameters, we pursued a patient specific airway stent. The patient's CT scan of the chest was used to create a 3D reconstruction in a proprietary web-based software package (Visionair LLC, Cleveland, OH, USA) and a patient specific stent prescription (Fig. **5**). A silicone Y stent was manufactured to seat in the bronchus intermedius to right main stem with a right upper lobe limb (Fig. **6**). With rigid bronchoscopy, the patient specific 3D printed silicone stent (PS3DS) was deployed into the right main stem using standard instruments (Rigid silicone stent deployment tools Bryan-Dumon, Woburn, MA, USA) (Fig. **7a**). We oriented the right upper lobe limb into its proper location with the aid of rigid and flexible forceps. Balloon dilation was performed to aid with seating the stent. After maneuvering, the stent was seated in the correct orientation, however, there was partial occlusion of the posterior segment of the right upper lobe deemed of minimal clinical significance (Fig. **7b**). CT Chest shows the position of the PS3DS post-implantation (Fig. **8**).

Complications

Partial occlusion of the posterior segment of the right upper lobe, moderate mucostasis.

Post-Intervention

The patient experienced significant subjective benefit in shortness of breath and cough. However, she had mucostasis typical of silicone stents. Treatment included increased frequency in the nebulization of albuterol and saline from twice to three times a day with added guaifenesin and use of a mucous clearance device as is our local stepwise practice in the absence of strong data.

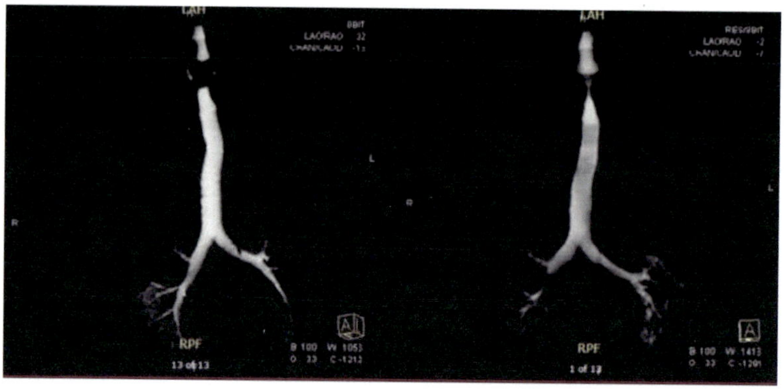

Fig. (1). Computer Tomography based tracheobronchial tree with inspiration (Left) and exhalation images (Right) showing residual collapse of bronchus intermedius.

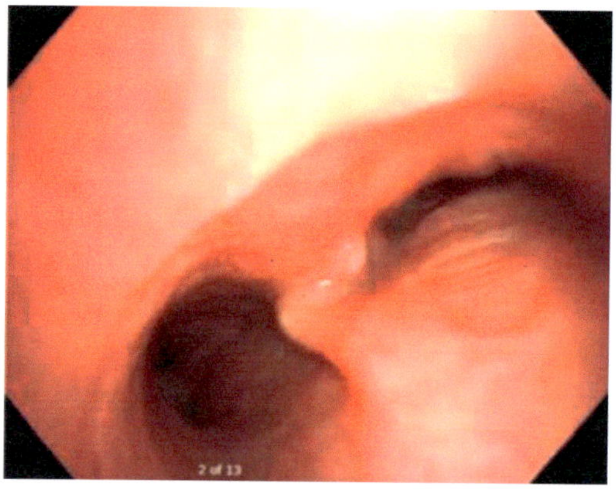

Fig. (2). Bronchoscopy showing severe malacia in native airway.

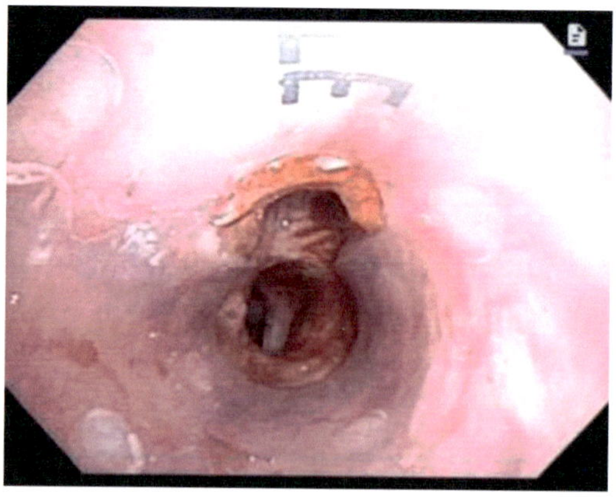

Fig. (3). Previous silicone tubular stent placement, silicone stent in RMSB with notch for RUL.

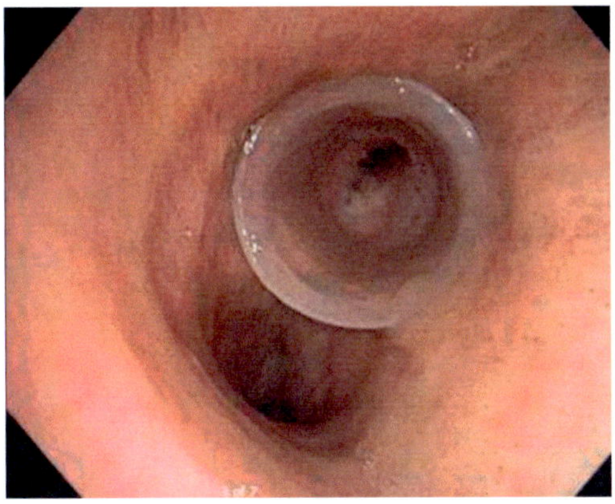

Fig. (4). Poorly fitting silicone tube stent with slight proximal migration.

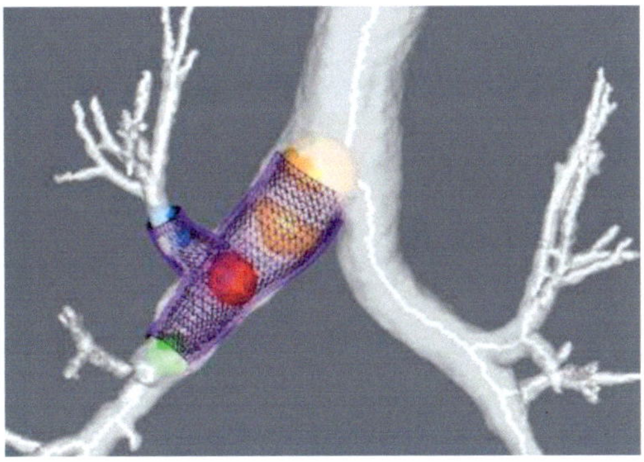

Fig. (5). 3D Airway reconstruction software designing patient specific stent prescription, the native airway seems to extend beyond the stent since the airway is flattened by malacia.

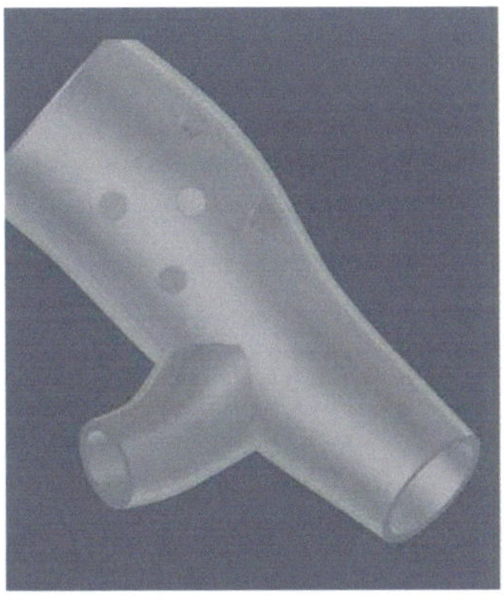

Fig. (6). Patient Specific Y stent fitting right mainstem to bronchus intermedius with right upper lobe limb.

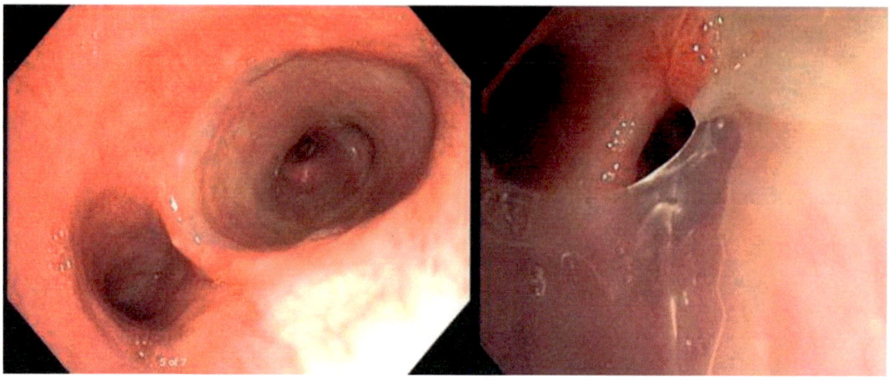

Fig. (7). (a) (Left) Patient specific stent well seated in the right mainstem-bronchus intermedius. **(b)** (Right) Minimal occlusion of the posterior segment of the right upper lobe after 2 months.

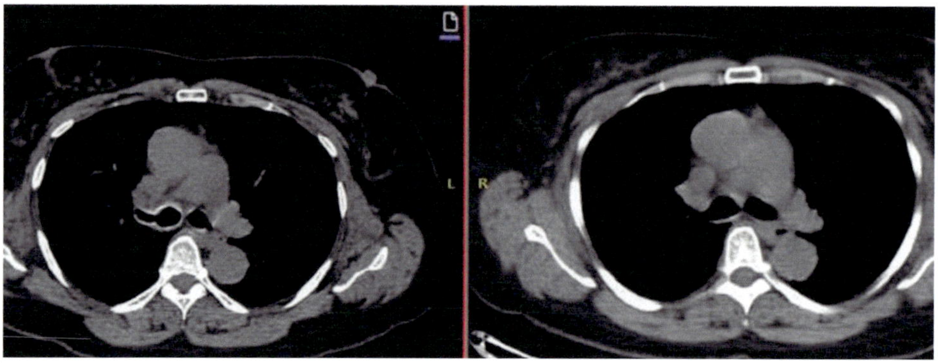

Fig. (8). CT Chest axial cut of right mainstem. The left image shows the increased lumen size and the stent branch in the right upper lobe. The CT on the right is prior to implant of the PS3DS.

Learning Points

- Complex benign airway disease may be treated with airway stenting as an option of last resort when conservative measures have failed. Due to significant variability among size and shape of the tracheobronchial tree among individuals, standard stents do not always provide an adequate fit. In this case, the unusual nature of the focal area of bronchomegaly and malacia may have been worsened by years of stent oversizing as part of initial treatment. The ability to more precisely size and position a stent improved symptoms in this patient and have been durable. While studies are lacking to delineate pathologies best suited for this technology and exactly how to size patient specific stents and to define the durability of treatment outcomes, this therapy helped this patient with prior failed treatment with standard stents [1, 2].

CONSENT FOR PUBLICATION

Not applicable

CONFLICT OF INTEREST

Dr. Azevedo declares no conflict of interest, financial or otherwise.

Cleveland Clinic and Cleveland Clinic Institutional Officials/Leaders have an equity interest in NEW Custom Orthopaedic Solutions (COS)/Visionair) and are entitled to royalty payments from the company for technology developed at Cleveland Clinic. NEWCOS/Visionair is the manufacturer of the stents. Dr. Gildea is the inventor and may be entitled to royalty payments from the company in accordance with Cleveland Clinic policy.

ACKNOWLEDGEMENT

Declared none.

REFERENCES

[1] Alraiyes AH, Avasarala SK, Machuzak MS, Gildea TR. 3D printing for airway disease. AME Med J 2019; 4: 14.
[http://dx.doi.org/10.21037/amj.2019.01.05] [PMID: 31650103] [PMCID: PMC6812574]
[2] Gildea TR, Young BP, Machuzak MS. Application of 3D printing for patient-specific silicone stents: 1-year follow-up on 2 Patients. Respiration 2018; 96(5): 488-94.
[http://dx.doi.org/10.1159/000489669] [PMID: 30212834]

Case 27

Patient Specific 3D Printed Stent for Treatment of Central Airway Disease due to IgG-Related Lung Disease

Prince Ntiamoah[1,2], **Alejandro Aragaki**[1,2], **Christopher Radchenko**[1,2], **Sadia Benzaquen**[3] and **Thomas R. Gildea**[1, 2,*]

[1] *Department of Pulmonary, Allergy and Critical Care Medicine & Transplant Center, Cleveland Clinic, Cleveland, Ohio, USA*

[2] *Department of Pulmonary, Critical Care and Sleep Medicine, University of Cincinnati, Ohio, USA*

[3] *Einstein Medical Center, Jefferson University, Philadelphia, Pennsylvania, USA*

Keywords: 3D printing, Airway stenting, Bronchomalacia, Tracheal stenosis, Y-stent.

Presentation

A 66-year-old woman, nonsmoker, presented with a non-productive cough, hoarseness, wheezing and dyspnea on exertion. No family or occupational history, or personal history of autoimmune disease or malignancy.

Comorbidities

She had been diagnosed with idiopathic tracheal stenosis 22 years ago and had tracheal resection which later manifested as multifocal airway disease and was eventually diagnosed with IgG4-related lung disease. During the following 10 years, she underwent multiple airway procedures including cryospray, balloon dilation and attempts at stenting. She remained symptomatic except for a short time following each bronchoscopy.

Chest Imaging

Chest computed tomography (CT) showed significant circumferential thickening of the right main stem bronchus (RMSB) and bronchus intermedius (BI), as well as moderate stenosis of the left main stem bronchus (LMSB).

* **Corresponding author Thomas R. Gildea:** Department of Pulmonary, Allergy and Critical Care Medicine & Transplant Center, Cleveland Clinic, Cleveland, Ohio, USA; Department of Pulmonary, Critical Care and Sleep Medicine, University of Cincinnati, Ohio, USA; E-mail: gildeat@ccf.org

Jamalul Azizi Abdul Rahaman & Tinku Joseph (Eds.)

Intervention

Prior attempts at placing silicone Y stents were unsuccessful due to asymmetric airway size and non-standard main carina morphology. The tracheobronchial mucosa appeared very waxy and friable. There was 75 percent stenosis of the bronchus intermedius (BI) and left main stem bronchus (LMSB) with a long segment malacia of the LMSB (Figs. **1a-d**). The patient's CT scan of the chest was used to create a 3D reconstruction in a proprietary web-based software package (Visionair LLC, Cleveland, OH, USA) and a patient specific stent prescription (Figs. **2a** and **b**). A silicone Y stent was manufactured to seat in the trachea, right mainstem to the bronchus intermedius bypassing the right upper lobe and then a branch into a long portion of the left main bronchus. A hole was made for the right upper lobe with the hole punch device (Bryan-Dumon, Woburn, MA, USA). With rigid bronchoscopy, the patient specific 3D printed silicone stent (PS3DS) was deployed using standard instruments (Rigid silicone stent deployment tools (Bryan-Dumon, Woburn, MA, USA) (Figs. **3a-e**).

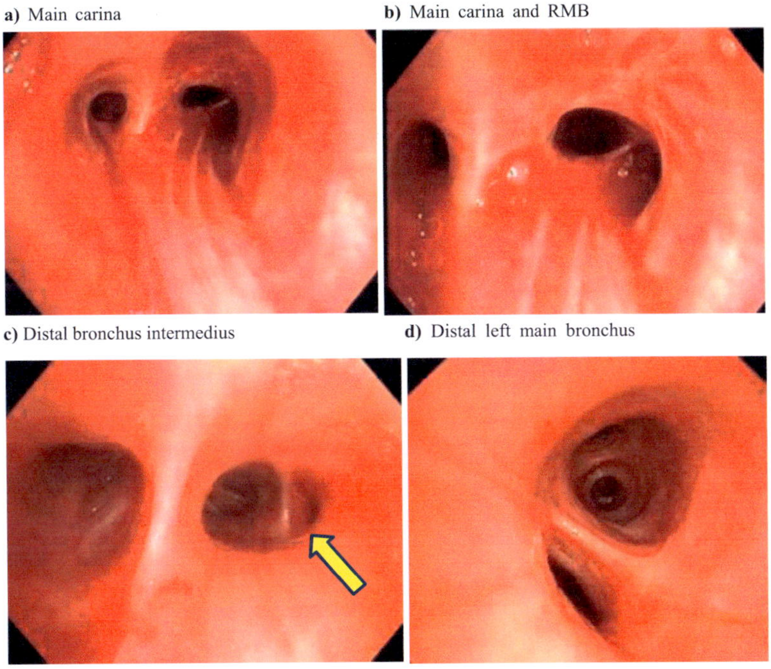

Fig. (1). (a-d) Bronchoscopy images of airway prior to stenting. Note Main carina is distorted, there is a major size difference between the left and right main bronchus. The RMB is very short, the distal bronchus intermedius is normal but the superior segment is narrow (arrow).

Complications

She had mucostasis as common in silicone stenting, but this did improve over time with saline nebulizers.

Post-Intervention

Immediately after patient specific stent insertion, the patient's shortness of breath improved. The patient is currently tolerating her customized stent for over 10 months now.

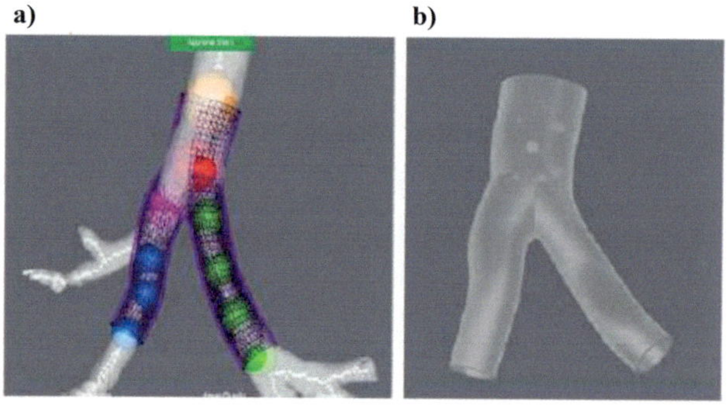

Fig. (2). (**a** and **b**) Patient specific silicone Y stent was designed using 3D airway reconstruction software, to account for the complex geometry.

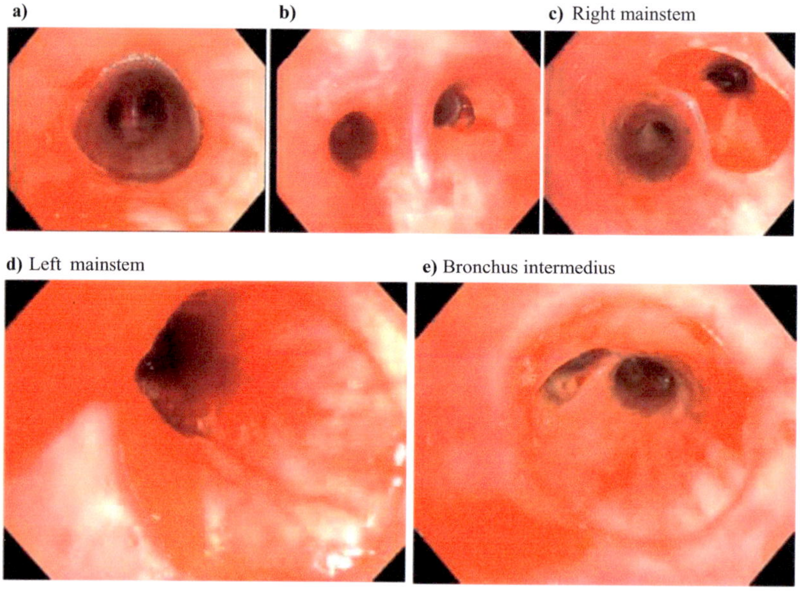

Fig. (3). **(a-e)** A patient specific Y-stent (Visionair, Cleveland OH USA) designed and deployed into the trachea, LMSB, RMSB, and BI. A hole was made for the right upper lobe (RUL).

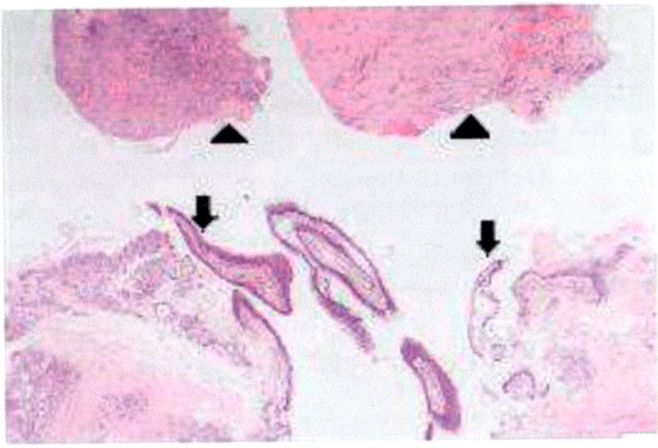

Fig. (4). (a) 2x magnification Fragments of bronchial wall (arrow). Fragments of polypoid granulation tissue (arrowhead).

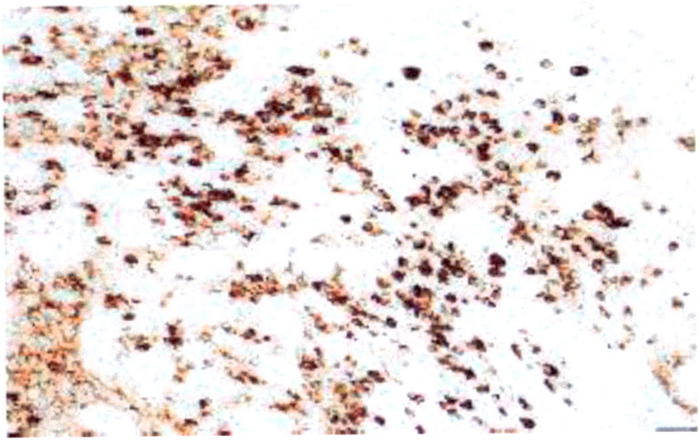

Fig. (4). (b) 40X- Predominance of plasma cells focally in clusters.

Learning Points

- IgG4-related disease (IgG4-RD) is an autoimmune disorder characterized by substantial infiltration of plasma cells with IgG4 in target organs with pulmonary involvement being a relatively new and unique clinical entity [1]. IgG4-related lung disease (IgG4-RLD) implies a series of clinical, radiological, and histopathological characteristics with a tissue biopsy needed to confirm the diagnosis (Figs. **4a** and **b**). It is primarily composed of four clinical pulmonary syndromes: inflammatory lung pseudotumor, central airway disease, interstitial pneumonia, and pleuritis. Patients may present with cough (dry), chest pain, exertional dyspnea while others may present with abnormal finding in chest imaging, with a lack of respiratory findings. Over 12 years of medical therapy, surgery and minimally invasive bronchoscopic techniques including cryospray and standard silicone stents were attempted prior to considering patient specific airway stenting after securing the diagnosis of IgG4-RLD. Patients with unusual airway anatomy and even more unusual underlying disease such as IgG4-RLD refractory to medical or even standard airway procedures may be reasonable candidates for patient specific airway stents [2]. The 3D reconstruction, atypical size and shape can be managed with this technique. Even the PS3DS required post processing modification of a hole punch for the right upper lobe as previously described for silicone stents [3]. Standard stent management of mucostasis is still important.

CONSENT FOR PUBLICATION

Not applicable.

CONFLICT OF INTEREST

Drs. Ntiamoah, Aragaki, Radchenko or Benzaquen declare no conflict of interest, financial or otherwise.

Cleveland Clinic and Cleveland Clinic Institutional Officials/Leaders have an equity interest in NEW Custom Orthopaedic Solutions (COS)/Visionair) and are entitled to royalty payments from the company for technology developed at Cleveland Clinic. NEWCOS/Visionair is the manufacturer of the stents. Dr. Gildea is the inventor and may be entitled to royalty payments from the company in accor dance with Cleveland Clinic policy.

ACKNOWLEDGEMENT

Declared none.

REFERENCES

[1] Raj R. IgG4-related lung disease. Am J Respir Crit Care Med 2013; 188(5): 527-29. [http://dx.doi.org/10.1164/rccm.201306-1121ED] [PMID: 23992587]

[2] Alraiyes AH, Avasarala SK, Machuzak MS, Gildea TR. 3D printing for airway disease. AME Med J 2019; 4: 14. [http://dx.doi.org/10.21037/amj.2019.01.05] [PMID: 31650103] [PMCID: PMC6812574]

[3] Breen DP, Dutau H. On-site customization of silicone stents: towards optimal palliation of complex airway conditions. Respiration 2009; 77(4): 447-53. [http://dx.doi.org/10.1159/000205396] [PMID: 19246883]

Case 28

Excessive Dynamic Airway Collapse/Tracheo-bronchomalacia

A Non-Invasive Treatment of Excessive Dynamic Airway Collapse

Khai Lip Ng[1], **Mona Zaria Nasaruddin**[1] and **Jamalul Azizi Abdul Rahaman**[1,*]

[1] *Department of Pulmonology, Serdang Hospital, Selangor, Malaysia*

Keywords: Choke point, Continous positive airway pressure, Excessive dynamic airway collapse, Non -invasive, Obstructive sleep apnea.

Presentation

A 75-year-old female presented with recent onset of wheezing for 2 months, shortness of breath and reduced effort tolerance and snoring at night. STOPBANG score was 6. Diagnosed as late-onset asthma and prescribed standard asthma medication. However, symptoms persisted.

Comorbidities

Diabetes, hypertension, vascular dementia, complete heart block on permanent pacemaker. A lifetime non-smoker. A few hospitalizations for pneumonia. BMI 36. Significant weight gain over the past 3 years. Normal thyroid function test.

Chest Imaging

HRCT thorax revealed posterior indentation of the mid and distal tracheal wall with significant luminal narrowing (Fig. **1**). She couldn't follow instructions for dynamic chest CT because of vascular dementia.

Flexible bronchoscopy under conscious sedation showed near total collapse (more than 80 percent) of the distal trachea, left mainstem bronchus and right mainstem bronchus on forced expiration consistent with excessive dynamic airway collapse (EDAC) (Fig. **2**). The patient desaturated and had to be reversed with flumazenil.

Partial polysomnogram confirmed severe OSA with AHI of 58/h. The lowest oxygen saturation documented was 51 percent (Fig. **3**).

*Corresponding author Jamalul Azizi Abdul Rahaman: Department of Pulmonology, Serdang Hospital, Selangor, Malaysia; E-mail: jamalulazizi@gmail.com

Intervention

cPAP prescription. cPAP trial under flexible bronchoscopy was not performed in view of desaturation during the first diagnostic bronchoscopy.

Complications

None.

Post-Intervention

AHI reduced to 1/h on cPAP at 11cm H_2O. Wheezing, dyspnea and snoring improved and there was cognitive improvement. Oxygen saturation was maintained at night (Fig. **4**).

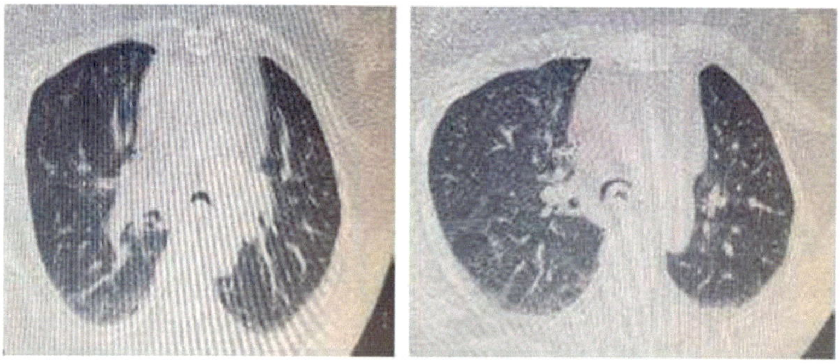

Fig. (1). Axial HRCT thorax shows excessive invagination of posterior tracheal wall at mid and distal trachea with significant luminal narrowing.

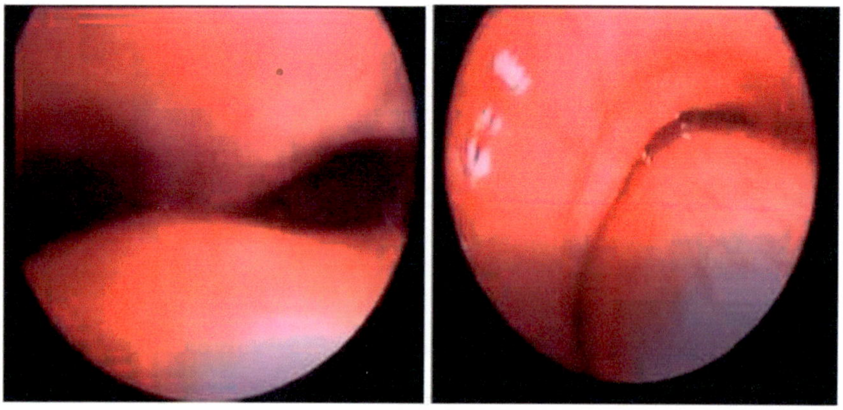

Fig. (2). (Left) Flexible bronchoscopy: Patent airway during inspiration. (Right) Total airway collapse during expiration.

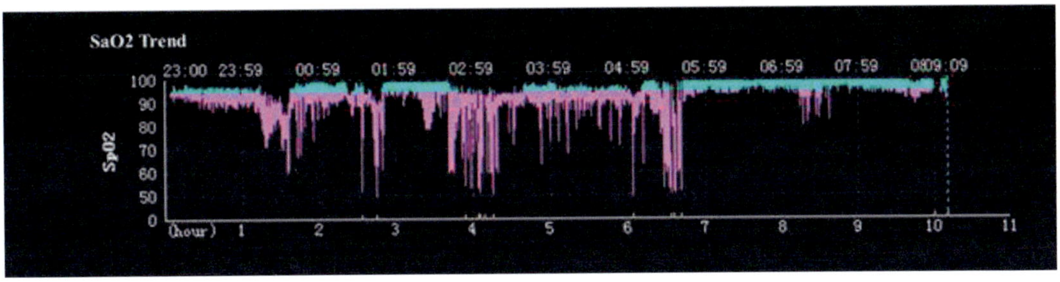

Fig. (3). Oxygen saturation trend before cPAP.

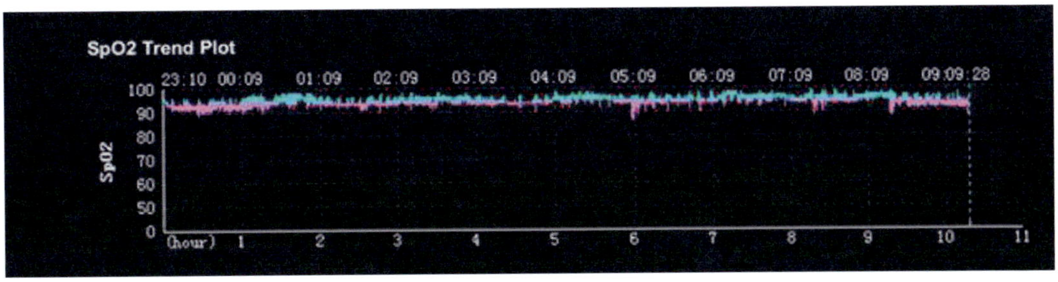

Fig. (4). Oxygen saturation trend after cPAP.

Learning Points

- EDAC is a rare condition that can mimic asthma. Dynamic airway CT thorax and functional bronchoscopy are the main investigations to diagnose EDAC. However, the choice of investigations and treatments need to be tailored to patient's condition. Due to her age and many comorbidities, a dynamic CT could not be done. cPAP trial under bronchoscopy to confirm response could not be done for the same reason. She is not an ideal candidate for a stent trial or tracheobronchoplasty. cPAP works as a pneumatic airway stent, is non-invasive and can improve exercise capacity in patients with EDAC [1].

Video

Near total collapse of the distal trachea, left mainstem bronchus and right mainstem bronchus on forced expiration during flexible bronchoscopy.

CONSENT FOR PUBLICATION

Not applicable.

CONFLICT OF INTEREST

The authors declare no conflict of interest, financial or otherwise.

ACKNOWLEDGEMENT

Declared none.

REFERENCE

[1] Razakamanantsoa L, Chahine B, Goument L, *et al*. Portable CPAP benefits on exercise capacity in patients with excessive dynamic airway collapse (EDAC). Eur Respirat J 2019; 54: PA672.

Case 29

Tracheobronchomalacia

Alex Chee[1,*] and **Elaine Dumoulin**[1]

[1] *Department of Medicine, University of Calgary, Calgary, Canada*

Keywords: Rigid bronchoscopy, SEMS, Self expanding metal stents, Tracheomalacia, Tracheobronchomalacia.

Presentation

A 72-year-old woman presented with a lifelong history of dyspnea on exertion and a diagnosis of asthma but lack of benefit from bronchodilators. She had a chronic barking cough and frequent episodes of coughing fits.

Comorbidities

Atrial fibrillation, asthma. Pulmonary Function Testing: Spirometry did not show obstruction and the flow volume loop was normal. FEV1 was 76% predicted. Her DLCO was 100% predicted.

Chest Imaging

Dynamic CT chest was performed showing full patency of the central airways on inspiration but near-complete crescentic collapse of the distal trachea, right mainstem bronchus, and left mainstem bronchus on forced expiration (Fig. **1**).

Flexible bronchoscopy: Dynamic bronchoscopy was performed under light sedation. There was greater than 90 percent collapse of the distal trachea, left mainstem bronchus, right mainstem bronchus and 70 percent collapse of the bronchus intermedius on forced expiration (Fig. **2**). There were no mucosal abnormalities but there were thin secretions throughout the airways.

Intervention

A one-week stent trial was carried out. Under general anesthesia and rigid bronchoscopy, self-expanding uncovered metal stents were placed in the distal trachea and left mainstem bronchus (Fig. **3**). The right mainstem bronchus was too

*Corresponding author Alex Chee: Department of Medicine, University of Calgary, Calgary, Canada; E-mail: Alex.chee@ahs.ca

short to maintain a stent and after stenting the distal trachea, it was determined that the right mainstem bronchus had re-established patency. The patient had significant improvement in her breathing and cough symptoms with the stent trial so a tracheobronchoplasty was performed. After a right thoracotomy and tracheal dissection, a cellular matrix mesh was shaped to the trachea and mainstem bronchi, and plicated to the posterior trachea and bronchi.

Complications

None.

Post-Intervention

After recovery from surgery, she felt significant improvement in her breathing and a change from her frequent, barking cough to a dry, inter mittent cough.

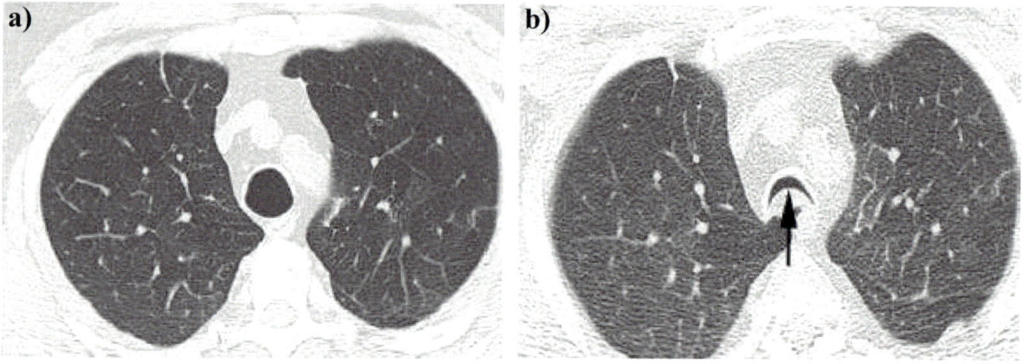

Fig. (1). Dynamic CT, performed on inhalation **(a)** and forced expiration **(b)** showing dynamic collapse of trachea on expiration.

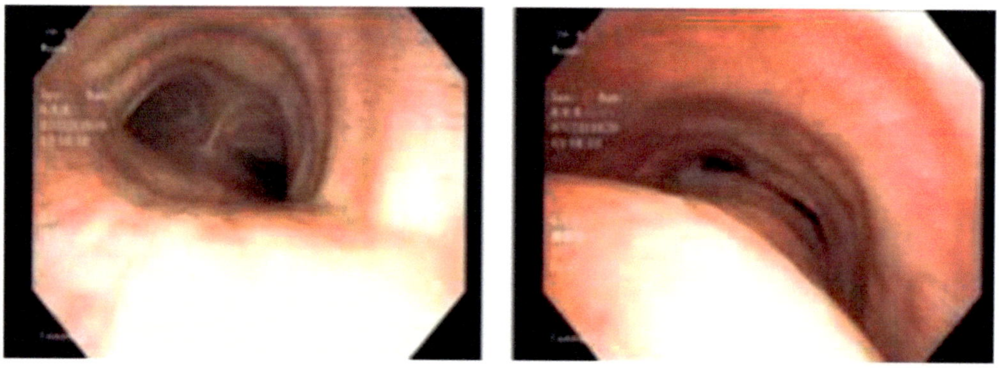

Fig. (2). Dynamic bronchoscopy and visualization of trachea on inspiration and forced expiration.

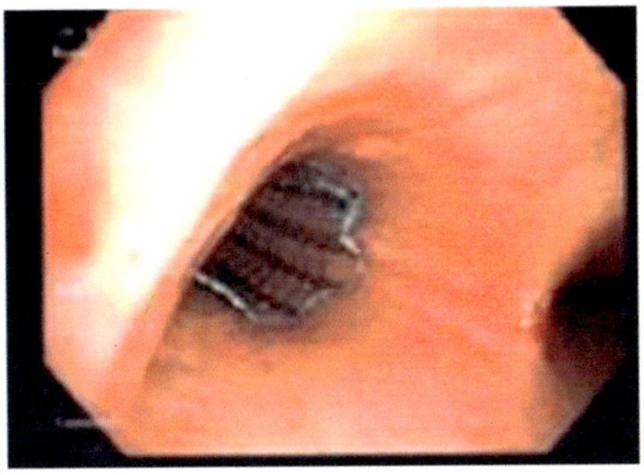

Fig. (3). Uncovered metal stent trial, stent visualized in left mainstem bronchus.

Learning Points

- Tracheobronchomalacia (TBM) is a central airway disease that is often misdiagnosed as asthma or other chronic obstructive airway diseases [1]. The typical symptoms include a chronic, barking cough and dyspnea on exertion (Buitrago *et al.*, 2017). Spirometry is unreliable for the diagnosis of TBM and diagnostic modalities include dynamic computed tomography and dynamic bronchoscopy to identify central airway collapse on expiration. Tracheobronchoplasty is the gold standard therapy for TBM and a short-term stent trial is often used as a surrogate to assess whether correction of the central airway collapse resolves symptoms.

CONSENT FOR PUBLICATION

Not applicable.

CONFLICT OF INTEREST

The authors declare no conflict of interest, financial or otherwise.

ACKNOWLEDGEMENT

Declared none.

REFERENCE

[1] Buitrago DH, Wilson JL, Parikh M, Majid A, Gangadharan SP. Current concepts in severe adult tracheobronchomalacia: evaluation and treatment. J Thoracic Dis 2017; 9(1): E57. [http://dx.doi.org/10.21037/jtd.2017.01.13] [PMID: 28203438]

Case 30

Photodynamic Therapy

Photodynamic Therapy for Endobronchial Carcinoma *in Situ* (CIS)

Kai Swenson[1], **Juan P. Uribe**[1] and **Adnan Majid**[1,*]

[1] *Section of Interventional Pulmonology, Division of Thoracic Surgery, Beth Israel Deaconess Medical Center, Harvard Medical School, Boston, MA, USA*

Keywords: Airway tumor, Carcinoma *in Situ*, Early lung cancer, Photodynamic therapy, Squamous cell carcinoma, Tracheal rumour.

Presentation

Bronchial squamous cell carcinoma *in situ* (CIS) diagnosed on surgical margins after left upper lobe (LUL) sleeve resection for squamous cell carcinoma.

Comorbidities

A 76-year-old woman, former smoker, history of LUL sleeve resection for stage IA squamous cell carcinoma.

Chest Imaging

Status post LUL sleeve resection.

Intervention

Bronchoscopy with white light revealed multiple endobronchial nodules and narrow band images showed evidence of neovascularization (dotted and tortuous vessels) in the distal left mainstem bronchus (Fig. **1**). Radial endobronchial ultrasound with balloon sheath revealed tumor which appeared confined to the epithelial layer without evidence of further tissue invasion to the cartilage (Fig. **2**) [1], and endobronchial biopsies and brushings of the lateral and medial wall demonstrated squamous cell carcinoma *in situ*. The patient received IV Photofrin 2mg/kg on day 1. This was followed on day 3 by a flexible bronchoscopy and photodynamic therapy light activation using a flexible 1.0cm quartz diffusing fiber and 200 Joules/ cm were delivered over 500 seconds (Fig. **3**).

*__Corresponding author Adnan Majid:__ Section of Interventional Pulmonology, Division of Thoracic Surgery, Beth Israel Deaconess Medical Center, Harvard Medical School, Boston, MA, USA; E-mail: amajid@bidmc.harvard.edu

Complications

None.

Post-Intervention

The patient underwent cleanout bronchoscopy *via* rigid bronchoscope on day 5 with mechanical debridement of the treated region (Fig. **4**) using a flexible forceps. Follow up bronchoscopy using white light and narrow band imaging at 6 weeks revealed no residual endobronchial nodularity, with endobronchial biopsies and brushings negative for malignancy.

Surveillance bronchoscopy was done at 3-month intervals during the first year, and then every 6 months until 5 years.

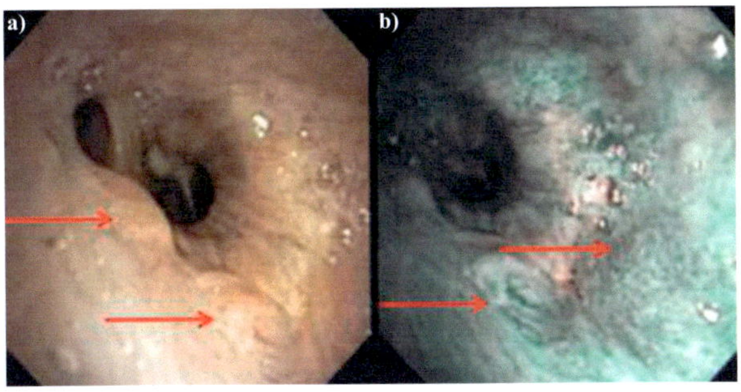

Fig. (1). Bronchoscopy with white light **(a)** & narrow band imaging **(b)** demonstrating endobronchial nodules (red arrows).

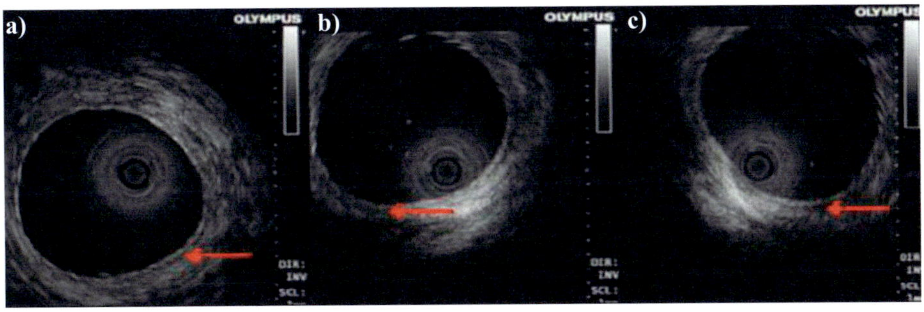

Fig. (2). (a, b and **c)** Radial probe endobronchial ultrasound (R-EBUS) demonstrating submucosal thickening with preservation of the cartilage (hypoechoic layer – red arrows), suggesting carcinoma *in situ*.

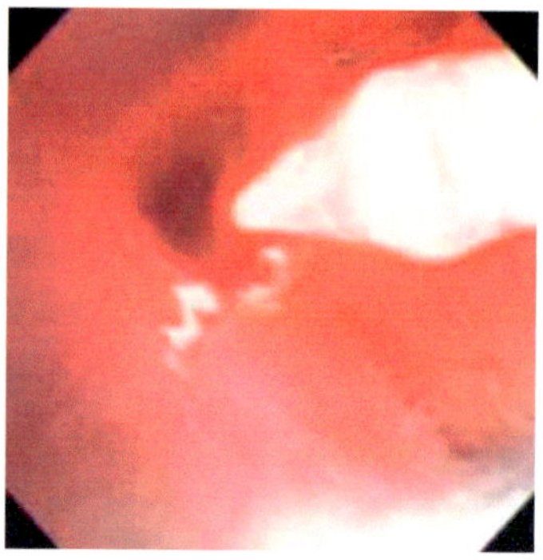

Fig. (3). Endobronchial photodynamic therapy using a flexible 1.0cm quartz diffusing fiber was placed adjacent to the nodules.

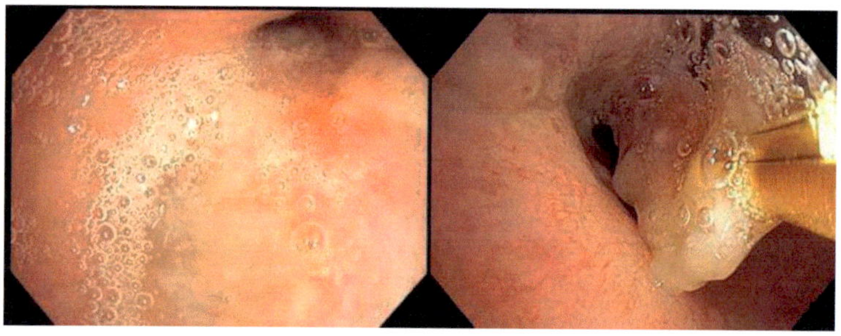

Fig. (4). Mechanical debridement of necrotic tumor was performed using a flexible forceps 48 hours after photodynamic therapy.

Learning Points

- Endobronchial photodynamic therapy can be curative as an adjunctive therapy for residual endobron chial malignancy in highly selected patients after surgical resection [2, 3].

CONSENT FOR PUBLICATION

Not applicable.

CONFLICT OF INTEREST

The author declares no conflict of interest, financial or otherwise.

ACKNOWLEDGEMENT

Declared none.

REFERENCES

[1] Miyazu Y, Miyazawa T, Kurimoto N, *et al.* Endobronchial ultrasonography in the assessment of centrally located early-stage lung cancer before photodynamic therapy. Am J Respir Crit Care Med. 2002; 165(6): 832-37.
[http://dx.doi.org/10.1164/ajrccm.165.6.2108092] [PMID: 11897652]

[2] Ernst A, Garland R, Beamis JF. Photodynamic treatment in lung cancer. J Bronchol 1996; 6: 285–8.
[http://dx.doi.org/10.1097/00128594-199910000-00013]

[3] Moghissi K, Dixon K, Andrew J, *et al.* Photodynamic therapy in early central lung cancer: a treatment option for patients ineligible for surgical resection. Thorax 2007; 62: 391–5.
[http://dx.doi.org/10.1136/thx.2006.061143] [PMID: 17090572]

Case 31

Photodynamic Therapy for Tracheal Adenoid Cystic Carcinoma

Kai Swenson[1], **Juan P. Uribe**[1] and **Adnan Majid**[1,*]

[1]*Section of Interventional Pulmonology, Division of Thoracic Surgery, Beth Israel Deaconess Medical Center, Harvard Medical School, Boston, MA, USA*

Keywords: Adenocystic carcinoma, Airway tumor, Airway obstruction, Photodynamic therapy, Tracheal tumor.

Presentation

A 37-year-old man, never smoker with progressive dyspnea, cough, stridor, dysphagia, and weight loss; spirometry flow loops demonstrating fixed obstruction with FEV1 34% predicted. Adenoid cystic carcinoma of the trachea status post prior bronchoscopic resection and external beam radiation therapy, with local recurrence.

Comorbidities

History of radiation-induced hypothyroidism.

Chest Imaging

Airway CT scan and PET/CT demonstrating hypermetabolic circumferential proximal tracheal lesion with luminal intrinsic compression (Fig. **1**).

Intervention

Initial flexible and rigid bronchoscopy revealed severe subglottic tracheal narrowing (Fig. **2a**) which was debrided with cryotherapy, balloon dilated and stented with a fully covered self-expanding metallic airway stent (14x30 mm Bonastent, Thoracent Inc) (Fig. **2b**). Endobronchial ultrasound guided needle aspiration revealed adenoid cystic carcinoma. Unfortunately, within 3 weeks, significant granulation tissue and tumor ingrowth had developed at the proximal end of the metallic stent (Figs. **2c** and **d**); therefore, a repeat rigid bronchoscopy

***Corresponding author Adnan Majid:** Section of Interventional Pulmonology, Division of Thoracic Surgery, Beth Israel Deaconess Medical Center, Harvard Medical School, Boston, MA, USA; E-mail: amajid@bidmc.harvard.edu

Jamalul Azizi Abdul Rahaman & Tinku Joseph (Eds.)

was performed with stent removal (Fig. **3a**), cryodebridement and percutaneous tracheostomy distal to the obstruction. Two weeks following this, IV Photofrin 2mg/ kg was administered on day 1 and photodynamic therapy light activation was applied on day 3. Using a 2cm rigid diffuser, a total of 200 Joules/cm were administered over 500 seconds. Since the lesion was 3.3cm in length, the treatment was divided into two, with 100 Joules/cm applied to the distal end of the lesion followed by 100 Joules/cm administered at the proximal end with a 7 mm overlap. The patient underwent two activation sessions (Fig. **3b**) and each was followed by mechanical debridement two days after (Figs. **3c** and **d**).

Complications

Granulation tissue formation at the site of metallic stent.

Post-Intervention

Two weeks following PDT therapy, a repeat rigid bronchoscopy was performed which demonstrated necrotic-appearing tissue at the site of prior PDT treatment (Fig. **4a**); cryodebridement was again performed and a Montgomery T-tube was placed [1]. Following this, the patient noted resolution of prior dyspnea, improved phonation, and improved swallowing ability and was able to gain weight. Immunotherapy was initiated. At three months post procedure, the Montgomery T tube was in place without compression by tumor or granulation tissue formation (Figs. **4b** and **d**).

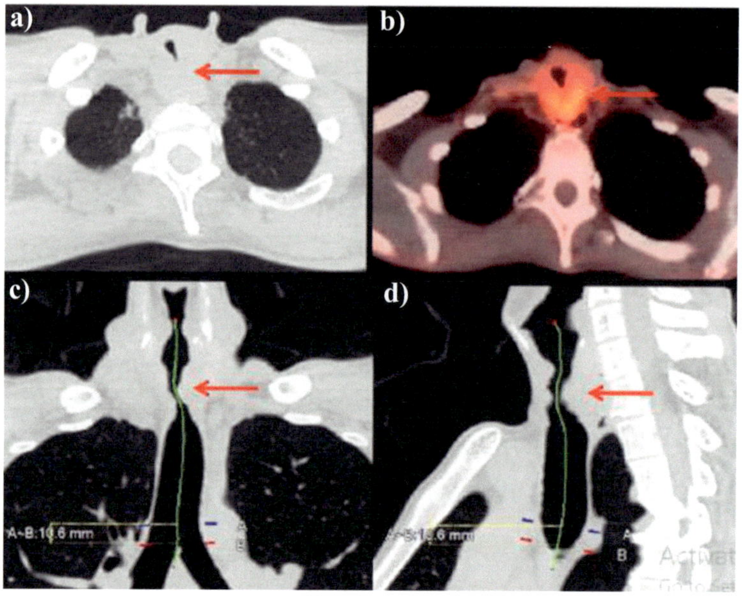

Fig. (1). Airway CT demonstrated a circumferential lesion in the proximal trachea with intrinsic compression of the tracheal lumen **(a, c** and **d)** and moderate FDG avidity on PET/CT **(b).**

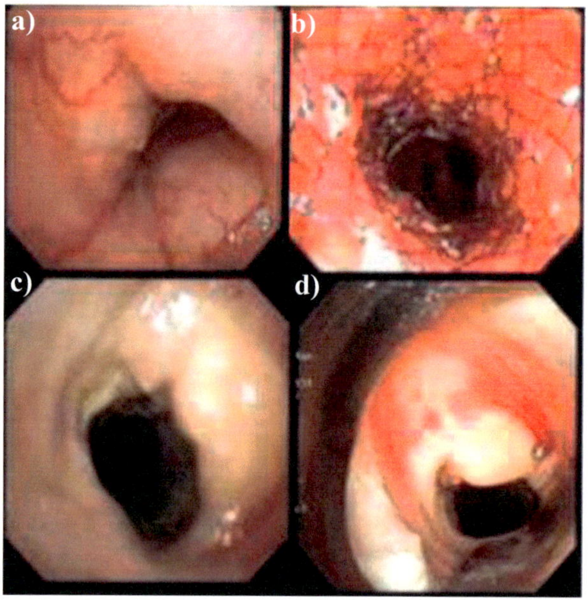

Fig. (2). Initial bronchoscopy revealed significant subglottic tracheal narrowing with intrinsic tumor involvement **(a),** status post debridement, balloon dilation and stenting **(b).** However, granulation tissue developed within 3 weeks at the proximal end of the stent with recurrent narrowing **(c** and **d).**

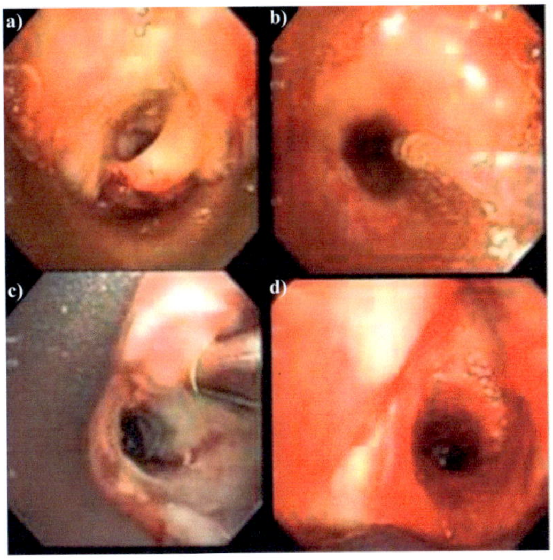

Fig. (3). Tumor and granulation tissue proximal to tracheal stent **(a).** Tracheal stent removal and debridement were performed, followed by 2 PDT activations separated by 48 hours **(b).** Two days after the second treatment, further mechanical debridement was performed to reveal a relatively preserved subglottic tracheal lumen **(c** and **d).**

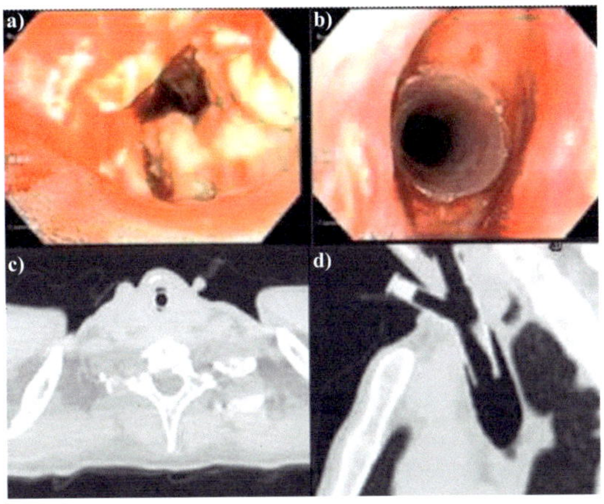

Fig. (4). Post-intervention results. Repeat bronchoscopy, 2 weeks after treatment demonstrated significant necrotic tissue proximal to the tracheal stoma **(a)** which was debrided and a custom designed Montgomery T-tube was placed. Follow up at 3 months showed patent airway **(b, c** and **d).**

Learning Points

- Photodynamic therapy can be an essential component of multimodal therapy to stabilize the airway in complex tracheal malignancy [2-4].

Video

Video of initial PDT treatment on Day 1 (0:06-0:43), clean out bronchoscopy with cryoablation and mechanical debridement on Day 3 followed by PDT reactivation (0:44-2:12), and repeat debridement on Day 5 (2:13-2:26), with tracheal patency maintained using Montgomery T tube placement (still images, 2:27-2:34).

CONSENT FOR PUBLICATION

Not applicable.

CONFLICT OF INTEREST

The author declares no conflict of interest, financial or otherwise.

ACKNOWLEDGEMENT

Declared none.

REFERENCES

[1] Cheng GZ, Folch E, Brik R, *et al.* Three-dimensional modeled T-tube design and insertion in a patient with tracheal dehiscence. Ches 2015; 148(4): e106-e108. [http://dx.doi.org/10.1378/chest.15-0240] [PMID: 26437816]

[2] Moghissi K, Dixon K, Andrew J, *et al.* Photodynamic therapy in early central lung cancer: a treatment option for patients ineligible for surgical resection. Thorax 2007; 62: 391–5. [http://dx.doi.org/10.1136/thx.2006.061143] [PMID: 17090572]

[3] Diaz-Jimenez JP, Martinez-Bellarin JE, Llunell A, *et al.* Efficacy and safety of photodynamic therapy versus Nd:YAG laser resection in NSCLC with airway obstruction. Eur Respir J 1999; 14: 800–5. [http://dx.doi.org/10.1034/j.1399-3003.1999.14d13.x] [PMID: 10573224]

[4] Santos RS, Raftopoulos Y, Keenan RJ, *et al.* Bronchoscopic palliation of primary lung cancer. Single or multimodality therapy? Surg Endoscopy 2004; 18: 931–6.

Case 32

Photodynamic Therapy for a Left Lower Lobe Bronchial Carcinoid Tumor

Kai Swenson[1], **Juan P. Uribe**[1] and **Adnan Majid**[1,*]

[1] *Section of Interventional Pulmonology, Division of Thoracic Surgery, Beth Israel Deaconess Medical Center, Harvard Medical School, Boston, MA, USA*

Keywords: Airway tumor, Airway obstruction, Bronchial carcinoid, Photodynamic therapy, Tracheal tumours.

Presentation

A left lower lobe (LLL) endobronchial lesion was incidentally noted on CT chest performed for evaluation of emphysema. Flexible bronchoscopy demonstrated an endobronchial lesion obstructing the LLL bronchus (Fig. **1a**); endobronchial biopsy was consistent with typical carcinoid with fewer than 2 mitoses per high power field. The patient was referred for consideration of endoscopic treatment.

Comorbidities

A 68-year-old man, former smoker, with a history of severe COPD (FEV1 45% predicted, DLCO 40% predicted).

Chest Imaging

CT chest demonstrated a 1.0cm LLL endobronchial lesion.

Intervention

Initially, the endobronchial component of the tumor was excised using a 2.4 mm cryoprobe (Fig. **1b**), with complete recanalization of the LLL bronchus (Fig. **1c**) This was followed by electrocautery to achieve hemostasis (Fig. **1d**). Follow up bronchoscopy at 6 weeks demonstrated a small LLL endobronchial lesion (Fig. **2a**) compatible for a small focus of residual carcinoid tumor, 0.2cm in the greatest dimension. Following IV Photofrin 2mg/kg, at day 3, a 1cm flexible diffuser was

*Corresponding author Adnan Majid: Section of Interventional Pulmonology, Division of Thoracic Surgery, Beth Israel Deaconess Medical Center, Harvard Medical School, Boston, MA, USA; E-mail: amajid@bidmc.harvard.edu

Jamalul Azizi Abdul Rahaman & Tinku Joseph (Eds.)

used for the activation (Fig. **2b**), followed by rigid bronchoscopy with cryodebridement on day 5.

Complications

None.

Post-Intervention

At 3 months follow up, there was no evidence of LLL bronchial obstruction, and flexible bronchoscopy with endobronchial biopsies and brushings of the LLL bronchus were negative for malignancy. Surveillance bronchoscopy was done at 3-month intervals during the first year and then every 6 months until 10 years.

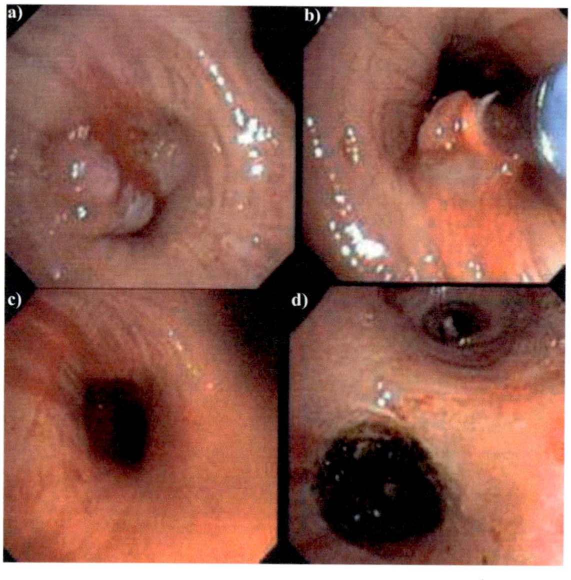

Fig. (1). Left lower lobe bronchus obstruct ed by endobronchial lesion **(a)** with pathology consistent with typical carcinoid; with cryodebridement **(b)**, the LLL was recanalized successfully **(c),** followed by electrocautery ablation to the region **(d).**

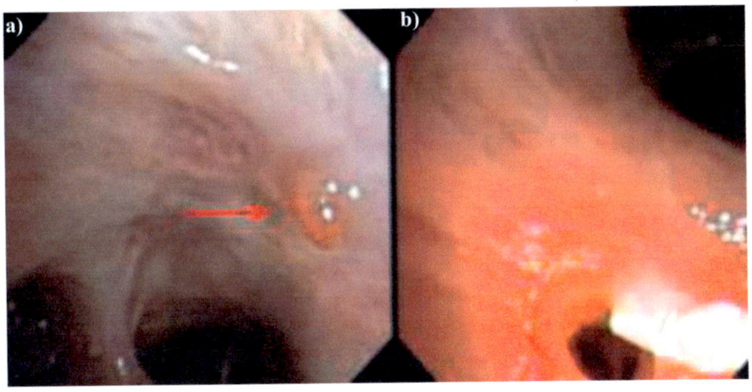

Fig. (2). Repeat bronchoscopy at 6 weeks after initial excision and ablation revealed a small endobronchial polypoid lesion **(a**, red arrow) with endobronchial biopsies consistent with small foci of residual typical carcinoid. Using a 1cm flexible diffuser, photodynamic therapy (200J - 500 seconds) was applied to the region of the proximal LLL bronchus **(b)** followed by debridement at 48 hours.

Learning Points

- Endobronchial photodynamic therapy with curative intent can be an option for treatment of typical endobronchial carcinoid tumors in highly selected patients who are not surgical candidates [1, 2].

CONSENT FOR PUBLICATION

Not applicable.

CONFLICT OF INTEREST

The author declares no conflict of interest, financial or otherwise.

ACKNOWLEDGEMENT

Declared none.

REFERENCES

[1] Sutedja TG, Schreurs AJ, Vanderschueren RG, *et al*. Bronchoscopic therapy in patients with intraluminal typical bronchial carcinoid. Chest 1995; 107(2): 556-58. [http://dx.doi.org/10.1378/chest.107.2.556] [PMID: 7842794]

[2] Moghissi K, Dixon K, Gibbins S. Photodynamic therapy for bronchial carcinoid tumours: complete response over a 10-year follow-up. Eur J Cardiothorac Surg 2013;43(6):1254-56. [http://dx.doi.org/10.1093/ejcts/ezs660] [PMID: 23284100]

Case 33

Microwave Ablation

Electromagnetic Navigation Bronchoscopy Cone-Beam CT Guided Lung Lesion Biopsy and Microwave Ablation

Joyce W.Y. Chan[1], **Rainbow W.H. Lau**[1] and **Calvin S.H. Ng**[1,*]

[1]*Department of Surgery, The Chinese University of Hong Kong, N.T., Hong Kong SAR*

Keywords: Ablation, Cone-Beam CT, Electromagnetic navigation bronchoscopy, Lung cancer, Microwave.

Presentation

An 83-year-old man with multiple comorbidities had a 1.5x0.5cm new suspicious lung lesion in the right lung apex.

Comorbidities

History of perforated sigmoid cancer with Hartmann's operation done, post-operatively complicated with sepsis, seizures and respiratory failure. Walked with quadstick slowly and declined any major surgery.

Chest Imaging

CT scan shows a right lung apical lesion (Fig. **1a**).

Intervention

Electromagnetic navigation bronchoscopy (ENB) biopsy of the lung lesion was performed in the hybrid operating room with cone-beam CT, and frozen section reported "adenocarcinoma". In the same operative session, ENB microwave ablation was performed by exchanging the localization tool with ablation catheter (Figs. **1b** and **c**).

*__Corresponding author Calvin S.H. Ng:__ Department of Surgery, The Chinese University of Hong Kong, N.T., Hong Kong SAR; E-mail: calvinng@surgery.cuhk.edu.hk

Jamalul Azizi Abdul Rahaman & Tinku Joseph (Eds.)

Complications

None.

Post-Intervention

The patient was discharged on post-operative day 2. At post-operative 1 month, 3 months and 1 year, follow up CT did not show local disease progression (Figs. **2** and **3**).

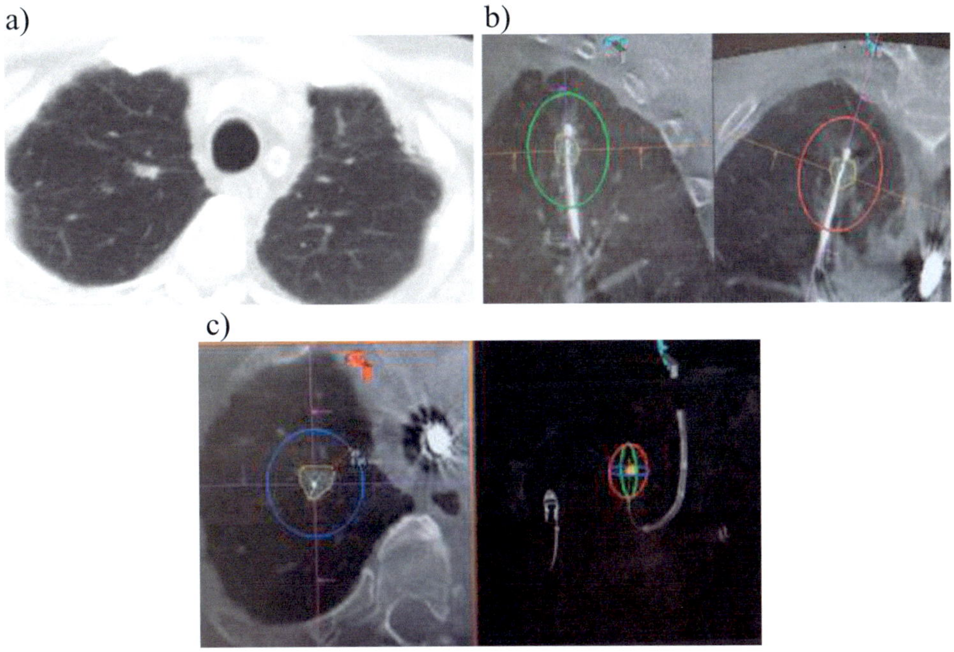

Fig. (1). (a) Shows the right upper lobe lung lesion with positive bronchus sign. **(b)** Shows the predicted ablation margin in 3 axes marked by green, red and blue circles. **(c)** The ablation catheter accurately punctures the target lesion, which is marked by yellow tracing.

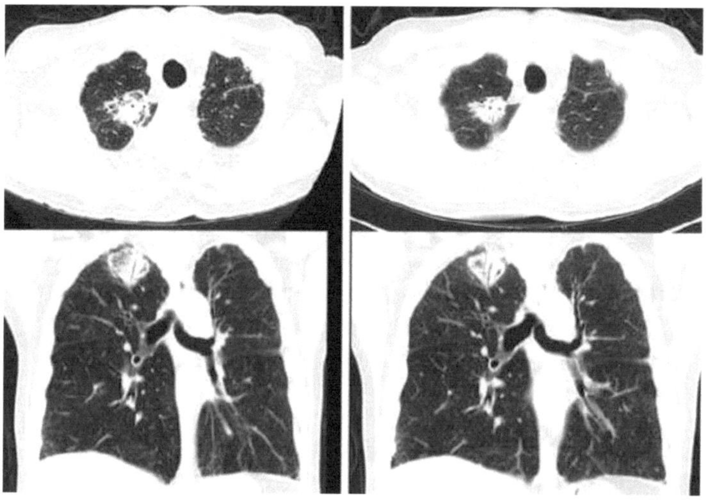

Fig. (2). Left side panels show the ablated region (represented by ground glass opacities with central air bronchogram) at 1 month post-ablation; while the right side panels show that at 3 months post-ablation, with contraction of ablated region.

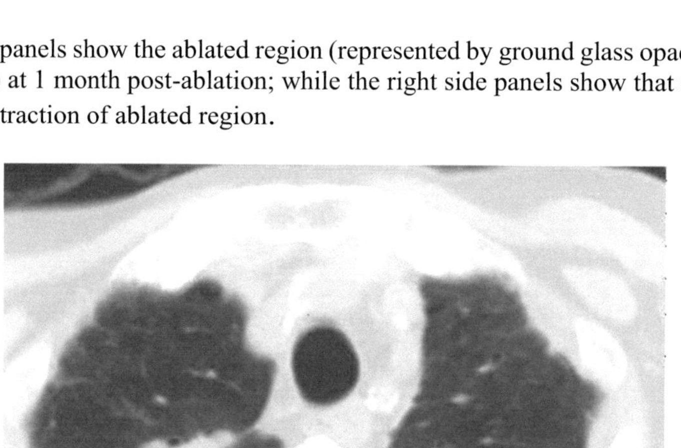

Fig. (3). The ablated region involutes after 1 year to become a scar-like soft tissue density.

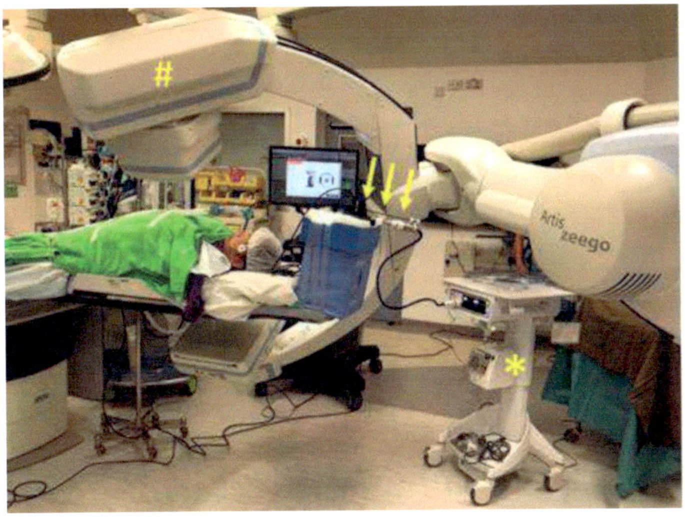

Fig. (4). Set up of ENB microwave ablation in the hybrid operating room is shown. Patient lies supine and the ENB bronchoscope enters airways *via* the endotracheal tube. Cone-beam CT (#) confirms accurate placement of instruments within target lung lesion. The microwave ablation catheter (arrows) is positioned within target lung lesion *via* ENB and connected to the microwave control console (*) externally.

Learning Points

- ENB in the hybrid operating room (Fig. **4**) is able to provide one-stop diagnosis and local treatment of lung malignancies, especially for patients who are not surgical candidates [1-4]. ENB microwave ablation is a novel technique with promising medium-term local control rates [5-8].

CONSENT FOR PUBLICATION

Not applicable.

CONFLICT OF INTEREST

The author declares no conflict of interest, financial or otherwise.

ACKNOWLEDGEMENT

Declared none.

REFERENCES

[1] Ng CSH, Zhao ZR, Lau RWH. Tailored Therapy for Stage I Non-small Cell Lung Cancer. J Clin Oncol 2017; 35(3): 268-70. [http://dx.doi.org/10.1200/JCO.2016.70.4718] [PMID: 27937087]

[2] Zhao ZR, Lau RW, Ng CS. Catheter-based alternative treatment for early-stage lung cancer with a high-risk for morbidity. J Thorac Dis 2018; 10(Suppl 16): S1864-70. [http://dx.doi.org/10.21037/jtd.2018.03.151] [PMID: 30026973]

[3] Chan JW, Yu PS, Lau RW, Ng CS. Hybrid Operating Room – One stop for Diagnosis, Staging and Treatment of Early Stage NSCLC. J Thorac Dis 2020; 12(2): 123-31. [http://dx.doi.org/10.21037/jtd.2019.08.36] [PMID: 32190362]

[4] Chan JWY, Lau RWH, Ng CSH. Image-Guided Ablative Therapies for Lung Tumors. In Park HS, ed. Lung Cancer - Modern Multidisciplinary Management. IntechOpen 2020. [http://dx.doi.org/10.5772/intechopen.94216]

[5] Chan JWY, Lau RWH, Ngai JCL, *et al.* Transbronchial microwave ablation of lung nodules with electromagnetic navigation bronchoscopy guidance – a novel technique and initial experience with 30 cases. Transl Lung Cancer Res 2021; 10(4): 1608-22. [http://dx.doi.org/10.21037/tlcr-20-1231]

[6] Chan JWY, Lau RW, Ng CS. 64MO Early experience of bronchoscopic transbronchial microwave ablation of lung nodules in the hybrid operating room. J Thorac Oncol 2021; 16(4), S730. [https://doi.org/10.1016/S1556-0864(21)01906-7]

[7] Chan JWY, Lau RWH, Ng CSH. Transbronchial Microwave Ablation of Malignant Lung Nodules – Outcomes, Challenges and Perspective. IASLC Lung Cancer News (ILCN) 2021 Aug. https://www.iaslc.org/iaslc-news/ilcn/transbronchial-microwave-ablation-malignant-lung-nodules-outcomes-challenges-and

[8] Ng CSH. Exploring a novel approach to lung cancer treatment. www.researchoutreach. org. https://researchoutreach.org/articles/exploring-novel-approach-lung-cancer-treatment / [http://dx.doi.org/10.32907/RO-125-1640818600]

Case 34

Bronchoscopic Microwave Ablations for Patients with Multiple Lung Nodules and Previous Lobectomy

Joyce W.Y. Chan[1], **Rainbow W.H. Lau**[1] and **Calvin S.H. Ng**[1,*]

[1]*Department of Surgery, The Chinese University of Hong Kong, N.T., Hong Kong SAR*

Keywords: Ablation, Cone-Beam CT, Electromagnetic navigation bronchoscopy, Lung cancer, Microwave.

Presentation

A 57-year-old lady had stage IB lung adenocarcinoma in the left upper lobe with lobectomy in 2013. Subsequent CT scan in 2019 showed new and enlarging left lower lobe (LLL) apical segment nodule (13mm) and right lower lobe (RLL) ground glass opacity (27mm). CT-guided biopsy of both lesions yielded adenocarcinoma with EGFR mutation (deletion of exon 19). There were no distant metastases on PET/CT scan. The patient will not be able to tolerate further LLL and RLL lung resections due to inadequate lung function.

Comorbidities

History of dyspepsia.

Chest Imaging

CT scan shows LLL and RLL nodules.

Intervention

Bronchoscopic microwave ablations of the two lung lesions were performed in two separate sessions in March and April 2019, under electromagnetic navigation bronchoscopy (ENB) guidance in the hybrid operating room (Fig. **1**) [1, 2].

*__Corresponding author Calvin S.H. Ng:__ Department of Surgery, The Chinese University of Hong Kong, N.T., Hong Kong SAR; E-mail: calvinng@surgery.cuhk.edu.hk

Complications

None.

Post-Intervention

At 1.5 years follow up, CT showed complete response of the LLL lung cancer (pure cyst with thin wall) (Fig. **2**) and partial response of the RLL lung cancer (smaller area of consolidated/collapsed lung) (Fig. **3**).

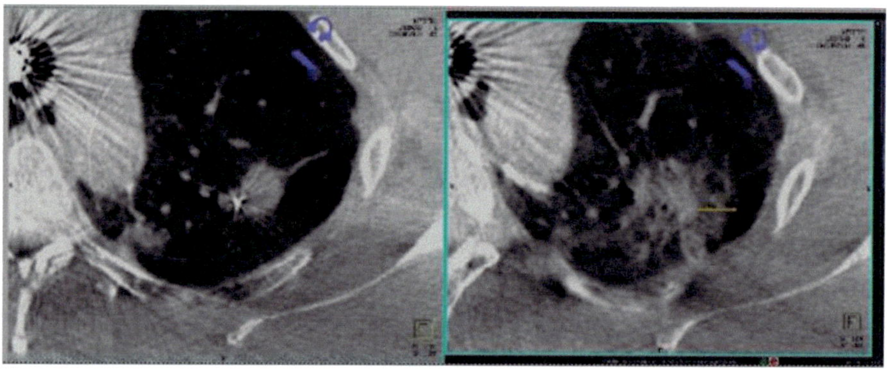

Fig. (1). Comparison of pre- (left) and post-ablation (right) intra-operative cone-beam CT of left lower lobe lesion is shown. The radiopaque bright spot (left) represents the ablation catheter. The ablated region (right) is represented by concentric ground-glass opacity, which covers the target lesion completely.

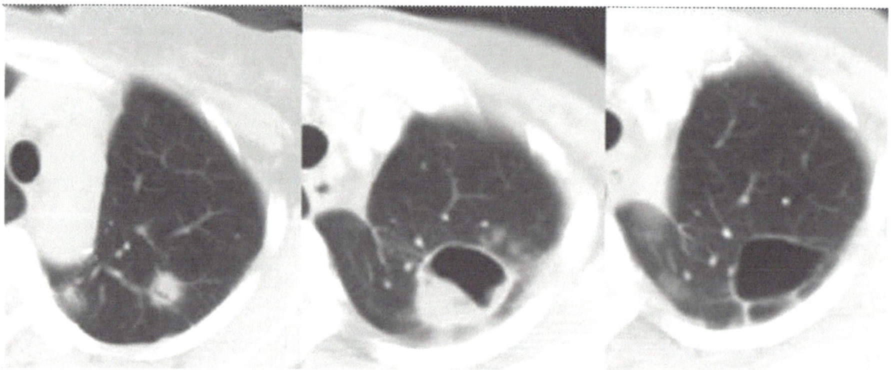

Fig. (2). CT scans showing the left lower lobe lung lesion pre-operatively (left), 1 month post-ablation with large cavity and internal soft tissue (middle), and 1.5 years post-ablation with simple pneumatocele, signifying complete response (right).

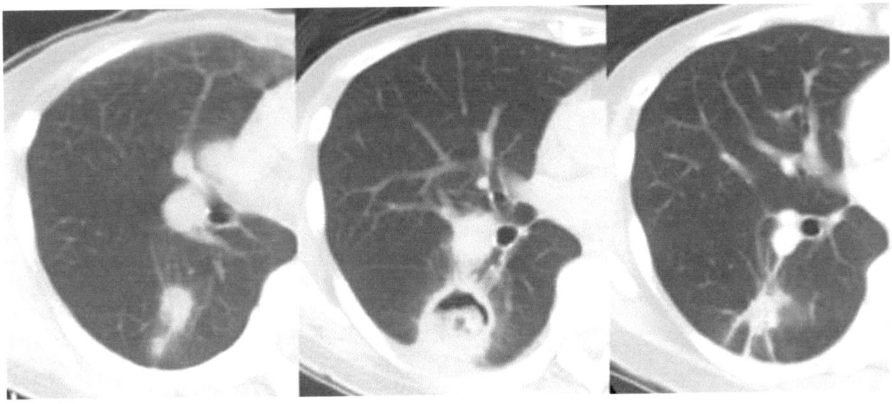

Fig. (3). CT scans showing the right lower lobe lesion pre-operatively (left), 1month post-ablation with thick- walled cavity and internal soft tissue (middle), and 1.5-years post-ablation with a shrunken soft tissue density scar (right).

Learning Points

- ENB guided microwave ablation is an invaluable lung-preserving treatment modality for patients with multi-focal disease and/or previous major lung resection [3-8]. Long term follow-up with CT is required to ensure no local recurrence.

CONSENT FOR PUBLICATION

Not applicable.

CONFLICT OF INTEREST

The author declares no conflict of interest, financial or otherwise.

ACKNOWLEDGEMENT

Declared none.

REFERENCES

[1] Ng CSH, Zhao ZR, Lau RWH. Tailored Therapy for Stage I Non-small Cell Lung Cancer. J Clin Oncol 2017; 35(3): 268-70.
[http://dx.doi.org/10.1200/JCO.2016.70.4718] [PMID: 27937087]

[2] Zhao ZR, Lau RW, Ng CS. Catheter-based alternative treatment for early-stage lung cancer with a high-risk for morbidity. J Thorac Dis 2018; 10(Suppl 16): S1864-70.
[http://dx.doi.org/10.21037/jtd.2018.03.151 PMID: 30026973]

[3] Yu PSY, Chu CM, Lau RWH, Ng CSH. Hybrid theatre facilitates lung-preserving multimodal treatment for multiple pulmonary metastases. Ann Thorac Surg 2021; 111(2): e89-92. [http://dx.doi.org/10.1016/j.athoracsur.2020.05.098]
[4] Chan JWY, Lau RWH, Ng CSH. Image-Guided Ablative Therapies for Lung Tumors. In Park HS, Ed. Lung Cancer - Modern Multidisciplinary Management. IntechOpen 2020. Available from: [http://dx.doi.org/10.5772/intechopen.94216]
[5] Chan JWY, Lau RWH, Ngai JCL, *et al.* Transbronchial microwave ablation of lung nodules with electromagnetic navigation bronchoscopy guidance – a novel technique and initial experience with 30 cases. Transl Lung Cancer Res 2021; 10(4): 1608-22. [http://dx.doi.org/10.21037/tlcr-20-1231]
[6] Chan JWY, Lau RW, Ng CS. Early experience of bronchoscopic transbronchial microwave ablation of lung nodules in the hybrid operating room. J Thorac Oncol 2021; 16(4), S730, 64MO. [https://doi.org/10.1016// S1556-0864(21)01906-7]
[7] Chan JWY, Lau RWH, Ng CSH. Transbronchial Microwave Ablation of Malignant Lung Nodules – Outcomes, Challenges and Perspective. IASLC Lung Cancer News (ILCN), 2021. Aug. https://www.iaslc.org/iaslc-news/ilcn/transbronchial-microwave-ablation-malignant-lung-nodules-outcomes-challenges-and
[8] Ng CSH. Exploring a novel approach to lung cancer treatment. Res Outreach 2021; 125. www.researchoutreach.org. https://researchoutreach.org/articles/exploring-novel-approach-lung-cancer-treatment [https://doi.org/10.32907/RO-125-1640818600]

Case 35

Bronchial Thermoplasty

Sustained Effect Beyond 5 Years with Good Asthma Control in Pregnancy

Nai-Chien Huan[1], **Mona Zaria Nasaruddin**[1] and **Jamalul Azizi Abdul Rahaman**[1,*]

[1] *Department of Pulmonology, Serdang Hospital, Selangor, Malaysia*

Keywords: Asthma in pregnancy, Bronchoscopy, Bronchial thermoplasty, Non-pharmacological, Severe asthma, Thermal energy.

Presentation

In 2013, a 24-year-old lady with a background history of severe asthma (diagnosed at the age of 14; had 4 intubations in the past 2 years for severe exacerbations of asthma). Her asthma was difficult to control despite on various inhalers (high dose inhaled corticosteroids, long-acting muscarinic antagonist, long-acting beta2 agonist), oral corticosteroids, theophylline and montelukast.

Comorbidities

None.

Chest Imaging

CXR was normal.

Spirometry showed FEV1 1.97L (86% predicted), FVC 1.99L (83% predicted), FEV1/FVC ratio 99%.

Intervention

She underwent three bronchial thermoplasty (BT) sessions (Alair™ Bronchial Thermoplasty System, Boston Scientific, Marlborough, USA). The first session involved a total of 55 activations in the right lower lobe. 3 weeks later, she had the second BT session which delivered 49 activations in the left lower lobe. A month

*Corresponding author Jamalul Azizi Abdul Rahaman: Department of Pulmonology, Serdang Hospital, Selangor, Malaysia; E-mail: jamalulazizi@gmail.com

later, a third BT session delivered 64 activations in both upper lobes. All the three BT sessions were conducted under general anaesthesia *via* an 8.5mm endotracheal tube.

Complications

All three sessions were uneventful. She did not experience exacerbations immediately after BT.

Post-Intervention

Her asthma symptoms continued to persist immediately post-BT. However, 3 months post-BT, she started to show improvements in her asthma control. She had only one admission post-BT in 2015 during the South East Asian haze but was not intubated. She gave birth to a pair of twins in 2016 and managed to further her post-graduate studies as a nurse focusing on child health in 2019. She managed to be taken off oral corticosteroids and enjoyed reduction in dosages of her inhaled corticosteroids. She remained well 7 years post-BT.

Learning Points

- BT is a non-pharmacological treatment of patients with severe asthma by delivering thermal energy into the airways *via* flexible bronchoscopy. The efficacy of BT in severe asthma has been demonstrated in the Asthma Intervention Research 2 (AIR 2) trial. The AIR2 extension study supports the sustained effect of BT in reducing severe exacerbations and emergency room visits out to 5 years [1].

Video

Bronchial thermoplasty procedure at Serdang Hospital, Selangor, Malaysia.

CONSENT FOR PUBLICATION

Not applicable.

CONFLICT OF INTEREST

The author declares no conflict of interest, financial or otherwise.

ACKNOWLEDGEMENT

Declared none.

REFERENCE

[1] Wechsler ME, Laviolette M, Rubin AS, *et al.* Bronchial thermoplasty: Long-term safety and effectiveness in patients with severe persistent asthma. J Allergy Clin Immunol 2013; 132(6): 1295-302.
[http://dx.doi.org/10.1016/j.jaci.2013.08.009] [PMID: 23998657] [PMCID: PMC4114404]

Case 36

Going Strong 6 Years Post-Bronchial Thermoplasty after Failure of Live Fish Treatment

Nai-Chien Huan[1], **Mona Zaria Nasaruddin**[1] and **Jamalul Azizi Abdul Rahaman**[1,*]

[1] *Department of Pulmonology, Serdang Hospital, Selangor, Malaysia*

Keywords: Bronchoscopy, Bronchial thermoplasty, Non-pharmacological, Severe asthma, Thermal energy.

Presentation

A 56-year-old gentleman presented to our centre in 2014. He has a background history of brittle asthma since the age of 43 with multiple exacerbations necessitating hospitalization, including one admission to the intensive care unit in 2013 where he was intubated for respiratory failure. In 2012, he went to Hyderabad, India in an attempt to seek a cure for his asthma where he swallowed live fish but there was no improvement. His asthma remained uncontrolled despite on optimum medical therapy.

Comorbidities

None.

Chest Imaging

CXR was normal.

Spirometry is consistent with obstructive ventila tory defect with FEV1 1.28L (50% predicted), FVC 2.41L (88% predicted), FEV1/FVC ratio of 53%.

Intervention

Three BT sessions (Alair™ Bronchial Thermoplasty System, Boston Scientific, Marlborough, USA). The first session involved a total of 58 activations in the right

*Corresponding author Jamalul Azizi Abdul Rahaman: Department of Pulmonology, Serdang Hospital, Selangor, Malaysia; E-mail: jamalulazizi@gmail.com

Jamalul Azizi Abdul Rahaman & Tinku Joseph (Eds.)

lower lobe, followed by 46 activations in the left lower lobe a month later and finally 64 activations in both upper lobes a month after the second session. All sessions were conducted under general anaesthesia *via* an 8.0mm endotracheal tube.

Complications

All three sessions were uneventful. He did not experience exacerbations post-BT.

Post-Intervention

The patient reported dramatic improvements in asthma control post-BT. He no longer had emer gency room visits or admissions. He has remained active and is able to exercise and walk as far as 5km, 3 times per week without feeling short of breath. He remained well 6 years post-BT.

Learning Points

- The patients demonstrated sustained benefits of BT beyond 5 years. These results were in line with the AIR2 extension study, where reductions in exacerbation rates and emergency department visits were maintained out to at least 5 years post-BT in patients with severe asthma [1]. Further studies will provide more clues in identifying potential clinical predictors of BT response among patients with severe asthma. BT can safely be performed in patients with reduced lung function [2].

Video

BT catheter delivering 4 activations in the LB8 subsegment.

CONSENT FOR PUBLICATION

Not applicable.

CONFLICT OF INTEREST

The author declares no conflict of interest, financial or otherwise.

ACKNOWLEDGEMENT

Declared none.

REFERENCES

[1] Wechsler ME, Laviolette M, Rubin AS, *et al.* Asthma Intervention Research 2 Trial Study Group. Bronchial thermoplasty: Long-term safety and effectiveness in patients with severe persistent asthma. J Allergy Clin Immunol 2013; 132(6): 1295-302. [http://dx.doi.org/10.1016/j.jaci.2013.08.009] [PMID: 23998657]

[2] Langton D, Ing A, Fielding D, Hersch N, *et al.* Safety and Effectiveness of Bronchial Thermoplasty When FEV1 Is Less Than 50. Chest 2020; 157(3): 509-15. [http://dx.doi.org/10.1016/j.chest.2019.08.2193] [PMID: 31525358]

Case 37

The Bronchial Thermoplasty Revolution in the Treatment of Severe Asthma

Anantham Devanand[1,*] and **Tay Chee Kiang Melvin**[1]

[1] *Sing Health Duke-NUS Lung Centre, Singapore*

Keywords: Bronchial Thermoplasty, Catheter-based therapy, Radiofrequency energy, Severe asthma, Smooth muscle ablation.

Presentation

Our patient was a 57-year-old Chinese male, non-smoker with a long standing history of asthma and recurrent admissions for asthma exacerbations. He had a family history of atopy and multiple drug allergies. Diagnosis of asthma was made on the basis of clinical history and positive bronchoprovocation testing. Triggers for asthma exacerbations include viral upper respiratory tract infections, smoke and perfume fragrances. Asthma medications at the time of referral included high dose inhaled steroids with long-acting bronchodilator combination therapy (Salmeterol/Fluticasone), Montelukast and Tiotropium. Asthma control test score was 9/25 and peak flow reading was 450 litres/minute.

Comorbidities

The patient's co-morbid conditions included allergic rhinitis, nasal polyposis, recurrent sinusitis, gastro-esophageal reflux disease. The patient was also being treated with intranasal steroids and proton-pump inhibitors.

Chest Imaging

CXR was normal. CT thorax reported no evidence of bronchiectasis. There was mild, but diffuse bronchial wall thickening in both lower lobes that was attributed to be due to inflammation with a suggestion of mucus plugging in several areas.

Spirometry showed a FEV1 of 97% predicted with mild obstructive physiology and a positive methacholine bronchoprovocation test (Figs. **1** and **2**). Blood eosinophil counts were 150 cells/µL. Aspergillus specific IgE was not detected. Anti-

*Corresponding author Anantham Devanand: Sing Health Duke-NUS Lung Centre, Singapore; E-mail: anantham.devanand@singhealth.com.sg

Jamalul Azizi Abdul Rahaman & Tinku Joseph (Eds.)

neutrophilcytoplasmic antibodies (ANCA) testing was negative for eosinophilic granulomatosis with polyangiitis.

Intervention

Bronchial Thermoplasty (BT).

Session 1

BT was performed *via* an endotracheal tube size 8.5 under general anaesthesia using an intravenous in fusion of propofol. The airways were normal on airway inspection. Catheter was introduced *via* the working channel of the bronchoscope and advanced until the distal end was seen. Then the catheter was expanded until the 4 electrodes were in contact with the airway wall.

After each activation, the electrodes were collapsed and repositioned proximally such that it was moved 1 black line marking at a time. Each activation took 10 seconds. 60 activations were delivered to the right lower lobe.

Session 2

BT was performed 3 weeks later *via* endotracheal tube size 8.5 under general anaesthesia with 79 activations to the left lower lobe.

Session 3

BT was performed 3 weeks later *via* endotracheal tube size 8.5 under general anaesthesia. On inspection, the left lower lobe was plugged with copious white secretions. Airway toilet was done prior to procedure by suctioning and 54 activations were delivered to the right upper lobe. The thermoplasty catheter was kinked by angulation into apical segment of the right upper lobe and needed replacement. Subsequently, 49 activations were delivered to the left upper lobe and lingular segments.

All procedures were performed with a diagnostic flexible bronchoscope (4.9mm outer diameter) that has a 2.0mm working channel.

Complications

During the second session, endoscopically visible bronchospasm was detected during the procedure. There was no pulse oximetry desaturation and the bronchospasm was aborted with 1ml of topical adrenaline at 1: 10 000 dilution. The thermoplasty procedure continued uneventfully after aborting the bronchospasm.

Post-Intervention

The patient was continued on oral prednisolone and weaned off supplemental oxygen in the recovery area. He was discharged with the contact number of our asthma nurse coordinator in case of emergencies and was reviewed in the outpatient clinic on Day 7 before being scheduled for his subsequent procedure. Asthma was re-evaluated in the 3 months after the last of the three thermoplasty procedures. Asthma control test was 21/25 and peak flow was 450 litres/minute. His Tiotropium was discontinued, but he was kept on the Salmeterol/Fluticasone inhaler.

FEVI (L)	**3.10**	**2.19**	**3.01**	**97**
FVC (L)	**4.22**	**3.00**	**4.53**	**107**
FEVI/FVC (%)	**80**	**72**	**66**	**83**
FEF Max (L/sec)	**8.36**		**7.90**	**95**

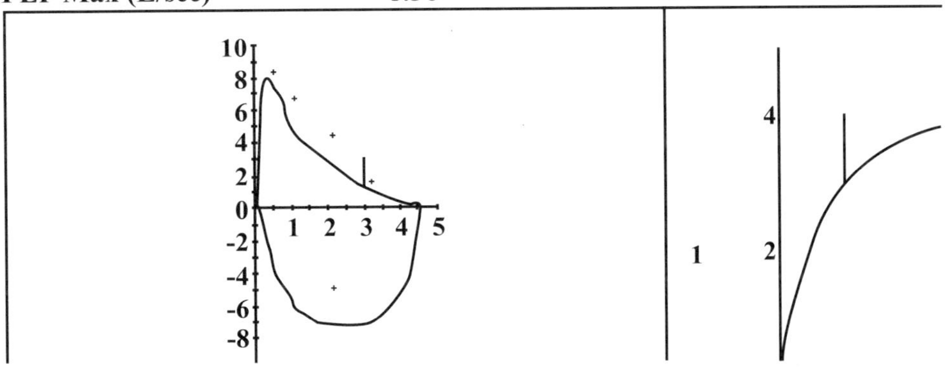

Fig. (1). Spirometry showing mild obstructive physiology.

	FEV1	FVC
Baseline value	3.01 2.99 2.95	4.56 4.55 4.53
Low dose (5mg/ml) 1 puff	2.61 2.61 2.55	4.39 4.34 4.32
4 puffs	2.18 2.17 2.10	4.03 4.01 3.87
Regular dose (25mg/ml) 1 puff		
4 puffs		
After bronchodilator	2.99 2.94 2.89	4.64 4.61 4.60
Max fall% of baseline	27.57%	11.62%

Fig. (2). Methacholine bronchoprovocation testing showing bronchial hyper-responsiveness.

Learning Points

- Bronchial Thermoplasty delivers radiofrequency energy to endoscopically visible airways to ablate smooth muscle. This is a therapeutic option for patients with poorly controlled asthma despite optimum medical therapy.
- Prior to considering BT, ensure that inhaler technique and compliance are checked, the diagnosis of asthma is confirmed, allergen exposure is minimized, and co-morbid conditions are controlled. These issues should be addressed before resorting to any interventional procedures. Alternative diagnoses such as eosinophilic granulomatosis with polyangiitis and allergic bronchopulmonary aspergillosis should also be excluded.
- When consent is taken, patients should have realistic expectations that the response to BT may take several weeks and that they will have to continue to take inhaled steroids after the procedure. There is unlikely to be any improvement in pulmonary function testing. The expected benefits from BT are improved symptom control and reduced exacerbations that require hospitalization.
- BT consists of 3 procedures performed 3 weeks apart. Typically, the right lower lobe istreated in the first session followed by the left lower lobe in the next and finally both upper lobes in the final session. The right middle lobe is

traditionally excluded from treatment to avoid the risk of right middle lobe syndrome [1].

- Exacerbation of asthma is a common complication of BT. Patients are pre-treated with oral prednisolone 50mg/day starting three days before the procedure and ending one day after (Total duration 5 days). Prior to the procedure, ensure that the patient has not had a recent exacerbation or upper respiratory tract infection. If so, postpone the procedure. Some centres perform peak flow or spirometry on the day of the procedure to ensure that the patient is at baseline lung function before proceeding.
- Prior to activation of the BT catheter, the airways should be endoscopically inspected for bronchomalacia and if present, that segment of the airway should be excluded from treatment. Mucus should also be suctioned out prior to activation.
- The airway should be anesthetized to minimize coughing and the endoscopist may need to 'surf' with respiratory movements to maintain the position of the catheter. Do not extend the Thermoplasty catheter beyond what is endoscopically visible and ensure that both sides of each sub-carina are treated.
- Keeping track of activations, a thorough understanding of airway anatomy is critical. It is helpful to have a systematic approach and a dedicated assistant to record activations. False activations can occur if there is inadequate contact between the catheter probe and the airway wall. This is why it is necessary to keep the catheter clean of debris and mucus. An audible error sequence sound from the device will alert the endoscopist of any false activation. Intraprocedural complications include bronchospasm (as seen in our patient) and bleeding.
- Besides asthma exacerbations, mucous impaction and atelectasis can occur post procedure. Most problems arise within 24 – 48 hours and resolve in 7 days. For this reason, there should be a low threshold to admit patients post procedure for observation. Patients need re-assessment in the outpatient clinic before listing for the next BT procedure.

Video

Bronchial thermoplasty of the left upper lobe anterior segment. The airway is inspected for bronchomalacia and cleared of secretions before the catheter is advanced until the distal end is barely visible. Then the catheter is expanded until the 4 electrodes are in contact with the airway wall. After each activation, the electrodes are collapsed and repositioned proximally such that the catheter is moved 1 black line marking at a time.

CONSENT FOR PUBLICATION

Not applicable.

CONFLICT OF INTEREST

The author declares no conflict of interest, financial or otherwise.

ACKNOWLEDGEMENT

Declared none.

REFERENCE

[1] Tan LD, Yoneda KY, Louie S, Hogarth DK, Castro M. Bronchial Thermoplasty: A Decade of Experience: State of the Art. J Allergy Clin Immunol Pract 2019; 7(1): 71-80. [http://dx.doi.org/10.1016/j.jaip.2018.08.017] [PMID: 30193939]

Case 38

Bronchoscopic Lung Volume Reduction (BLVR)

Bronchoscopic Lung Volume Reduction for Lower Lobe Emphysaema

Mohd Faizul Abu Samah[1] and **Jamalul Azizi Abdul Rahaman**[1,*]

[1] *Department of Pulmonology, Serdang Hospital, Selangor, Malaysia*

Keywords: Bronchoscopic lung volume reduction (BLVR), Endobronchial valve, Emphysema, Pneumothorax, Lower lobe.

Presentation

A 75-year-old gentleman with COPD (GOLD Class D), was referred for worsening dyspnea on minimal exertion despite on maximum medical therapy. His modified Medical Reseach Council (mMRC) Dyspnoea Scale was 3. His full lung function test showed severe obstructive ventilatory defect, hyperinflation and air trapping with reduced DLCO consistent with emphysema: FEVI 10.81L (41% predicted), FVC 2.69L (92% predicted), FEV1/FVC 30%, TLC 9.21L (215% predicted), VC 2.69L (92% predicted), RV 6.53L (349% predicted), RV/TLC 71%, DLCO 49% predicted.

Comorbidities

Ischaemic heart disease, Type 2 diabetes mellitus, hypertension, allergic rhinitis, benign prostatic hyper plasia. Ex-smoker of 13 pack years.

Chest Imaging

CXR showed bilateral hyperinflated lungs (Fig. **1**).

HRCT thorax showed predominantly paraseptal emphysaema in bilateral upper lobes and panlobular emphysema in lower lobes (Fig. **2**). The most emphysematous area was the left lower lobe. All fissures were intact.

[*]**Corresponding author Jamalul Azizi Abdul Rahaman:** Department of Pulmonology, Serdang Hospital, Selangor, Malaysia; E-mail: jamalulazizi@gmail.com

Jamalul Azizi Abdul Rahaman & Tinku Joseph (Eds.)

Intervention

Zephyr EBV (endobronchial valve) treatment of the left lower lobe was performed in August 2019 under general anaesthesia after Chartis® measurement to exclude collateral ventilation. Zephyr EBVs were deployed at LB8, LB9, LB10 and LB6. The entire procedure took 36 minutes.

Complications

Left-sided pneumothorax 4 hours post-procedure requiring tube thoracostomy (Fig. **3**).

Post-Intervention

Pneumothorax resolved after 5 days on chest tube and CXR showed left lower lobe collapse (Fig. **4**). Patient was discharged well.

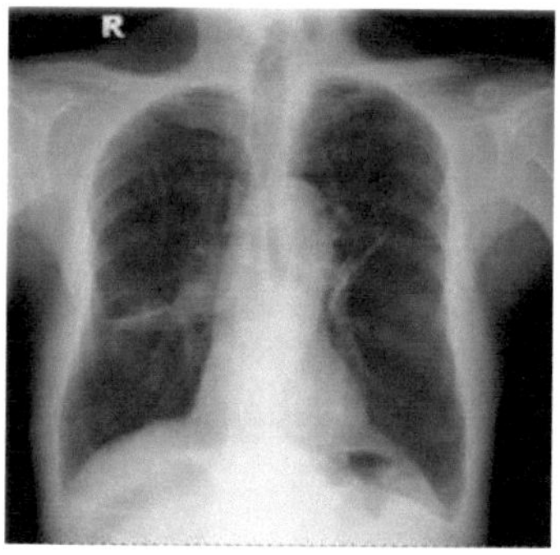

Fig. (1). CXR pre-procedure showed bilateral hyperinflated lungs.

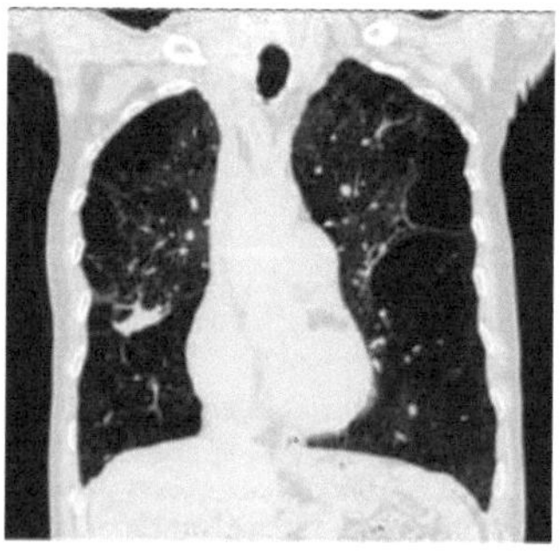

Fig. (2). Coronal HRCT Thorax showed predominantly paraseptal emphysaema in both upper lobes and panlobular emphysaema in lower lobes.

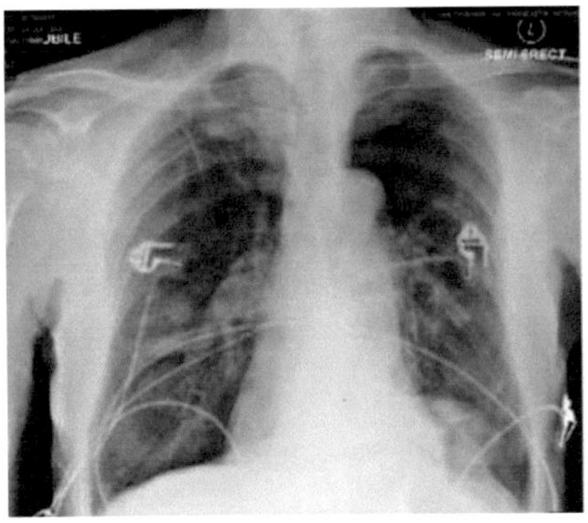

Fig. (3). CXR 4 hours post-procedure shows left-sided pneumothorax.

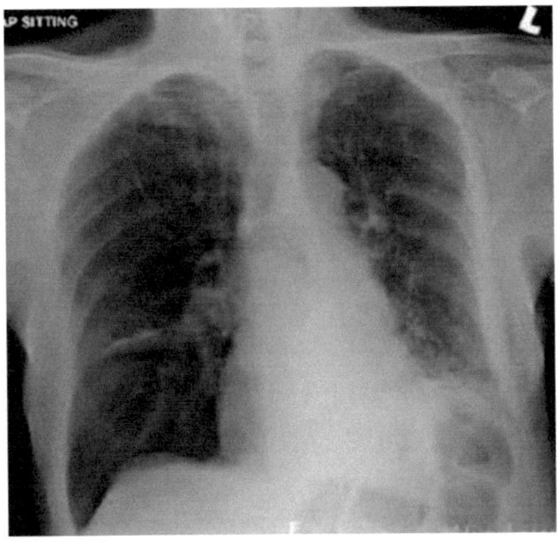

Fig. (4). CXR 5 days post-procedure showed left lower lobe collapse and resolution of pneumothorax.

Learning Points

- Current medical treatment is suboptimal for advanced emphysema. Bronchoscopic lung volume reduction (BLVR) has been shown to improve physiologic function, QOL and functional capacity in selected emphysema patients [1]. The primary complication of BLVR with EBV is pneumothorax with a reported incidence of 20 to 31 percent [2]. Potential patients should be referred to an experienced center for consideration of BLVR with EBV. Unlike lung volume reduction surgery (LVRS) which is only suitable for upper lobe predominant emphysaema, EBV can be offered to patients with lower lobe emphysaema.

Video

Balloon of the Chartis® catheter to assess for collateral ventilation and the subsequent deployment of Zephyr EBVs in the left lower lobe.

CONSENT FOR PUBLICATION

Not applicable.

CONFLICT OF INTEREST

The author declares no conflict of interest, financial or otherwise.

ACKNOWLEDGEMENT

Declared none.

REFERENCES

[1] Dransfield MT, Garner JL, Bhatt SP, *et al.* Effect of Zephyr Endobronchial Valves on Dyspnea, Activity Levels, and Quality of Life at One Year. Results from a Randomized Clinical Trial. Ann Am Thorac Soc 2020; 17(7): 829-38. [http://dx.doi.org/10.1513/AnnalsATS.201909-666OC] [PMID: 32223724]

[2] Abia-Trujillo D, Johnson MM, Patel NM, *et al.* Bronchoscopic Lung Volume Reduction. Mayo Clin Proc 2021; 96(2): 464-72. [http://dx.doi.org/10.1016/j.mayocp.2020.03.027] [PMID: 32829903]

Case 39

Sustained Benefits Out to 5 Years in an Emphysema Patient Following Zephyr Endobronchial Valve Therapy

Nai-Chien Huan[1], **Mona Zaria Nasaruddin**[1] and **Jamalul Azizi Abdul Rahaman**[1,*]

[1] *Department of Pulmonology, Serdang Hospital, Selangor, Malaysia*

Keywords: Chronic obstructive pulmonary disease, Collateral ventilation, Endobronchial valve, Emphysema, Non-pharmacological.

Presentation

A 53-year-old gentleman with COPD (GOLD class D). Still feeling short of breath despite on maximal medical therapy. His modified Medical Research Council (mMRC) Dyspnoea Scale was 2; FEV1 28% predicted; RV 515% pre dicted; TLC 200% predicted.

Comorbidities

Ex-smoker of 40 pack years.

Chest Imaging

CT thorax demonstrated heterogenous predominantly upper lobe emphysema with intact fissures. The left upper lobe was worse than the right upper lobe.

Intervention

Zephyr EBV (endobronchial valve) treatment of the left upper lobe was performed in December 2015 after Chartis measurement to exclude collateral ventilation. The entire procedure took 45 minutes.

[*]**Corresponding author Jamalul Azizi Abdul Rahaman:** Department of Pulmonology, Serdang Hospital, Selangor, Malaysia; E-mail: jamalulazizi@gmail.com

Jamalul Azizi Abdul Rahaman & Tinku Joseph (Eds.)

Complications

Procedure was uneventful.

Post-Intervention

Successful intentional atelectasis of the target lobe (left upper lobe) was achieved post-procedure as demonstrated by CXR (Fig. **1**). CT thorax in 2017 (2 years post-EBV insertion) showed collapse of anterior segment of left upper lobe with EBV *in situ* (Fig. **2**).

More importantly, the patient reported sustained improvement in the quality of life, reduction in dyspnoea with improvement in serial lung function tests (Table **1**).

Table 1: The Improvement in FEV1, RV and TLC from 2015 to 2020.

Year	FEV1	RV	TLC
2015	28% predicted	515% predicted	200% predicted
2017	36% predicted	242% predicted	114% predicted
2020	55% predicted	167% predicted	110% predicted

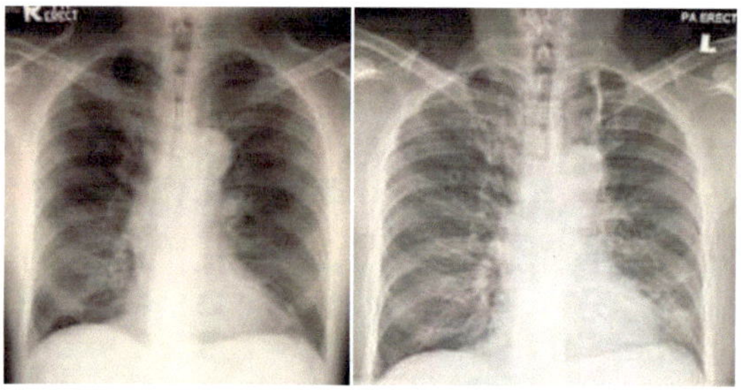

Fig. (1). CXR pre-EBV (left) and post-EBV (right).

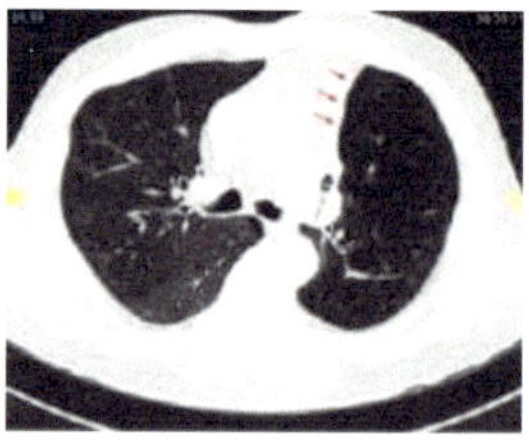

Fig. (2). CT thorax in 2017 (2 years post-EBV insertion) demonstrating collapse of anterior segment of left upper lobe (red arrows). EBV, shown as a dense tubular structure (green arrow) is *in situ*.

Learning Points

- Medical treatment is ineffective in very advanced emphysaema. EBV treatment has been shown to improve lung function, exercise capacity and quality of life in a subset of COPD patients with emphysema phenotype out to at least 12 months [1]. It is less invasive than Lung Volume Reduction Surgery (LVRS).

Video

The valves in the left upper division and lingula after deployment in this patient.

CONSENT FOR PUBLICATION

Not applicable.

CONFLICT OF INTEREST

The author declares no conflict of interest, financial or otherwise.

ACKNOWLEDGEMENT

Declared none.

REFERENCE

[1] Criner GJ, Sue R, Wright S, *et al.* A Multicenter Randomized Controlled Trial of Zephyr Endobronchial Valve Treatment in Heterogeneous Emphysema (LIBERATE). Am J Respir Crit Care Med 2018; 198(9): 1151-64. [http://dx.doi.org/10.1164/rccm.201803-0590OC] [PMID: 29787288]

Case 40

Segmental Bronchoscopic Lung Volume Reduction with Thermal Vapour Ablation

Anantham Devanand[1,*] and **Tay Chee Kiang Melvin**[1]

[1] *SingHealth Duke-NUS Lung Centre, Singapore*

Keywords: Heterogeneous emphysema, Segmental lung volume reduction, Sequential treatment, Thermal vapour ablation, Upper lobe predominant.

Presentation

Our patient was a 55-year-old, Malay male who was an ex-smoker having quit for 12 months following a 40 pack-year history. He had been diagnosed with Chronic Obstructive Pulmonary Disease (COPD) based on exertional dyspnea and pulmonary function testing. He was classified as Group D according to the GOLD classification system. There had been 4 hospitalizations for acute exacerbations of COPD in the past including an occasion of type 2 respiratory failure necessitating non-invasive mechanical ventilation. At the time of presentation, he was followed up at a multi-disciplinary COPD clinic and was undergoing outpatient pulmonary rehabilitation. Medications include combination bronchodilator therapy with tiotropium and olodaterol, as well as inhaled fluticasone 250 Micrograms bid. He was current with pneumococcal and influenza vaccinations and did not require long-term supplemental oxygen therapy.

Comorbidities

He had a previous history of intravenous heroin use and had a vascular pseudoaneurysm that had been treated surgically.

Chest Imaging

CT Thorax showed severe centrilobular emphysema that was predominantly in both upper lobes (Fig. **1**).

Transthoracic echocardiogram revealed an ejection fraction of 55 percent, estimated pulmonary systolic pressure of 21mm Hg and no evidence of regional

*__Corresponding author Anantham Devanand:__ SingHealth Duke-NUS Lung Centre, Singapore; E-mail: anantham.devanand@singhealth.com.sg

wall motion abnormalities. Pulmonary function testing showed severe obstructive pattern on spirometry with severely reduced diffusion coefficient and evidence of air trapping when lung volumes were measured on plethysmography. RV/TLC was 66% (Fig. **2**). The 6-minute walk test distance was 160 metres.

Intervention

Bronchoscopic thermal vapour ablation (BTVA) Procedure.

Planning

Non-contrast CT scan with a slice thickness of 1.0mm (0.5–1.25mm are acceptable) was performed to characterize the emphysema severity, emphysema distribution and interlobar fissure integrity. Based on the CT data, the planning software derived a measure of emphysema disease severity termed the tissue- to-air ratio. The tissue-to-air ratio is calculated based on the Hounsfield units of each lung segment. The heterogeneity index is derived by comparing the tissue-to-air ratio of the upper lobe with the lower lobe. The ideal target segments are the segments with the highest disease severity, the highest heterogeneity index and the highest segmental volume. For each bronchopulmonary segment, the planning software calculates treatment times which indicate the effective vapor dose required *i.e.* 8.5 calorie per gram. In this patient, the LB3 segment was selected to be the target for treatment.

Treatment 1

The BTVA generator generates precise amounts of the heated water vapor from sterile water. The heated water vapor from the generator is delivered to the target lung segment *via* a dedicated catheter. At the distal tip of the catheter, an inflatable silicone balloon is used to occlude the target airway during the treatment while the proximal end of the catheter is connected to the BTVA generator.

BTVA was performed in this patient under general anaesthesia using intravenous infusion of propofol with fentanyl to suppress the cough reflex. Bronchial washing was performed on the contralateral right upper lobe and was sent for bacterial Gram stain and aerobic culture to guide subsequent antibiotics if necessary. After endobronchial inspection and treatment of the LB3 segment by suctioning, the BTVA cath eter was advanced to the LB3a1 subsegment. After the airway was sealed by inflating the balloon, the heated water vapour was delivered for 5.4 seconds that had been calculated by the planning software. Thereafter, the balloon was deflated and the catheter was inserted into LB3a2 subsegment and vapour was delivered for 5.2 seconds as calculated during planning. The time that elapsed between the two va pour treatments was at least 3 minutes. The entire procedure was repeated for LB3b subsegment. The total procedure time for this session of BTVA was < 15 minutes.

Treatment 2

The second BTVA treatment was scheduled 12 weeks after the first one. The patient was asymptomatic following the first treatment. The same planning parameters were used and the LB1+2 segment was chosen this time for treatment. BTVA was again performed under general anaesthesia using intravenous infusion of propofol with fentanyl to suppress the cough reflex. Based on the endoscopic anatomy (Learning Point 6), it was decided to treat at the segmental level rather than the subsegmental level. BTVA catheter was advanced to the LB1+2 segment and the 100°C heated water vapour was delivered according to the 7.6 seconds that was calculated by the planning software.

All procedures were performed with a therapeutic flexible bronchoscope (6.0mm outer diameter) that had a 2.8mm working channel.

Complications

After the second procedure, the patient had blood-stained sputum that was self-limiting. The patient had been given amoxicillin/clavulanic acid as prophylactic antibiotic and this was continued for 14 days. However, the patient was re-admitted after 3 weeks for a COPD exacerbation with type 2 respiratory failure. He was managed with non-invasive ventilation, intravenous hydrocortisone and piperacillin/ tazobactam, as well as bronchodilators.

Post-Intervention

A CXR was performed following each procedure to exclude pneumothorax although this is a rare complication. As complications from the inflammatory reaction secondary to thermal vapour ablation typical ly occur during the first 2 to 4 weeks, the patient was discharged with the contact number of our COPD nurse coordinator in case of emergencies. He was reviewed in the outpatient clinic at 7, 14 and 28 days after treatment. Volume reduction following BTVA occurs gradually over a 4 to 6-week period (Figs. **3a-c**).

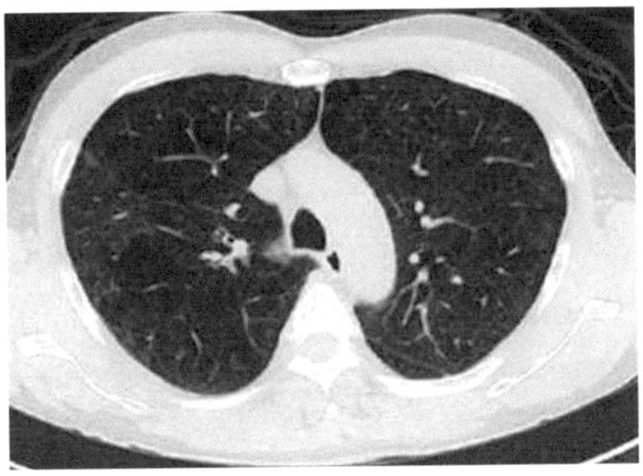

Fig. (1). CT Thorax showing upper lobe predominant severe emphysema.

--- SPIROMETRY ---	Pred	LLN	Actual	%Pred
FEVI (L)	2.92	2.01	1.04	36
FVC (L)	3.88	2.66	2.40	62
FEVI/FVC (%)	81	73	43	54

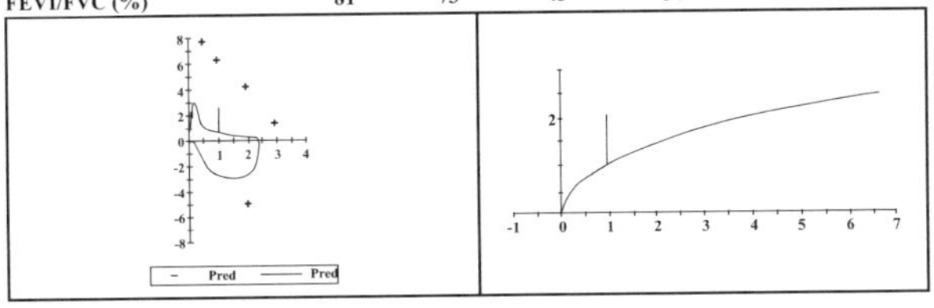

--- LUNG VOLUMES---	Pred	LLN	ULN	Actual	%Pred
RV (Pleth) (L)	1.66	0.92	2.40	4.40	265
TLC (Pleth) (L)	5.23	3.65	6.81	6.71	128
RV/TLC (Pleth) (%)	30	21	39	66	219

---- DIFFUSION----	Pred	ULN	LLN	Actual	%Pred
DLCOune (mm/min/kPa)	8.84	12.88	4.80	2.52	29
DLCOcor (mM/min/kPa)	8.84	12.88	4.80	2.40	27
DL/VA (mM/min/kPa/L)	1.69	2.17	1.21	0.49	29
Hgb (gm/dL)	12-18			16.5	

Fig. (2). Pulmonary function testing showing severe obstructive physiology with air trapping and reduced diffusion coefficient.

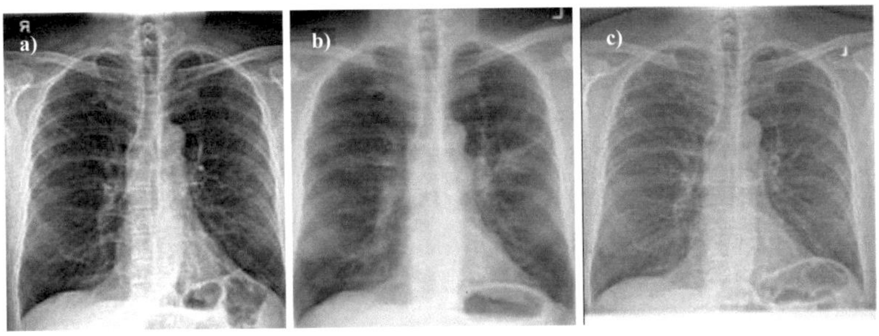

Fig. (3). Serial CXRs. **(a)** (Left) Baseline CXR with hyperinflated lung fields and flattened diaphragms. **(b)** (Middle) CXR 1 month after treatment of LB3 showing left upper zone infiltrates at the site of treatment. **(c)** (Right) CXR 3 months after treatment of LB3 showing resolution of left upper zone infiltrates and improved diaphragm curvature.

Learning Points

- Bronchoscopic Thermal Vapour Ablation (BTVA) is indicated for the treatment of heterogenous, upper lobe predominant emphysema in patients who are symptomatic despite optimal medical therapy. It is used for the selective and sequential treatment of emphysematous upper lobe segments. This aims to affect segmental lung volume reduction and reduce static hyperinflation.
- The sequential strategy towards segmental bronchoscopic lung volume reduction is to treat 1 emphysematous segment of an upper lobe during the first session, followed by BTVA of 1 or 2 segments during a second session performed 12 weeks later. The patient should have fully recovered prior to being scheduled for the second procedure.
- BTVA is a treatment option for advanced COPD that is of the emphysema predominant phenotype with severe hyperinflation. Patients aged 45–75 years with severe, upper lobe-predominant emphysema with a FEV1 between 20% and 45%, evidence of hyperinflation and post-rehabilitation 6-min walk test distance of > 140m can be considered.
- Potential candidates must have stable COPD with ≤ 3 COPD-related hospitalizations in past 12 months, no COPD-related hospitalization in past 3 months, and must not require regular use of systemic steroids. Acute COPD exacerbations, concomitant bronchiectasis, bacterial infections, significant sputum, or known microbiological colonization (*e.g., Pseudomonas aeruginosa*) are contraindications.

Other patients who should be excluded are those who are taking anticoagulation, who have had previous lung resection, and have either concomitant pulmonary hypertension or congestive cardiac failure. All candidates should have medical therapy optimized and have had pulmonary rehabilitation prior to consideration for BTVA [1].

- When consent is taken, patients should have realistic expectations that the response to BTVA may take several weeks and that they will have to continue to take inhalers after the procedure. There may not be any improvement in pulmonary function testing. The expected benefits from BTVA are improved symptom control resulting in improved quality of life. There is the potential for short term complications such as acute exacerbation of COPD, haemoptysis and pneumonia which can occur within a week of the procedure.
- Large bulla should not be treated with BTVA.
- During the procedure, application of the vapor induces a cough that can displace the balloon catheter. This can result in the thermal energy being applied to an

incorrect site. Therefore, controlling of cough and adequacy of anaesthesia are crucially important.

- When placing the balloon catheter, avoid placing it directly towards the sub carina or against the airway wall. These anatomical considerations should be factored into the decision as to whether to treat at the segmental or the sub-segmental level.
- When inflating the balloon on the treatment catheter, ensure that there is a good seal to deliver the full dose of the thermal energy into the targeted segment. Avoid over-inflating the balloon such that it herniates out of the orifice of the target airway. This may result in a poor seal.

Video

Bronchial Thermal Vapour Ablation of the anterior segment of the left upper lobe. After endobronchial inspection and toilet of the segment, the catheter is advanced to the LB3a1 subsegment. After the airway is sealed by inflating the balloon, heated water vapour is delivered according to what had been calculated by the planning software. Thereafter, the balloon is deflated and the catheter is inserted into LB3a2 subsegment before vapour is delivered again.

CONSENT FOR PUBLICATION

Not applicable.

CONFLICT OF INTEREST

The author declares no conflict of interest, financial or otherwise.

ACKNOWLEDGEMENT

Declared none.

REFERENCE

[1] Gompelmann D, Shah PL, Valipour A, Herth FJF. Bronchoscopic Thermal Vapor Ablation: Best Practice Recommendations from an Expert Panel on Endoscopic Lung Volume Reduction. Respiration 2018; 95(6): 392-400.
[http://dx.doi.org/10.1159/000489815] [PMID: 29895029]

Case 41

Persistent Air Leak

Successful Treatment of Persistent Air Leak with Zephyr Endobronchial Valve

Khai Lip Ng[1], **Mona Zaria Nasaruddin**[1] and **Jamalul Azizi Abdul Rahaman**[1,*]

[1] *Department of Pulmonology, Serdang Hospital, Selangor, Malaysia*

Keywords: Bullae, Endobronchial valve, Persistent air leak, Pneumothorax, Tuberculosis.

Presentation

A 37-year-old lady presented with progressive shortness of breath 2 months after completing anti-TB treatment. CXR showed a large left-sided pneumothorax requiring tube thoracostomy. The CXR showed full expansion of the left lung. However, the underwater seal drainage system was still bubbling after more than 5 days indicating persistent air leak. She had pneumothorax on the same side during the intensive phase of anti-TB treatment which resolved with tube thoracostomy. She was deemed not suitable for surgical management of persistent air leak in view of poor lung function.

Comorbidities

Diabetes mellitus, Pulmonary TB - completed 6 months of anti-TB treatment. History of ectopic pregnancy.

Chest Imaging

CXR showed full expansion of the left lung with chest tube *in situ* (Fig. **1**). The underwater seal drainage system was still bubbling. CECT thorax showed ruptured bullae in the left lung. No obvious broncho-pleural fistulae were seen.

Intervention

Zephyr endobronchial valve (EBV) deployment *via* rigid bronchoscopy under general anaesthesia. Chartis® System showed no collateral ventilation between the

*Corresponding author Jamalul Azizi Abdul Rahaman: Department of Pulmonology, Serdang Hospital, Selangor, Malaysia; E-mail: jamalulazizi@gmail.com

left upper lobe and left lower lobe. The under water seal drainage system stopped bubbling when the left upper lobe was blocked with the Chartis® balloon. 3 Zephyr EBVs were deployed in LB1, LB2 and LB3. 1 Zephyr EBV was deployed in the lingula (Fig. **2**). There was no bubbling seen in the under water seal drainage system at the end of the procedure (Fig. **3**).

Complications

None.

Post-Intervention

CXR remained expanded and there was no bubbling noted (Fig. **4**). Patient's symptoms improved. The chest tube was removed 4 days post-EBV. She was discharged well. She remained well 4 years post-intervention.

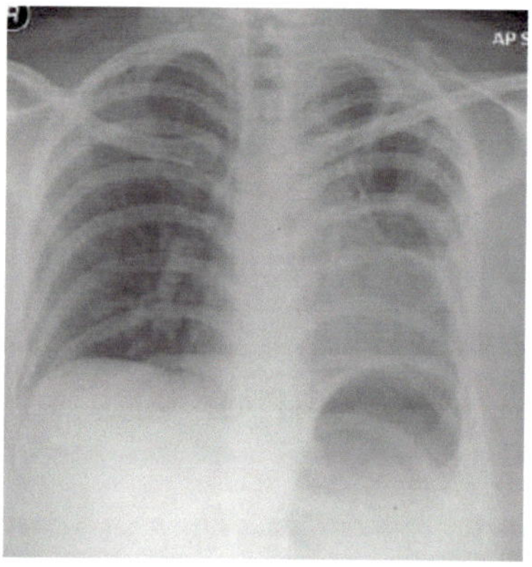

Fig. (1). CXR pre-EBV.

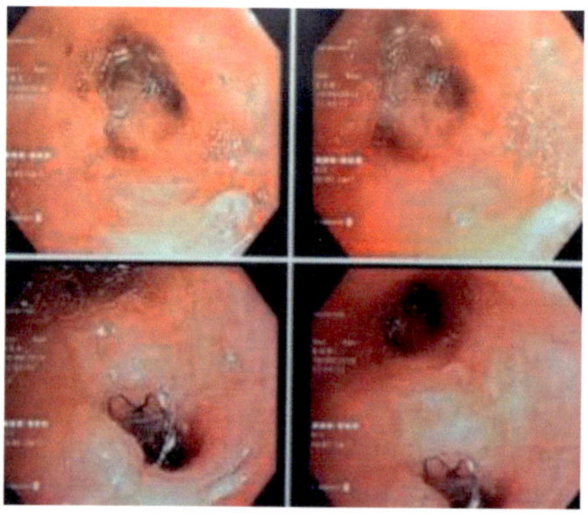

Fig. (2). Zephyr EBVs in the left upper lobe.

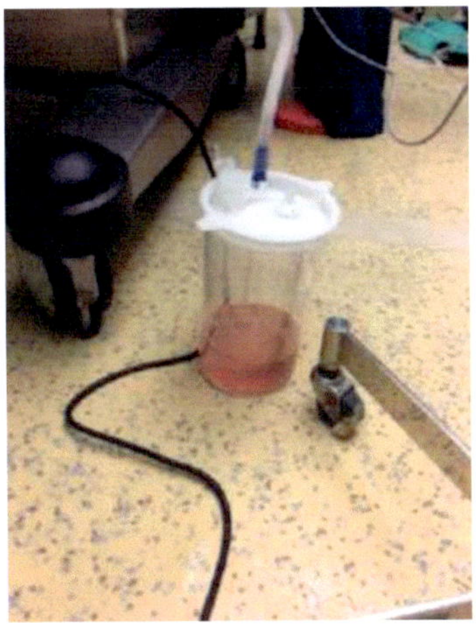

Fig. (3). Bubbling stopped after EBV placement.

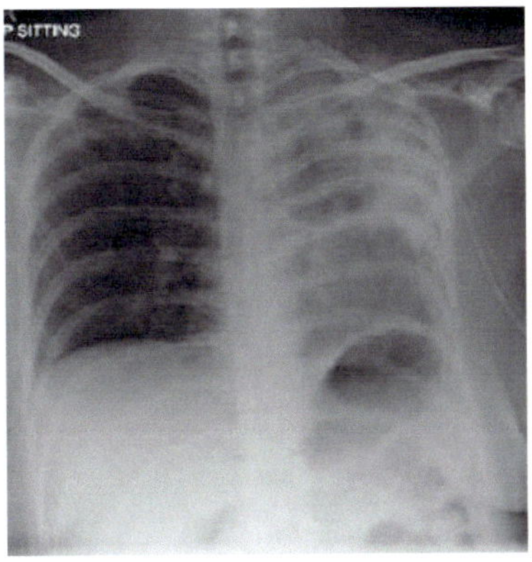

Fig. (4). CXR post-EBV (EBVs can be seen in the LUL).

Learning Points

- Persistent air leak is a common complication of spontaneous pneumothorax being treated by chest tube drainage. It is generally recommended that surgical intervention be considered when an air leak continues for 5 to 7 days after tube thoracostomy. Unfortunately, some patients are poor candidates for surgery or may refuse surgery. Prolonged chest tube *in situ* is undesirable because of an increased risk of complications, prolonged immobilisation and its consequences and increased duration of hospital stay.
- EBV can be used to treat persistent air leak complicating pneumothorax. The rationale is that air leakage will stop if air is prevented from entering the airway leading to the leak site. Predictors for success include intact interlobar fissures,

fewer medical comorbidities and immediate air leak cessation after completion of EBV implantation [1].

Video

Zephyr endobronchial valve (EBV) deployment in the left upper lobe. Balloon of the Chartis® catheter was used to confirm the absence of collateral ventilation.

CONSENT FOR PUBLICATION

Not applicable.

CONFLICT OF INTEREST

The author declares no conflict of interest, financial or otherwise.

ACKNOWLEDGEMENT

Declared none.

REFERENCE

[1] Yu WC, Yu ELM, Kwok HC, *et al.* Endobronchial valve for treatment of persistent air leak complicating spontaneous pneumothorax. Hong Kong Med J 2018; 24(2): 158-65. [http://dx.doi.org/10.12809/hkmj176823] [PMID: 29622759]

Case 42

Endobronchial Valves for Persistent Air Leak

Alex Chee[1,*] and **Elaine Dumoulin**[1]

[1] *Department of Medicine, University of Calgary, Calgary, Canada*

Keywords: Endobronchial valve, Bronchopleural fistula, Intrabronchial valve, Persistent air leak, Spiration.

Presentation

A 42-year-old gentleman with a history of an aspergilloma presented with a tension pneumothorax during spirometry. An urgent tube thoracostomy was performed and the patient was admitted to hospital. There was a brisk air leak on expiration and after one week of conservation management, there was no change in the air leak. Attempted wean of the chest tube from wall suction to gravity drainage failed so a decision was made to attempt endobronchial blockade to resolve the air leak.

Comorbidities

History of a right upper lobe lung cavity with subsequent aspergilloma. Bronchoscopic aspergilloma removal was carried out one month prior to spirometry.

Chest Imaging

CXR revealed right pneumothorax immediately after spirometry attempt. CT thorax was done after tube thoracostomy. Right apical cavity was the likely source of the air leak (Fig. **1**).

Intervention

The patient was taken for flexible bronchoscopy under moderate sedation. The chest tube output was monitored with a pleuro-vac and the degree of air leak was observed during the bronchoscopy. A 7F Fogarty balloon was placed through the working channel of the bronchoscope and inflated in the right upper lobe. There was a significant reduction in the air leak with balloon occlusion of the right upper lobe. The right upper lobe airway segments were measured with a calibrated

*Corresponding author Alex Chee: Department of Medicine, University of Calgary, Calgary, Canada; E-mail: Alex.chee@ahs.ca

Jamalul Azizi Abdul Rahaman & Tinku Joseph (Eds.)

balloon and one-way intrabronchial valves were placed in all segments of the right upper lobe, starting with the most anatomically angled apical segment (Fig. **2**).

Complications

None.

Post-Intervention

The air leak subsided, the patient was weaned off suction and the chest tube was removed after four days (Fig. **3**).

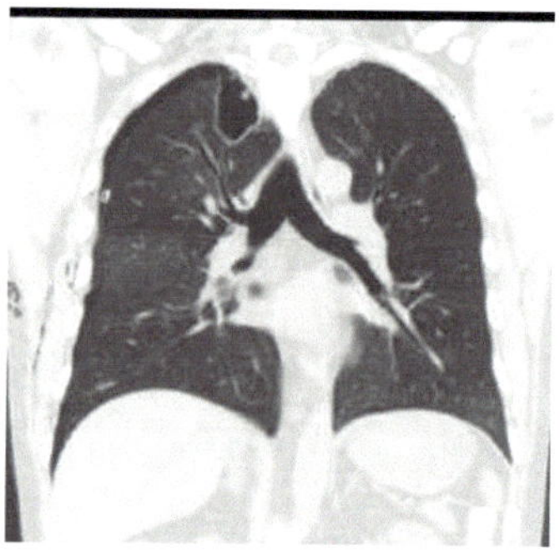

Fig. (1). Coronal CT thorax of pneumothorax with chest tube in place. Likely culprit of the air leak was the cavity in the right upper lobe.

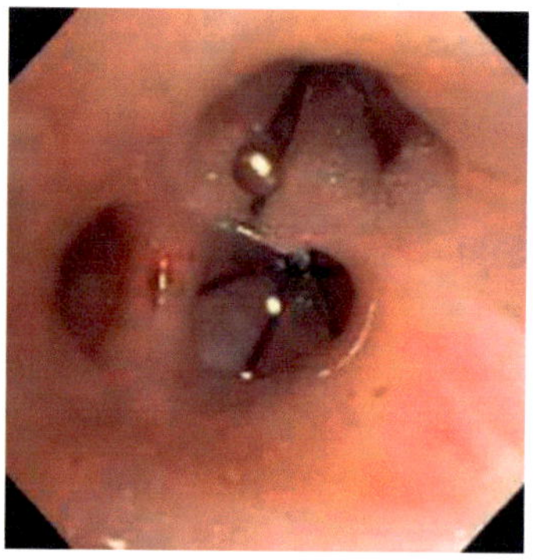

Fig. (2). Bronchoscopic image of Spiration (Olympus Corporation, USA) valves in the apical and posterior segments of the right upper lobe.

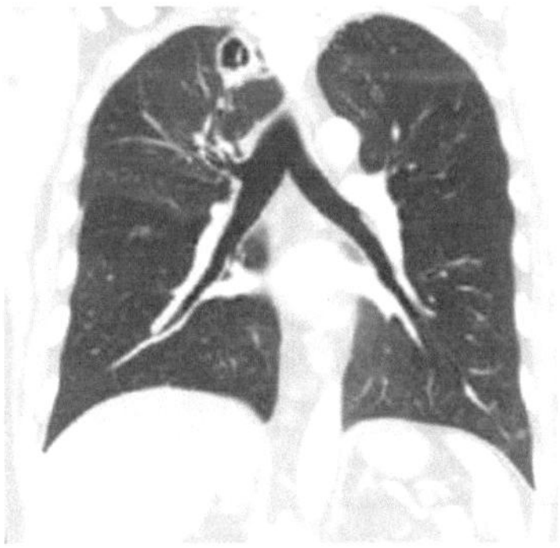

Fig. (3). CXR 2 weeks after valve placement. Partial atelectasis of right upper lobe. One intrabronchial valve is visible in the posterior segment.

Learning Points

- Pneumothorax with persistent air leak, defined as air leak after 5-7 days, can result in significant morbidity and mortality [1]. If conservative therapy with tube thoracostomy and watchful waiting do not heal the air leak, then more aggressive measures are often taken. Historically, surgical therapy with the removal of blebs or bullae along with pleurodesis have been performed.
- There has also been varying success with sealants, Watanabe spigots, as well as blood patches. Endobronchial valves have approval in North America to be used for persistent air leak after thoracic surgery, though valves have been used off-label for spontaneous pneumothorax. If an air leak persists despite valves, a reduction in the air leak may allow a patient to be transitioned to a Heimlich valve for outpatient management. Typically, endobronchial valves remain in place for six weeks to allow for healing of the pleural surface and then can be removed.

CONSENT FOR PUBLICATION

Not applicable.

CONFLICT OF INTEREST

The author declares no conflict of interest, financial or otherwise.

ACKNOWLEDGEMENT

Declared none.

REFERENCE

[1] Dugan KC, Laxmanan B, Murgu S, Hogarth DK. Management of Persistent Air Leaks. Chest 2017; 152(2): 417-23.
[http://dx.doi.org/10.1016/j.chest.2017.02.020] [PMID: 28267436]

Case 43

Giant Bullae

Treatment of Giant Bullous Emphysaema with Zephyr Endobronchial Valves

Khai Lip Ng[1], **Mona Zaria Nasaruddin**[1] and **Jamalul Azizi Abdul Rahaman**[1,*]

[1] *Department of Pulmonology, Serdang Hospital, Selangor, Malaysia*

Keywords: Collateral ventilation, Emphysema, Endobronchial valve, Giant bullae, Hyperinflation.

Presentation

A 60-year-old gentleman with underlying GOLD D COPD presented with markedly reduced effort tolerance and shortness of breath on minimal exertion despite on maximal medical therapy. On long term oxygen therapy, he was home bound since 2017.

Comorbidities

Ex-smoker of 15 pack years. Benign prostatic hyperplasia.

Chest Imaging

CT thorax showed bilateral hyperinflated lungs. Large thin-walled bulla obliterating the left upper lobe. 16.0cm x 15.9cm x 14.1cm (Fig. **1**). Smaller thin-walled bulla seen within the right upper lobe. Bronchiectatic changes seen at both lower lobes. Lung function test: FEV1- 0.54L (18% predicted), FVC - 1.33L (32% predicted), FEV1/FVC-38%, DLCO – 39% predicted. 6-minute walk test: 60m and oxygen saturation (SpO_2) dropped to 85%. He was deemed not suitable for surgical bullectomy in view of poor lung function and functional status.

Intervention

Zephyr endobronchial valve (EBV) inserted at LB1+2, LB3 and the lingula (Fig. **2**). Collateral ventilation assessment with the Chartis® System was not performed to shorten the procedure time in view of the very reduced lung reserve. The entire procedure took 30 minutes.

*__Corresponding author Jamalul Azizi Abdul Rahaman:__ Department of Pulmonology, Serdang Hospital, Selangor, Malaysia; E-mail: jamalulazizi@gmail.com

Complications

Patient had bronchospasm after the procedure. Bronchospasm resolved with nebulized bronchodilator. No pneumothorax after the procedure. Extubated the next day.

Post-Intervention

Upon review in the clinic, his exercise tolerance much improved, was able to leave the house and more active. Repeat CXR after 1 month and 6 months showed improvement in hyperinflation and reduced size of the left upper lobe bulla (Figs. **3a** and **b**). 6-minute walking test improved to 223m (from 60m). Patient only used oxygen occasionally at night. There was also improvement in his lung function testing; FEV1- 0.64L (20% predicted) FVC- 1.69L (38% predicted), FEV1/FVC- 38%, DLCO- 63% predicted.

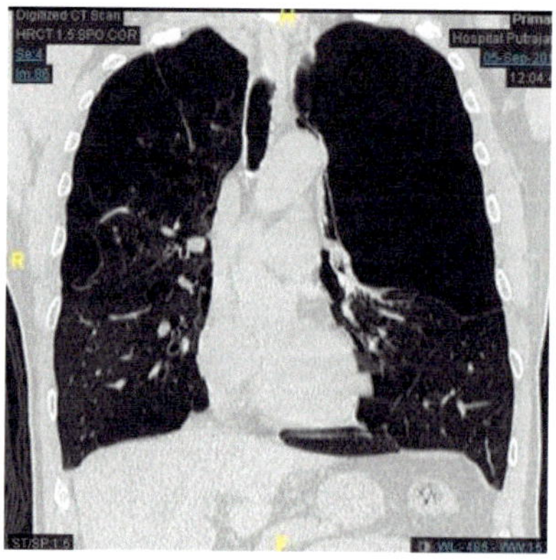

Fig. (1). Coronal CT thorax showing the left giant bulla.

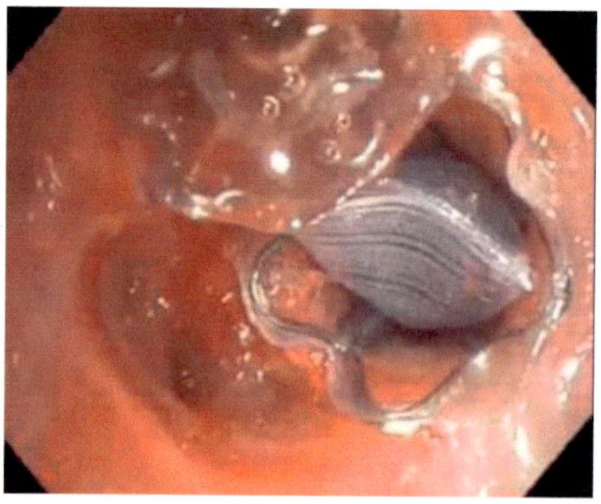

Fig. (2). EBVs placed at LB1+2, LB3 and the lingula.

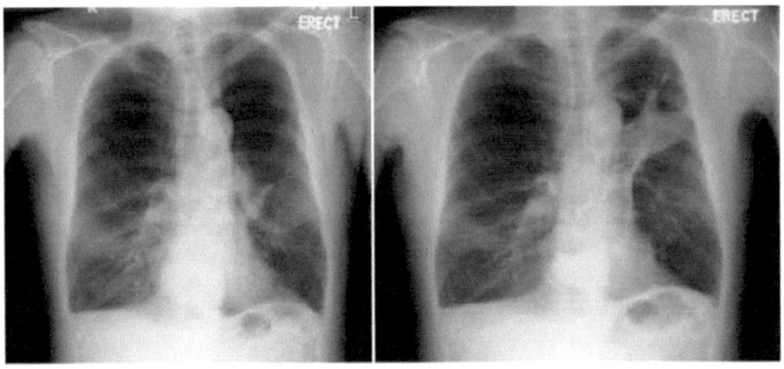

Fig. (3). (a) (Left) CXR 1 month post-EBV. **(b)** (Right) CXR 6 months post-EBV showing significant reduction of the bulla size.

Learning Points

- We report the successful and safe EBV treatment in a patient with a huge bullous emphysaema in the left upper lobe. Giant bullae are defined as greater than 5cm in diameter.
- Bronchoscopic lung volume reduction methods including EBV have been included in the GOLD guidelines for COPD (emphysaema phenotype) without collateral ventilation. However, the use of EBV to treat giant bullae is seldom reported.
- A new hypothesis suggests that the bullous emphysaema is associated with free airway communication caused by compliance higher than that of the surrounding lung [1]. For bullae that are not fed by an airway, EBV treatment will probably not be effective. However, when bullae are large, contained within a lobe and likely fed by an airway, reduction of the volume of bullae can be achieved similar to the lobar volume reduction in emphysaema.
- Our case supports recent suggestions that EBV can serve as a good alternative treatment for giant bullae in appropriately selected patients [2].

Video

The deployment of Zephyr EBVs in the left upper lobe.

CONSENT FOR PUBLICATION

Not applicable.

CONFLICT OF INTEREST

The author declares no conflict of interest, financial or otherwise.

ACKNOWLEDGEMENT

Declared none.

REFERENCES

[1] Klingman RR, Angelillo VA, DeMeester TR. Cystic and bullous lung disease. Ann Thorac Surg 1991; 52(3): 576-80.
[http://dx.doi.org/10.1016/0003-4975(91)90939-N] [PMID: 1898156]

[2] Eung gu Lee, Chin Kook Rhee. Bronchoscopic lung volume reduction using an endobronchial valve to treat a huge emphysaematous bullae: a case report. BMC Pulm Med 2019; 19: 92.
[http://dx.doi.org/10.1186/s12890-019-0849-z] [PMID: 31088437]

Case 44

Foreign Body Removal

Bronchoscopic Retrieval of an Impacted Fish Bone

Tinku Joseph[1,*] and **Sathish C. Reddy**[1]

[1] *Division of Interventional Pulmonology, Amrita Institute of Medical Sciences, Kochi, India*

Keywords: Cryoextraction, Cylindrical bronchiectasis, Foreign body aspiration, Foreign body removal, Rigid bronchoscopy.

Presentation

A 51-year-old male presented with complaints of cough with mucoid expectoration, exertional breathlessness of 4 months duration. He was initially admitted to another hospital for worsening breathlessness, cough with expectoration and treated with antibiotics, steroids and was further evaluated with CT chest which showed opacity in the right bronchus raising the suspicion of mucous plug or foreign body. Subsequently, he came to our center for further evaluation and management. He also had history of persisting symptoms since the last 3 years.

Comorbidities

None.

Chest Imaging

CXR: Right middle lobe collapse.

CECT Chest:

- High density foreign body in the right bronchus intermedius, with focal eccentric bronchial wall thickening - inflammation / mucous impaction (Fig. **1**).
- Atelectatic changes with areas of cylindrical bronchiectasis and air bronchogram seen in the medial segment of the right middle lobe with areas of acinar nodular opacities in the lateral segment of right middle lobe - likely to be secondary infection.

*__Corresponding author Tinku Joseph:__ Division of Interventional Pulmonology, Amrita Institute of Medical Sciences, Kochi, India; E-mail: tinkujoseph2010@gmail.com

Intervention

In view of suspicion of foreign body aspiration and long-standing history, plan was made to do rigid bronchoscopy and foreign body removal. The patient was intubated and ventilated with 12-13mm size rigid tracheoscope and flexible bronchoscopy done, which showed a foreign body (suspected chicken bone) in the right bronchus intermedius surrounded with granulation tissue (Fig. **2**). The foreign body was retrieved with the help of 1.9mm flexible cryoprobe and grasping forceps (Figs. **3-5**). Multiple granulation tissues were present at the site of the impacted foreign body and were debulked using a snare electrocautery and the remaining granulation tissues were cryo-ablated. Adequate hemostasis was achieved with bronchial blocker (5F Fogarty balloon), cold saline and adrenaline instillation locally. The patient tolerated the procedure well and he was extubated on the table.

Complications

No immediate post-procedure complications were noted.

Post-Intervention

The patient was discharged on tapering dose of oral corticosteroids for 2 weeks in view of minimal granulation tissue at the site of foreign body impaction. Surveillance bronchoscopy done after 4 weeks showed complete patency of the right middle lobe and lower lobe bronchus with no evidence of any residual granulation tissue.

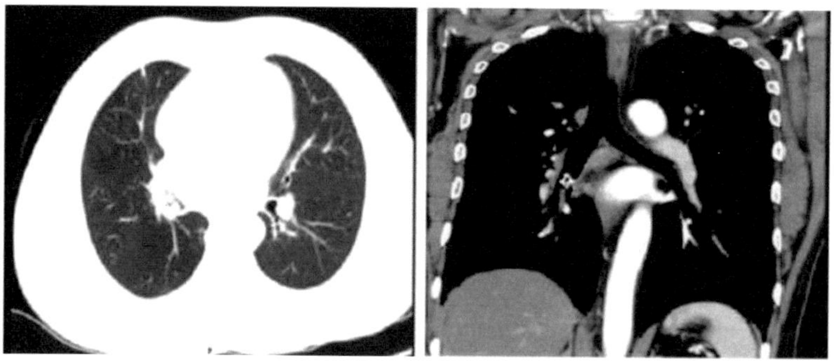

Fig. (1). Axial and coronal CECT chest: Impacted foreign body in right bronchus intermedius.

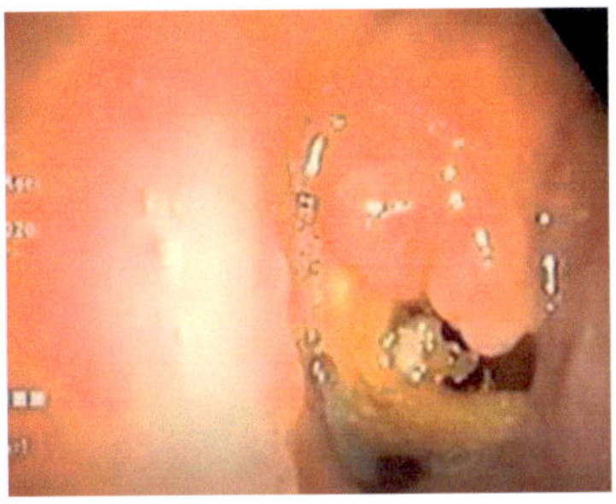

Fig. (2). Bronchoscopic image: Impacted foreign body in right bronchus intermedius.

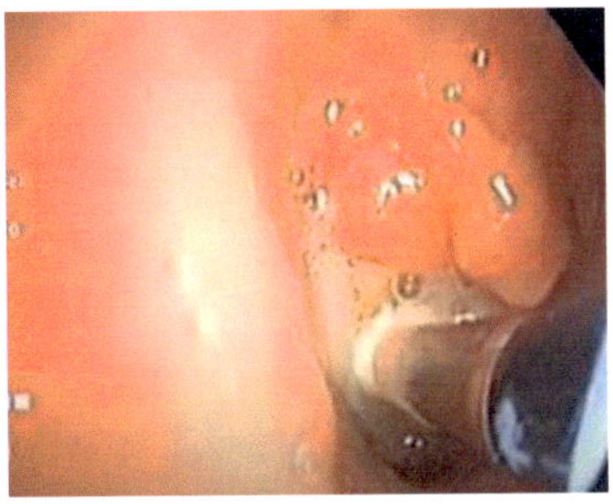

Fig. (3). Bronchoscopic image: Attempted cryoextraction of the foreign body.

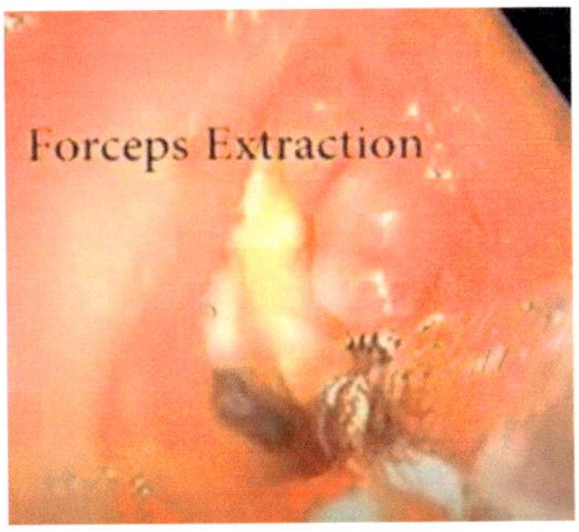

Fig. (4). Bronchoscopic image: Forceps extraction of impacted foreign body.

a) **b)**

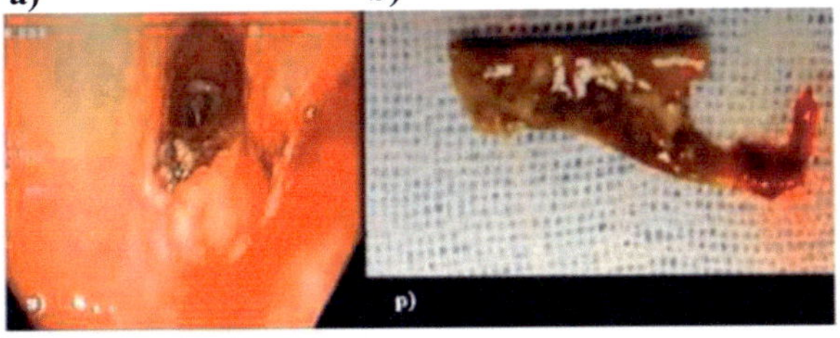

Fig. (5). Bronchoscopic image. **a**) Right bronchus intermedius after foreign body removal. **b**) Extracted foreign body (Fish bone).

Learning Points

- An aspirated foreign body should be considered as one of the differentials in non-resolving pneumonia.
- Cryo extraction is an extremely useful technique for removing impacted foreign bodies [1].

Video

Bronchoscopic retrieval of impacted fish bone.

CONSENT FOR PUBLICATION

Not applicable.

CONFLICT OF INTEREST

The author declares no conflict of interest, financial or otherwise.

ACKNOWLEDGEMENT

Declared none.

REFERENCE

[1] Agarwal R, Sehgal IS, Dhooria S, Behera D. Use of cryoprobe for removal of a large tracheobronchial foreign body during flexible bronchoscopy. Lung India 2016; 33(5): 543-5. [http://dx.doi.org/10.4103/0970-2113.188978] [PMID: 27625452]

Case 45

Hijab Pin in the Airway

Mohamed Faisal Abdul Hamid[1,*] , **Nik Nuratiqah Nik Abeed**[1], **Ng Boon Hau**[1] and **Andrea Ban Yu-Lin**[1]

[1] *Respiratory Unit, Faculty of Medicine, National University of Malaysia, Selangor, Malaysia*

Keywords: Airway, Foreign body, Flexible bronchoscopy, Hijab, Pin, Rigid bronchoscopy.

Presentation

A 22-year-old woman accidentally aspirated a hijab pin. It occurred when she was answering a phone call while holding the pin between her teeth. She only came to seek treatment 16 days later after she complained of chest discomfort and mild hemoptysis. On presentation, she was comfortable with stable vital signs.

Comorbidities

None.

Chest Imaging

Initial CXR revealed a radio-opaque linear opacity in the left lower zone (Fig. **1a**). CT thorax confirmed the location of the pin in the left lower lobe (Fig. **1b**).

Intervention

Flexible fibreoptic bronchoscopy (Olympus BF - IT260; EVIS LUCERA ELITE bronchovideoscope system) with a working channel of 2.8mm *via* a rigid bronchial tube (7.5mm, 43cm Karl Storz Endoskope system) under general anaesthesia. The pin was identified in the lateral segment of the left lower lobe (LB9) with surrounding granulation tissue. We used the Olympus V-Shape (FG-25C-1) grasping forceps to retrieve the pin. The sharp end of the pin was partially embedded in the bronchial mucosa. We gripped the shaft of the pin and pulled it out through the rigid bronchoscope. This required multiple attempts due to the

***Corresponding author Mohamed Faisal Abdul Hamid:** Respiratory Unit, Faculty of Medicine, National University of Malaysia, Selangor, Malaysia; E-mail: faisal.hamid@ppukm.ukm.edu.my

Jamalul Azizi Abdul Rahaman & Tinku Joseph (Eds.)

inadvertent slipping away of the pin. Upon removal, the pin was noted to be 4cm in length and bent at 120 degrees (Figs. **2a-c**).

Complications

Minimal mucosal bleeding.

Post-Intervention

The patient was extubated 2 days post-procedure. She completed 5 days of empirical intravenous amoxicillin-clavulanate acid 1.2g three times a day and 2 days of intravenous dexamethasone 4mg twice daily. She developed bronchospasm a day after the procedure which resolved with regular salbutamol nebuliser. She was discharged 4 days post-procedure. On follow-up one month later, she remained well with a normal CXR (Fig. **1c**).

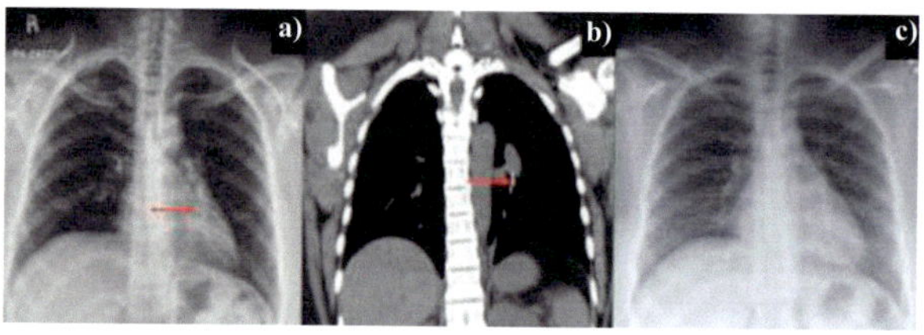

Fig. (1). (**a**) CXR revealed a radio-opaque linear opacity in the left lower zone. (**b**) Coronal CT thorax revealed the location of the pin in the left lower lobe. (**c**) CXR post-intervention was normal.

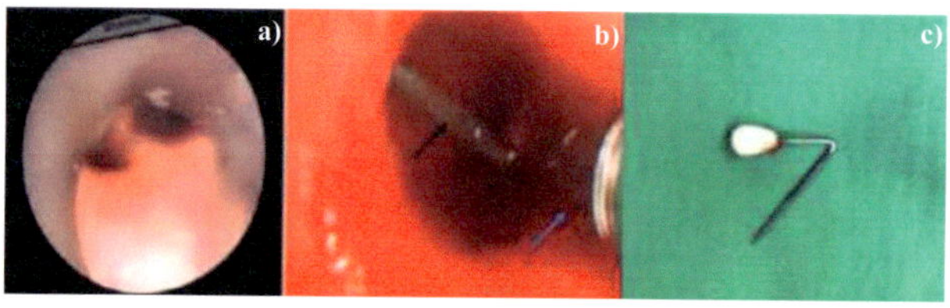

Fig. (2). (**a**) Rigid bronchoscopy (Karl Storz Endoskope system) was performed. (**b**) The pin (black arrow) which was embedded in the mucosa at the left lower lobe was identified using a flexible fibreoptic bronchoscope (Olympus BF - IT260; EVIS LUCERA ELITE bronchovideoscope system) via the rigid scope, and Olympus V-Shape (FG-25C-1) grasping forceps (blue arrow) was used to retrieve the pin. (**c**) The retrieved pin size was 4cm in length and bent at 120 degrees.

Learning Points

- Foreign body aspiration is life-threatening when the object is large enough to obstruct the central airway. The commonest cause is careless movement such as simultaneously talking, laughing or coughing whilst holding the pin between the teeth. The clinical presentation may vary ranging from acute airway obstruction, classical choking, haemoptysis and penetration syndromes (coughing, suffocation and dyspnoea) to no symptoms [1]. Owing to the metallic nature of the pin, radiological imaging such as chest radiograph can help localise the site of the pin. These pins usually settle in the left bronchial tree [2]. Hijab pins in the airway will require removal either with a rigid or flexible bronchoscope. Thoracotomy needs to be considered if the pin migrates to the smaller subsegmental bronchus. The interval between aspiration of the hijab pin and intervention is important. The delay in presentation or intervention will lead to migration and potential penetration of the bronchial wall.

Video

Foreign body removal in this patient *via* rigid bronchoscopy using a grasping forceps.

CONSENT FOR PUBLICATION

Not applicable.

CONFLICT OF INTEREST

The author declares no conflict of interest, financial or otherwise.

ACKNOWLEDGEMENT

Declared none.

REFERENCES

[1] Stool SE, Manning SC. Foreign bodies of the pharynx and esophagus. Pediatric otolaryngology 1996; 2: 1169-80.

[2] Zaghba N, Benjelloun H, Bakhatar A, Yassine N, Bahlaoui A. [Scarf pin: an intrabronchial foreign body who is not unusual]. Rev Pneumol Clin 2013; 69(2): 65-9. [http://dx.doi.org/10.1016/j.pneumo.2012.09.003] [PMID: 23347798]

Case 46

Localised Bronchiectasis Caused by Foreign Body Aspiration

Hema Yamini Ramarmuty[1,*]

[1]*Respiratory Department, Queen Elizabeth Hospital, Kota Kinabalu, Sabah, Malaysia*

Keywords: Bronchiectasis, Foreign body aspiration, Foreign body removal, Localised disease, Rigid bronchoscopy.

Presentation

A 55-year-old teacher presented with chronic productive cough for 3 years. There were no constitutional symptoms. She completed multiple courses of antibiotics with temporary relief.

Comorbidities

Asthma since childhood which was well controlled. She had COVID-19 infection 9 months earlier. She is a non- smoker.

Chest Imaging

CXR revealed right midzone and lower zone infiltrates. CECT thorax demonstrated right middle lobe bronchiectasis. There was a calcified, linear density with branching pattern within the right main bronchus extending into the right bronchus intermedius (Fig. **1**).

Intervention

We performed rigid bronchoscopy for exploration of the airways under total intravenous anaesthesia. Flexible fibreoptic bronchoscope was introduced through the rigid bronchoscope and airway assessment identified a linear foreign body with sharp edges, lodged longitudinally within the right main bronchus. Large amount of purulent secretions was present in the right bronchus intermedius. Attempts to extract the foreign body with a flexible alligator forceps failed.

*__Corresponding author Hema Yamini Ramarmuty:__ Respiratory Department, Queen Elizabeth Hospital, Kota Kinabalu, Sabah, Malaysia; E-mail: yamini8254@hotmail.com

Jamalul Azizi Abdul Rahaman & Tinku Joseph (Eds.)

A rigid forceps was then used but we could not get a firm grip. The distal end of the foreign body had become embedded in the bronchial wall, and it could not be removed. Thus, we used a snare to get a better grip around the foreign body and was able to dislodge it, however the snare with the foreign body could not be removed through the rigid bronchoscope barrel as the diameter of the distal end of the foreign body was too large to be passed through the rigid bronchoscope. Removing the foreign body en bloc with the rigid bronchoscope was not done to protect the vocal cords and the airways from potential injury.

The patient was placed in a Trendelenburg position to prevent the foreign body from moving distally. We then used the rigid forceps to fragment parts of the foreign body (piecemeal) till it became small enough to pass through the barrel of the rigid tube (Figs. **2a-f**).

Complications

Minimal bleeding was seen in the right bronchus intermedius after the removal of the foreign body using the snare but haemostasis was secured with instillation of cold saline and adrenaline (1:10000). She was extubated post-procedure and received antibiotics to treat the post-obstructive pneumonia.

Post-Intervention

The foreign body was noted to be of bony consistency. Although she was scheduled for a repeat bronchoscopy for airway reassessment, she was unable to come to the hospital for the procedure due to the movement restriction during the COVID-19 pandemic. She has, however, been under the observation of doctors in a nearby district hospital in the event of any complications.

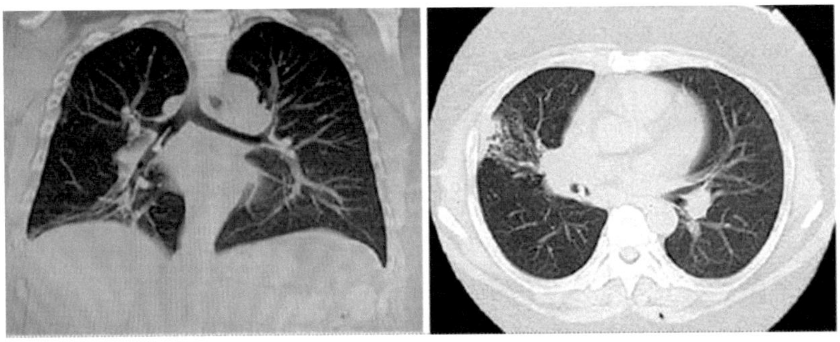

Fig. (1). Coronal and axial CT thorax showing right middle lobe bronchiectasis. There is a calcified, linear density in the right main bronchus extending into the bronchus intermedius suspicious for a foreign body.

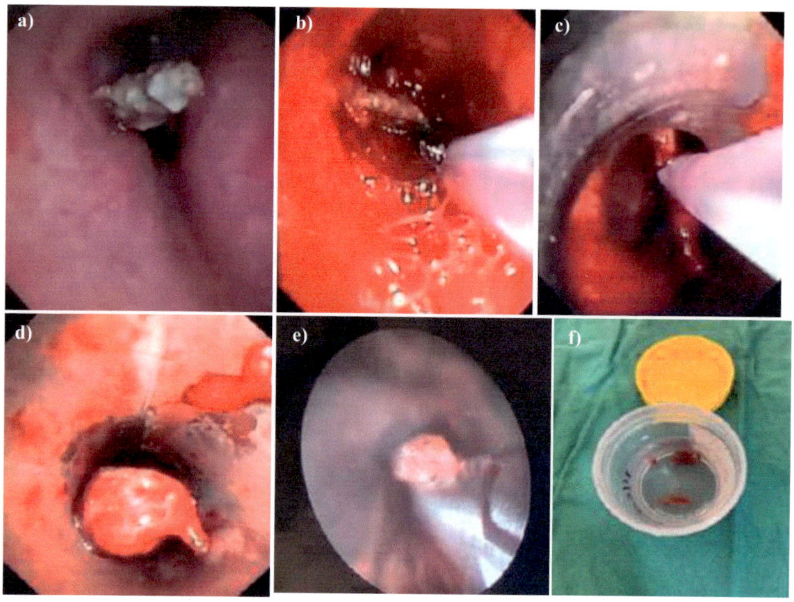

Fig. (2). (**a**) Endoscopic view of foreign body lodged in the right main bronchus with its distal end in the bronchus intermedius. (**b**) Foreign body is gripped using the snare. (**c**) Foreign body could not be passed through the rigid bronchoscope barrel when pulled using the snare. (**d**) The distal end with the largest diameter had been fragmented with rigid forceps and is able to fit through the rigid bronchoscope barrel. (**e**) Rigid forceps used to remove the fragmented pieces. (**f**) Fragmented pieces of the foreign body seen in the specimen pot.

Learning Points

- Localised bronchiectasis or non-resolving pneumonia should always prompt further assessment with bronchoscopy to rule out an endobronchial lesion or foreign body within the airways. Many a times foreign body retrieval can be performed using flexible fiberoptic bronchoscope with a reported success rate of 86% [1]. In cases where the foreign body has been lodged within the airways for a long duration of time, there may be development of granulation tissue, causing it to be embedded within the airway mucosa. This may lead to bleeding during removal. In such cases, removal with a flexible fiberoptic bronchoscope may be difficult, as suctioning blood while passing the grasping instruments through the working channel at the same time can be challenging.
- Rigid bronchoscope secures the airway and facilitates the extraction of large foreign bodies without injuring the laryngeal or airway wall. It also allows the use of a variety of larger instruments for foreign body removal. In our patient, the foreign body had sharp edges and its diameter was larger than the inner diameter of the rigid bronchoscope barrel. A good way to fragment it prior to

removal is by using rigid scissors which were not available to us. Another option is to use Nd: YAG laser [2].

CONSENT FOR PUBLICATION

Not applicable.

CONFLICT OF INTEREST

The author declares no conflict of interest, financial or otherwise.

ACKNOWLEDGEMENT

Declared none.

REFERENCES

[1] Blanco Ramos M, Botana-Rial M, García-Fontán E, Fernández-Villar A, Gallas Torreira M. Update in the extraction of airway foreign bodies in adults. J Thorac Dis 2016; 8(11): 3452-56. [http://dx.doi.org/10.21037/jtd.2016.11.32] [PMID: 28066626]

[2] Mahajan AK, Khandhar SJ. Successful bronchoscopic removal of a chicken bone lodged in airway for 4-years. Am J Respir Crit Care Med 2016; 194(7): e8-9.

[http://dx.doi.org/10.1164/rccm.201603-0637IM] [PMID: 27315452]

Case 47

Whole Lung Lavage for PAP

Whole Lung Lavage for Pulmonary Alveolar Proteinosis

Mohamed Faisal Abdul Hamid[1,*] and **Khairulamir Zainuddin**[2]

[1] *Respiratory Unit, Faculty of Medicine, National University of Malaysia, Selangor, Malaysia*

[2]*Anesthesiology Department, KPJ Selangor Specialist Hospital, Malaysia*

Keywords: Bronchoscopy, Crazy-paving, Diffuse parenchymal lung disease, Double-lumen tube, Pulmonary alveolar proteinosis, Whole lung lavage.

Presentation

A 41-year-old female presented in February 2011 with a 3-month history of cough and progressive shortness of breath on exertion. She was treated as asthma but there was no response to inhaled budesonide/for moterol. She had a history of recurrent pneumonia and required bilevel positive airway pressure (BiPAP) 6 months before the clinic review.

Physical examination revealed her oxygen saturation was 93% on room air. Chest examination revealed fine crepitations over right mid-lower zone with reduced air entry. There was no loud P2. Other systemic examinations were normal.

Comorbidities

None.

Chest Imaging

A CXR showed bilateral pulmonary reticulation (Fig. **1a**). CECT thorax showed bilateral pulmonary infiltrates and thickened interlobular septa ("crazy paving" pattern) (Fig. **1b**).

Bronchoscopy revealed normal airways and bronchoalveolar lavage shows plaques of granular amphophilic in a background containing numerous bronchial lining cells, alveolar macrophages, and occasional squamous cells. Subsequent VATS biopsy confirmed pulmonary alveolar proteinosis (PAP).

[*]**Corresponding author Mohamed Faisal Abdul Hamid:** Respiratory Unit, Faculty of Medicine, National University of Malaysia, Selangor, Malaysia; E-mail: faisal.hamid@ppukm.ukm.edu.my

Jamalul Azizi Abdul Rahaman & Tinku Joseph (Eds.)

General respiratory function test showed a severe restrictive ventilatory defect with total lung capacity (TLC) of 1.42L (38.8% predicted), forced vital capacity (FVC) 1.67L (63.4% predicted) and residual volume (RV) of 0.16L (14% predicted). DLCO (corrected for haemoglobin) was 1.06mL/min/mmHg (18% predicted).

Intervention

She required whole lung lavage (WLL) with saline solution in March 2012 (left lung 11.5L; right lung 13L), December 2012 (left lung 9L), March 2014 (left lung 13L; right lung 11L), and July 2019 (left lung 6L; right lung 6L). Steps for WLL are summarised below as well as in the video.

1. Generous pre-oxygenation before induction with general anesthesia.
2. Insertion of double lumen tube (DLT). Tracheal and bronchial balloons are inflated to isolate the lung.
3. Auscultation to confirm placement of DLT and lung isolation.
4. Confirmation of DLT placement with fiberoptic bronchoscope (FOB).
5. Insertion of Y-connecter connecting the DLT to the fluid and drainage system (Figs. **2a** and **b**).
6. Single lung ventilation applied while large volume lavages (warmed normal saline in 1L aliquots) are instilled into the non-ventilated lung while the patient in reverse Trendelenburg position.
7. After 1L of normal saline fluid instilled, the inflow tubing is clamped, positioning is changed to Trendelenburg position to help drain the lavaged fluid with application of low pressure wall suction.
8. Physiotherapy (chest percussion) and vibration during the procedure are done to improve the efficiency of the lung lavage for 4-5 minutes.
9. Once outflow diminishes, the outflow tract is clamped and steps 6-8 are repeated until the effluent becomes clear with careful monitoring of the fluid balance.
10. Once the procedure is done, DLT is changed to a single lumen tube and the patient ventilated in intensive care unit (ICU).

Complications

None

Post-Intervention

After each procedure, she was ventilated in ICU for a few hours for lung recruitment. After a few hours in ICU, she was extubated and discharged to the ward. A repeat WLL was done on the opposite lung a week later. She had a marked ventilatory and radiological improvement after each WLL (Fig. **3**). To date, she remains asymptomatic. Her latest lung function in 2019 showed FVC of 1.94L (72%) and DLCO (corrected for haemoglobin) was 14.3mL/min/mmHg (72% predicted).

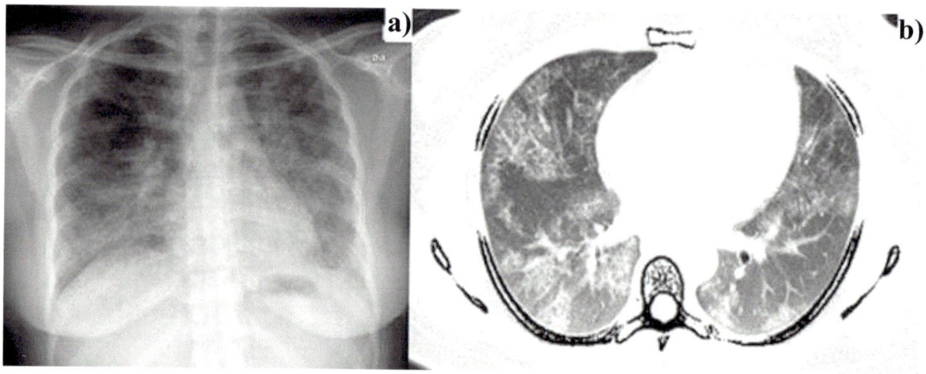

Fig. (1). Initial CXR (**a**) showed bilateral pulmonary infiltrates. Axial CT Thorax (**b**) showed bilateral pulmonary infiltrates and thickened interlobular septa, "crazy paving" pattern.

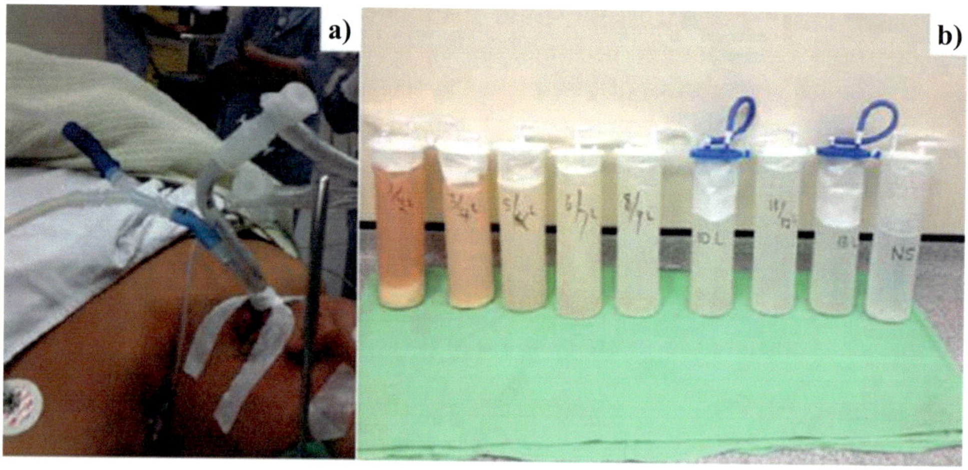

Fig. (2). Y-connector (**a**) inserted to connect the DLT to the fluid and drainage system. Effluents which were cloudy initially became clearer after 13L of warm saline instillation (**b**).

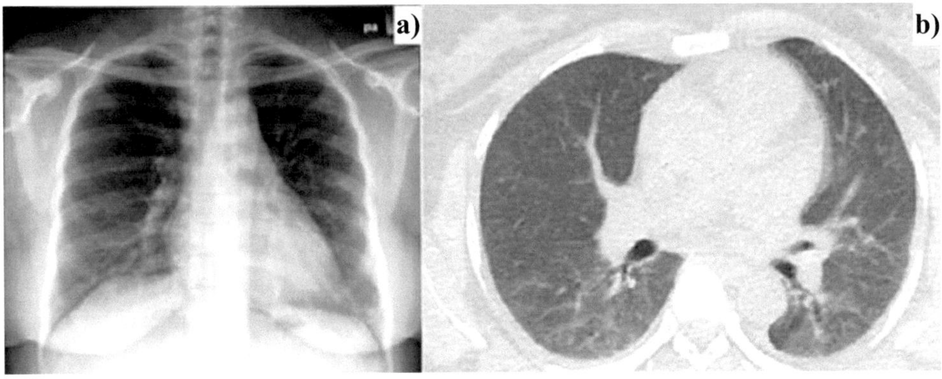

Fig. (3). Latest CXR (**a**) showed marked improvement of the pulmonary infiltrates. Axial CT Thorax (**b**) showed residual reticular opacities at the lower lobes.

Learning Points

- PAP is a form of diffuse parenchymal lung disease where there is accumulation of a surfactant in the alveoli consisting of a mixture of proteins and lipid resulting from mutations in surfactant proteins or granulocyte macrophage-colony stimulating factor (GM-CSF) receptor genes [1]. PAP may be congenital, primary (autoimmune) or secondary (*e.g.*, haematological disorders, inhalational disorders) [2]. The main treatment of PAP is WLL [1, 2]. For patients who cannot undergo WLL, do not respond to WLL or in centres without facilities for WLL, recombinant granulocyte macrophage-colony stimulating factor (GM-CSF, sargramostim) may be an alternative. Other therapies *e.g.*, Rituximab and plasmapheresis have been tried for resistant cases but are still under investigation and need further evidence.

Video

A step-by-step approach to perform whole lung lavage in PAP.

CONSENT FOR PUBLICATION

Not applicable.

CONFLICT OF INTEREST

The author declares no conflict of interest, financial or otherwise.

ACKNOWLEDGEMENT

Declared none.

REFERENCES

[1] Borie R, Danel C, Debray MP, *et al.* Pulmonary alveolar proteinosis. Eur Respir Rev 2011; 20(120): 98-107.
[http://dx.doi.org/10.1183/09059180.00001311] [PMID: 21632797]
[2] Suzuki T, Trapnell BC. Pulmonary alveolar proteinosis syndrome. Clin Chest Med 2016; 37(3): 431-40.
[http://dx.doi.org/10.1016/j.ccm.2016.04.006] [PMID: 27514590]

Case 48

A Case of Pulmonary Alveolar Proteinosis with Good Response to Whole Lung Lavage

Sameer Arbat[1,*]

[1] *One Healthcare, Nagpur, India*

Keywords: Bronchoscopic washing, Crazy paving pattern, Interventional pulmonology, Whole lung lavage, Pulmonary alveolar proteinosis.

Presentation

A 22-year-old male presented with dyspnoea and was noted to have hypoxia on examination.

Comorbidities

None.

Chest Imaging

HRCT thorax showed extensive areas of interlobar septal thickening along with ground glass opacities (GGO) giving rise to a crazy paving appearance in all lobes of both lungs (Fig. **1**).

Intervention

A whole lung lavage (WLL) of the left lung was performed under general anaesthesia with double lumen endotracheal tube. 6.8L of saline was infused in 9 cycles with approximately 5.4L recovered from the left lung. The lavage recovered showed turbid milky appearance characteristic of pulmonary alveolar proteinosis (PAP) with sequential collection showing decreased viscosity and protein sediments (Fig. **2**). Each cycle included 5 minutes of chest physiotherapy followed by drainage of fluid.

[*]**Corresponding author Sameer Arbat:** One Healthcare, Nagpur, India; E-mail: Dr.sameerarbat@gmail.com

Jamalul Azizi Abdul Rahaman & Tinku Joseph (Eds.)

Complications

None.

Post-Intervention

Repeat CXR showed significant resolution of the left lung GGO and the patient was discharged with substantial relief in dyspnoea (Fig. **3**). However, he was lost to follow-up and did not undergo WLL for the right lung.

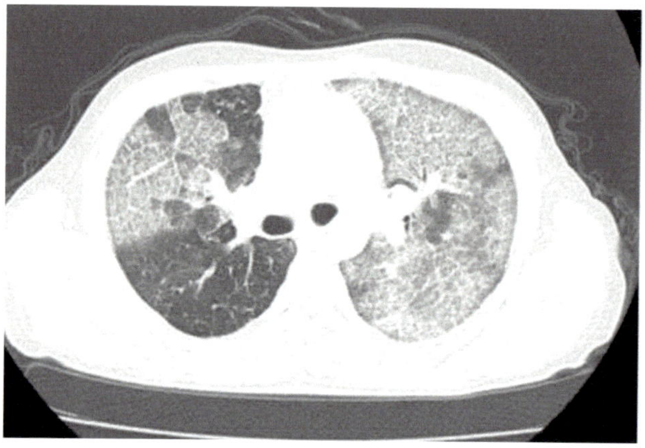

Fig. (1). Axial HRCT thorax showing extensive areas of interlobar septal thickening along with ground glass opacities giving a crazy paving appearance in all lobes of both lungs.

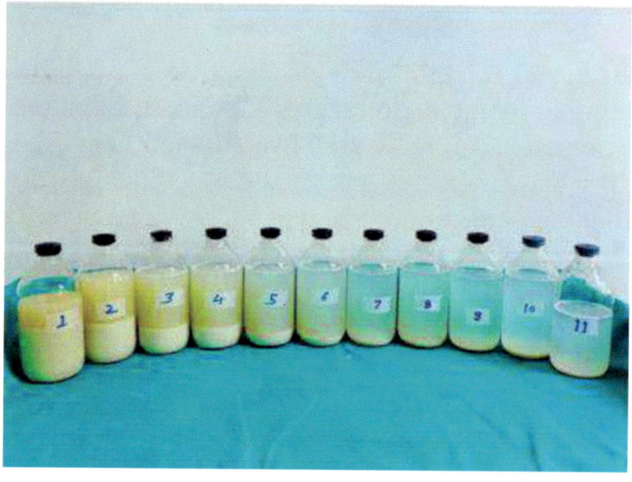

Fig. (2). Sequential collection of lavages showing decreased viscosity and protein sediments.

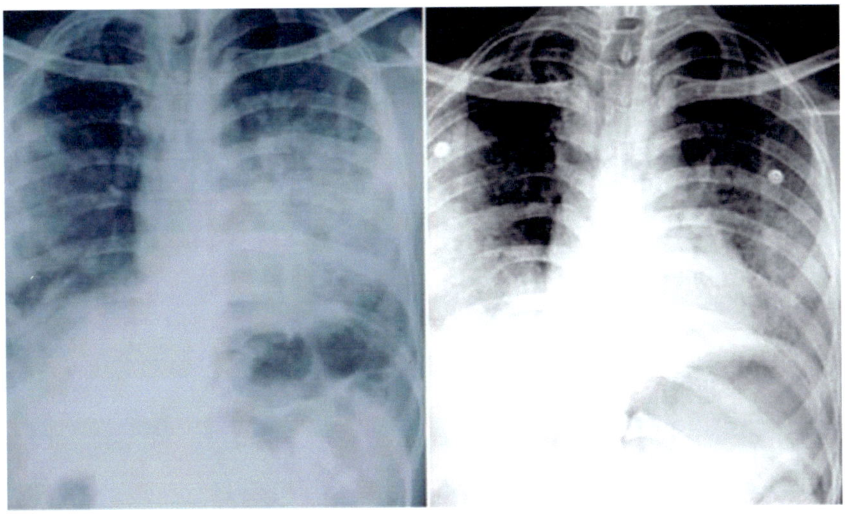

Fig. (3). CXR pre and post whole lung lavage of the left lung.

Learning Points

- WLL is an effective therapeutic procedure in PAP and requires a multidisciplinary team of pulmonologists, anesthesiologists and chest physiotherapists. WLL is a safe procedure and is the current standard of care treatment for patients with PAP [1].

Video

The whole lung lavage procedure in this patient.

CONSENT FOR PUBLICATION

Not applicable.

CONFLICT OF INTEREST

The author declares no conflict of interest, financial or otherwise.

ACKNOWLEDGEMENT

Declared none.

REFERENCE

[1] Beccaria M, Luisetti M, Rodi G, *et al.* Long-term durable benefit after whole lung lavage in pulmonary alveolar proteinosis. Eur Respir J 2004; 23(4): 526-31. [http://dx.doi.org/10.1183/09031936.04.00102704] [PMID: 15083749]

Section C

Pleural Procedures

Case 1

Pleuroscopy

Pleuroscopy: A Step by Step Approach

Hema Yamini Ramarmuty[1,*]

[1] *Respiratory Department, Queen Elizabeth Hospital, Kota Kinabalu, Sabah, Malaysia*

Keywords: Complications, Contra-indications, Indication, Pleuroscopy, Steps.

Pleuroscopy (sometimes referred to as medical thoracoscopy) is a procedure performed to examine the pleura and obtain biopsies from the parietal pleura by introducing an endoscope into the pleural cavity under direct vision [1]. It is also used to perform therapeutic interventions within the pleural cavity [2].

Indications

Diagnostic

- Undiagnosed pleural effusions.
- Suspected malignant effusions: for biopsy, staging and additional tests to identify driver mutations.
- To obtain biopsies for MTB culture and histology in tuberculous pleural effusions.

Therapeutic

- Pleurodesis (talc poudrage).
- Drainage and mechanical adhesiolysis in complex parapneumonic effusions and empyema.

*Corresponding author Hema Yamini Ramarmuty: Respiratory Department, Queen Elizabeth Hospital, Kota Kinabalu, Sabah, Malaysia; E-mail: yamini8254@hotmail.com

Jamalul Azizi Abdul Rahaman & Tinku Joseph (Eds.)

Contraindications

Absolute Contraindications

Lack of pleural space due to:

- Advanced empyema or extensive adhesions.
- Pleural thickening of unknown aetiology.
- Suspected mesothelioma where the visceral and parietal surfaces are fused.
- Previous pleurodesis.

Relative Contraindications

- Inability to tolerate lateral decubitus position.
- Hemodynamic instability.
- Presence of severe, uncorrectable hypoxaemia despite oxygen therapy.
- Bleeding diathesis.
- Pulmonary arterial hypertension.
- Refractory cough.
- Reduced general health status with short expected survival.

Equipment

Pleuroscopy can be performed using non-disposable rigid, semi-rigid or flexible instruments.

- Rigid thoracoscope and rigid trocar, or
- Semirigid fiberoptic video pleuroscope and flexible disposable trocar, or
- Flexible fiberoptic bronchoscope and flexible disposable trocar [3-5] (this is the practice in some hospitals in Malaysia).

Others

- Dressing set with sterile drapes
- Chlorhexidine solution/ Povidone Iodine
- Chest drain and underwater seal drainage system
- Normal Saline (NS) (0.9%) for flushing and drug dilution
- Forceps for dissection
- Scalpel
- 10-15ml Lignocaine 2%

Pre-Procedural Preparation and Patient Monitoring

1) Informed consent, pre-procedural blood workup.
2) Patient is instructed to fast 6-8 hours before the procedure.
3) A point of entry is chosen (Figs. **1a** and **b**).

- The patient is placed in the lateral decubitus position with the affected side facing up.
- A point of entry is then chosen under ultrasound guidance. In patients with minimal effusion, artificial pneumothorax can be created using various pneumothorax needles. However, a prerequisite for this is the presence of 'sliding sign' on USG.

4) Blood pressure, cardiac rhythm and oxygen saturation are monitored and recorded throughout the procedure.
5) Intravenous access obtained for the administration of sedatives and other drugs.
6) Nasal oxygen if required.

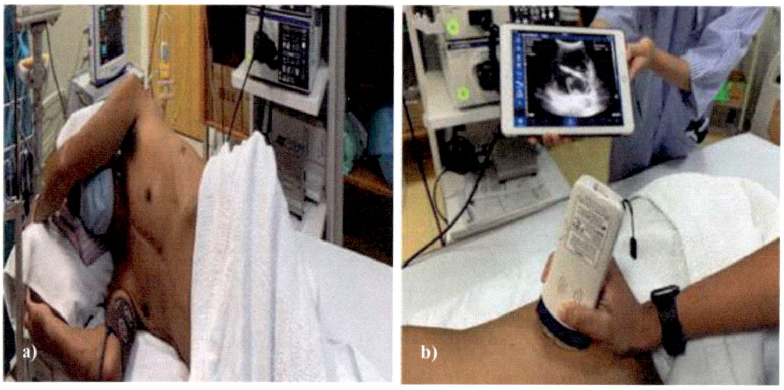

Fig. (1). (a) To choose a point of entry, patient is placed in a lateral decubitus position with affected side up. **(b)** USG performed to identify point of entry.

- Pleuroscopy is typically performed under 'conscious sedation' with the patient breathing spontaneously. Sedative drugs are titrated to provide the desired depth of sedation.
- Benzodiazepines: Intravenous midazolam is preferred as it has a rapid onset of action, easily reversible and is able to be titrated to provide desired depth of sedation.
- Opioid: Intravenous fentanyl, a short acting analgesic is given in combination with midazolam.

- Others: Propofol has a similar efficacy to midazolam. However, due to its narrow therapeutic index it should only be administered by those who are formally trained in its administration (*e.g.*, anaesthetists).

Steps

1) Patient is placed in the lateral decubitus position with the affected side up.
2) Predetermined point of entry cleaned and draped using sterile precautions (Figs. **2a** and **b**).

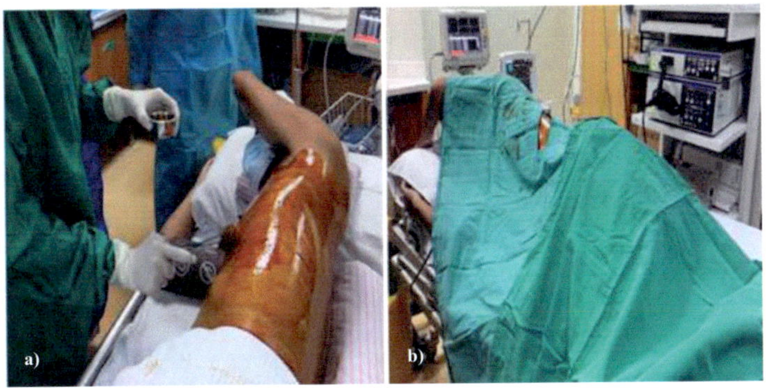

Fig. (2). (a) Predetermined area cleaned with povidone iodine. **(b)** Surgical drapes are used to maintain a sterile field.

3) Local Anesthesia (LA) is administered at the skin and further infiltrated in a perpendicular fashion into the subcutaneous tissue, intercostal muscles down to the parietal pleura (passing through the upper border of the lower rib) (Figs. **3a** and **b**) to ensure that the tip of the needle is not within a vessel, aspiration is performed before infiltration of lignocaine.

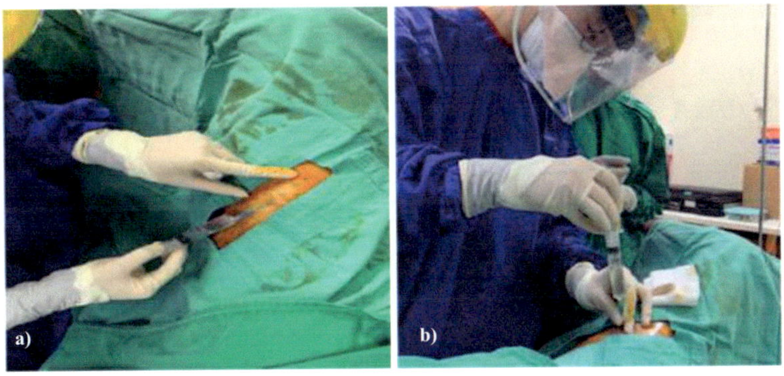

Fig. (3). (a) LA is administrated at the skin and subcutaneous tissue. **(b)** The LA is infiltrated in to the subcutaneous tissue, intercostal muscles down to the parietal pleura.

4) Once adequate anaesthesia is given, a 1-2cm skin incision is made at the selected intercostal space parallel to the rib (Fig. **4a**).
5) Blunt dissection of deeper tissues using forceps is performed till the pleural cavity is reached (Fig. **4b**).

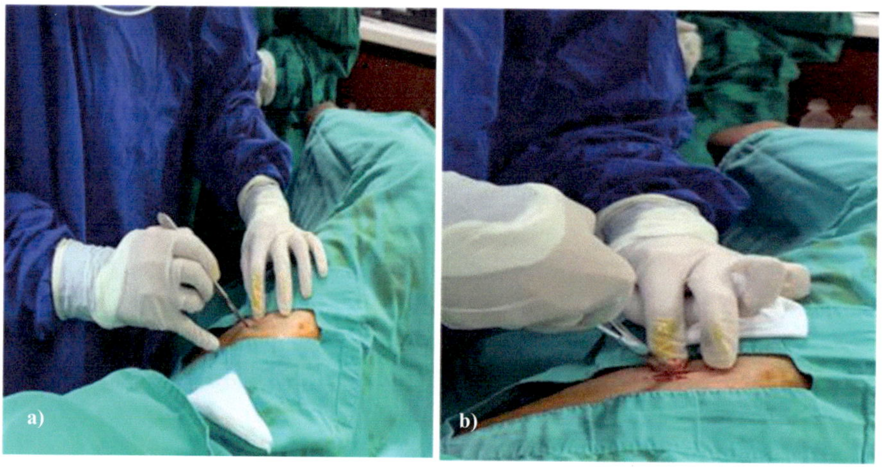

Fig. (4). (a) An incision is made with the scalpel through the skin and subcutaneous tissue. **(b)** Blunt dissection of the deeper tissues performed with forceps.

6) A trocar is then inserted in a corkscrew motion through the tract created by blunt dissection. The trocar is held using the palm with the index finger extended to limit the depth of insertion required to safely reach the pleural cavity (Fig. **5a**). The trocar is subsequently removed leaving the outer cannula within the pleural cavity.
7) The pleuroscope is then advanced under direct vision through the cannula into the pleural cavity (Figs. **5b** and **c**).

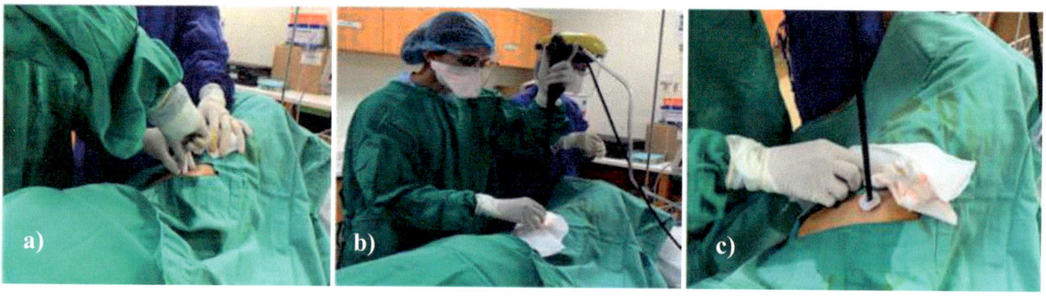

Fig. (5). (a) A flexible disposable trocar is inserted into the pleural cavity. (**b** and **c**) The semirigid pleuroscope is introduced through the outer cannula.

8) Once the pleural cavity is reached, pleural fluid is drained if present (Fig. **6a**).
9) A thorough examination of the pleural cavity is performed using the pleuroscope (Fig. **6b**).
10) Multiple biopsies (2-6 biopsies) are obtained from mainly the parietal pleura under direct vision (Fig. **6c**). Specimens are sent for histopathological examination and MTB culture (Fig. **6d**).

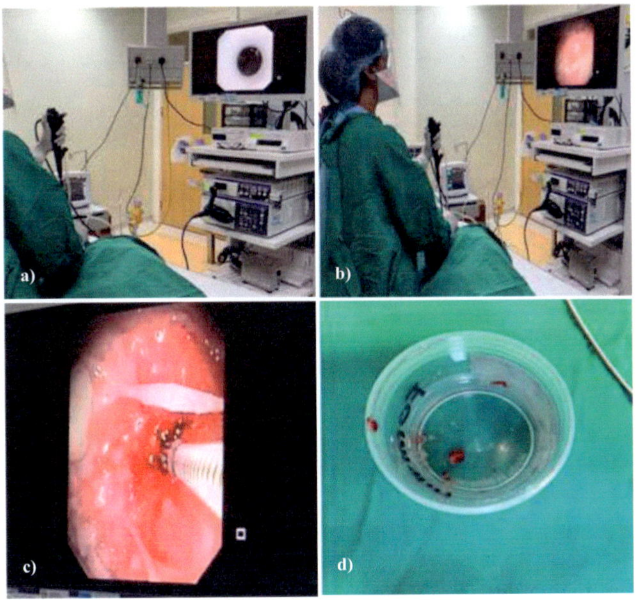

Fig. (6). **(a)** Pleural cavity is entered through the cannula under direct vision. **(b)** Pleural cavity is examined. **(c)** Biopsies obtained from the parietal pleura using flexible biopsy forceps. **(d)** Biopsy specimens were seen within the specimen pot.

11) If the patient is eligible for thoracoscopic talc poudrage, pleural fluid is drained completely after inspection. Talc insufflation is performed through a catheter placed at the working channel of the pleuroscope. The catheter is connected to a bottle containing talc and the talc is instilled into the pleural cavity. Uniform distribution of the talc can be confirmed through the endoscopic view.
12) At the end of the procedure, a chest drain (16-24Fr) is inserted to drain residual fluid or air, allowing the lung to re-expand. In cases where talc poudrage is performed, negative pressure suction (5 to 20cm H_2O) is applied.

Potential Complications

- Allergic reaction to sedatives/LA
- Pain
- Hypoxaemia

- Cardiac arrhythmia
- Hypotension
- Bleeding
- Injury to the lung and other organs
- Re-expansion pulmonary edema
- Subcutaneous emphysema
- Prolonged air leak
- Empyema
- Complications related to talc poudrage
- Seeding of chest wall by tumour cells in mesothelioma

CONSENT FOR PUBLICATION

Not applicable.

CONFLICT OF INTEREST

The author declares no conflict of interest, financial or otherwise.

ACKNOWLEDGEMENT

Declared none.

REFERENCES

[1] Ali MS, Light RW, Maldonado F. Pleuroscopy or video-assisted thoracoscopic surgery for exudative pleural effusion: a comparative overview. J Thorac Dis 2019; 11(7): 3207-16. [http://dx.doi.org/10.21037/jtd.2019.03.86] [PMID: 31463153]

[2] Loddenkemper R, Lee P, Noppen M, Mathur PN. Medical thoracoscopy/ pleuroscopy: step by step. Breathe 2011; 8: 156-67. [http://dx.doi.org/10.1183/20734735.011611]

[3] Yokoyama T, Toda R, Tomioka R, Aizawa H. Medical thoracoscopy performed using a flexible bronchoscope inserted through a chest tube under local anesthesia. Diagn Ther Endosc 2009; 2009: 1-4. [http://dx.doi.org/10.1155/2009/394817] [PMID: 19536345]

[4] Senno A, Moallem S, Quijano ER, Adeyemo A, Clauss RH. Thoracoscopy with the fiberoptic bronchoscope. J Thorac Cardiovasc Surg 1974; 67(4): 606-11. [http://dx.doi.org/10.1016/S0022-5223(19)40495-9] [PMID: 4818537]

[5] Williams T, Thomas P. The diagnosis of pleural effusions by fiberoptic bronchoscopy and pleuroscopy. Chest 1981; 80(5): 566-9. [http://dx.doi.org/10.1378/chest.80.5.566] [PMID: 7297147]

Case 2

Pleuroscopic Adhesiolysis for Complex Pleural Effusion

Kho Sze Shyang[1,2,*] and **Tie Siew Teck**[1]

[1] *Division of Respiratory Medicine, Sarawak General Hospital, Kuching, Malaysia*

[2] *Department of Pulmonology, Serdang Hospital, Selangor, Malaysia*

Keywords: Adhesiolysis, Complex pleural effusion, Medical thoracoscopy, Pleuroscopy, Therapeutic pleuroscopy.

Presentation

An 18-year-old man presented with a two-week history of fever and right pleuritic chest pain. No close TB contacts. The patient was febrile with a temperature of 39°C, reduced air entry and dullness to percussion over the right hemithorax. Total white cell on admission was 13.16×10^9/l.

Comorbidities

None.

Chest Imaging

Plain CXR demonstrated right pleural effusion (Fig. **1**). Transthoracic ultrasound over the right hemithorax confirmed complex right pleural collection with multiple fibrin strands and echogenic pleural fluid (Fig. **2**). Diagnostic thoracocentesis showed dark amber colored fluid with pleural fluid (Pf) pH of 7.231, Pf protein of 62 g/dl, Pf lactate dehydrogenase of 6024 U/l and Pf glucose of 3.8 mmol/l. Sputum direct smear for AFB was negative.

Intervention

Under conscious sedation (intravenous bolus of pethidine and midazolam), the pleural cavity was exposed with an 8mm flexible trocar (MAJ-1058, Olympus,

*Corresponding author **Kho Sze Shyang:** Division of Respiratory Medicine, Sarawak General Hospital, Kuching, Malaysia; E-mail: khosze@moh.gov.my

Jamalul Azizi Abdul Rahaman & Tinku Joseph (Eds.)

Japan) after blunt dissection. Upon entry into the pleural space with a semi-rigid pleuroscope (LTF-160, Olympus, Japan), the pleural space was severely restricted by dense adhesions which limited exploration and examination. Adhesions and fibrin strands were carefully separated and removed with a flexible forceps. Locules of fluid and fibrinopurulent materials were aspirated and sent for microbiological analysis (Fig. **3**). Upon completion of the procedure, the right lung was freed from adhesions from the parietal pleura and was expandable under direct visualization. Visualized parietal and visceral pleurae were severely thickened and inflamed. Total procedure time was 90 minutes.

Complications

Post-procedure, the patient was put on thoracic suction at -15m H_2O to aid lung expansion, no prolonged air leak was encountered. Intercostal chest tube was removed uneventfully after 48 hours of minimal drainage with adequate lung expansion. Repeat transthoracic ultrasound and CXR revealed minimal residual organized pleural collection at dependent area with pleural thickening (Fig. **4**).

Post-Intervention

HPE of the pleural tissue showed chronic necrotizing granulomatous inflammation highly suggestive of pleural TB. Pleural fluid and tissue culture were negative for Mycobacterium tuberculosis. The patient was initiated on standard anti-TB therapy and responded well with only minimal residual pleural thickening.

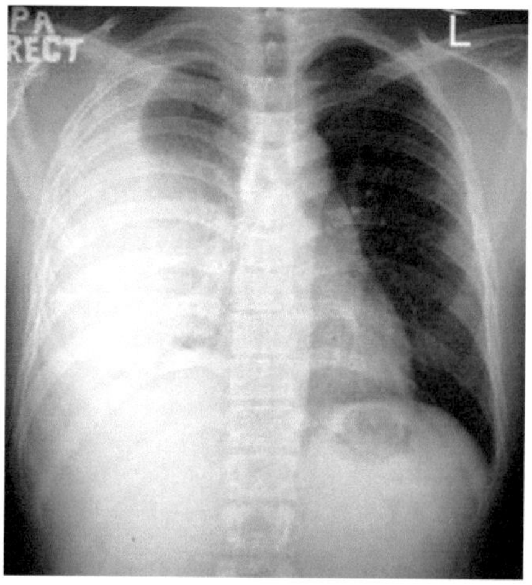

Fig. (1). Massive loculated pleural effusion on plain CXR upon presentation.

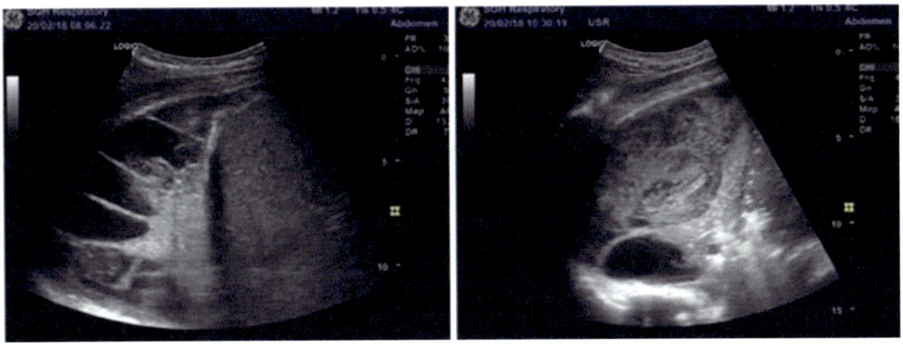

Fig. (2). Multiple fibrins and septation seen on transthoracic ultrasound, along with complex hyperechoic pleural fluid.

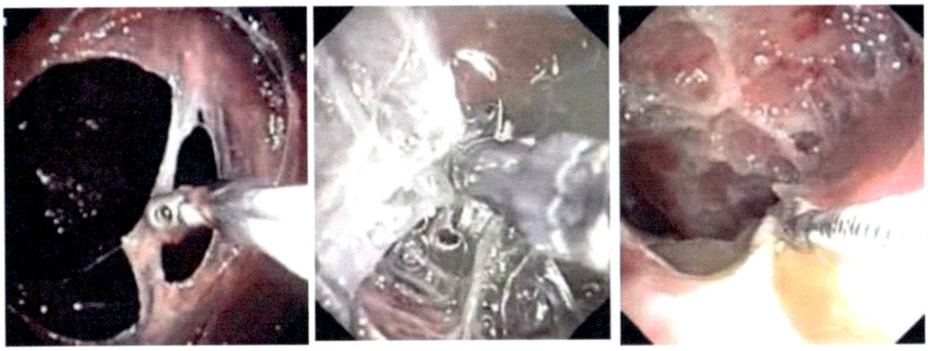

Fig. (3). Adhesions and fibrin strands were carefully separated and removed using flexible forceps while avoiding the visceral pleura. Locules of fluid and fibrinopurulent materials were aspirated and sent for microbiological analysis.

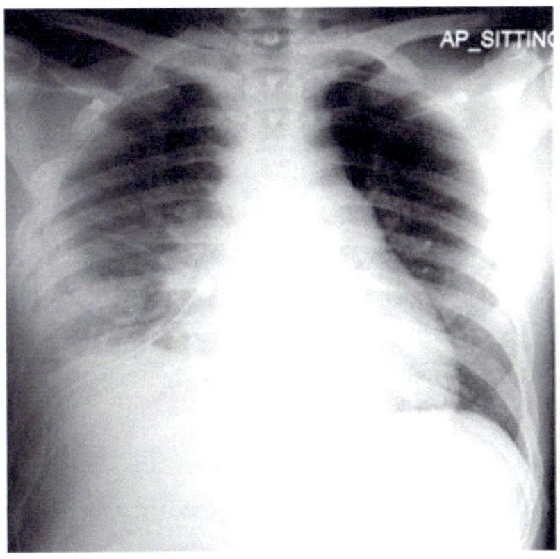

Fig. (4). Post-procedure CXR showed right lung aeration with pleural thickening.

Learning Points

- Pleuroscopic adhesiolysis maybe a feasible option when dealing with complex pleural effusion. In a randomized control trial comparing intrapleural fibrinolytic therapy *versus* pleuroscopy for treatment of pleural infection, patients who underwent pleuroscopy had shorter hospital stay compared with patients who received intrapleural fibrinolytic therapy [1]. Further studies to confirm its efficacy in comparison to standard of care (intrapleural fibrinolytic) are warranted.

Video

Adhesiolysis using flexible forceps during pleuroscopy.

CONSENT FOR PUBLICATION

Not applicable.

CONFLICT OF INTEREST

The author declares no conflict of interest, financial or otherwise.

ACKNOWLEDGEMENT

Declared none.

REFERENCE

[1] Kheir F, Thakore S, Mehta H, *et al*. Intrapleural fibrinolytic therapy versus early medical thoracoscopy for treatment of pleural infection: randomized clinical trial. Ann Am Thorac Soc 2020; 17(8): 958-64.
[http://dx.doi.org/10.1513/AnnalsATS.202001-076OC] [PMID: 32421353]

Case 3

Pleuroscopy in Malignant Effusion. Is Pleural Fluid Cytology Enough?

Hema Yamini Ramarmuty[1,*]

[1] *Respiratory Department, Queen Elizabeth Hospital, Kota Kinabalu, Sabah, Malaysia*

Keywords: Malignancy, Pleuroscopy, Pleural fluid cytology, Pleural biopsy, Thoracentesis.

Presentation

A 52-year-old, gentleman presented with a 2-month history of pleuritic chest pain, cough and breathlessness on exertion. He reported a weight loss of 5kg in 2 months. No family history of malignancy.

Comorbidities

The patient was an ex-smoker with a 10 pack-year smoking history. He had hypertension, for which he was under a district hospital follow-up. His ECOG (Eastern Cooperative Oncology Group) performance status was 1.

Chest Imaging

CXR revealed a large pleural effusion, occupying the left hemithorax (Fig. **1**). There multiple nodules of varying sizes seen bilaterally. USG thorax confirmed the presence of a large left pleural effusion. USG-guided thoracentesis revealed a straw-coloured, exudative pleural fluid. Pleural fluid gram stain and cultures were negative. Pleural fluid cytology showed atypical cells suspicious of malignancy but was inadequate for further analysis.

Intervention

We performed a pleuroscopic examination under conscious sedation (Fentanyl and Midazolam) using an Olympus LTF 160, semirigid pleuroscope. Once adequate local anaesthesia was given, a 1-2 cm skin incision was made in the middle of the

*Corresponding author Hema Yamini Ramarmuty: Respiratory Department, Queen Elizabeth Hospital, Kota Kinabalu, Sabah, Malaysia; E-mail: yamini8254@hotmail.com

Jamalul Azizi Abdul Rahaman & Tinku Joseph (Eds.)

selected intercostal space (parallel to the rib). Blunt dissection using artery forceps was performed till the pleural cavity was reached. A disposable 8mm flexible trocar was then inserted in a corkscrew motion through the tract created by the blunt dissection. The trocar was removed leaving the outer cannula. The semirigid pleuroscope was advanced under direct vision through the cannula into the pleural cavity.

Upon entering the pleural cavity, 1.6L of straw-coloured pleural fluid was drained. (Fig. **2a**). Whitish plaques were seen throughout the parietal pleura (Fig. **2b**). Collapsed left lung with anthracotic pigmentation was visualized on the visceral pleura. Random biopsies using flexible forceps were taken from the parietal pleura (Fig. **2c**). Specimens were sent for HPE.

An 18F chest tube was inserted after the procedure and was connected to underwater seal drainage. Talc pleurodesis was performed through the chest drain prior to discharge.

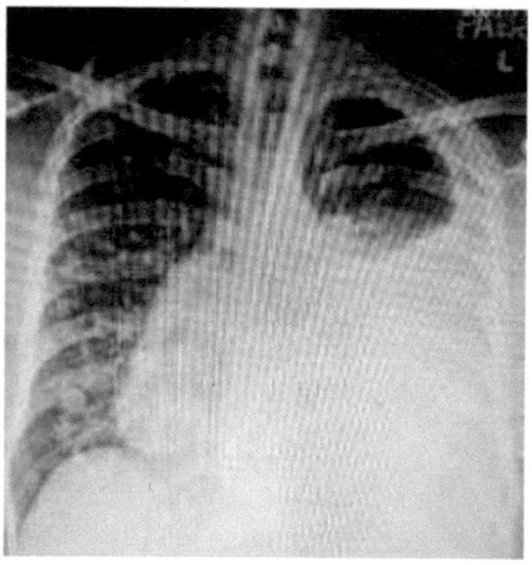

Fig. (1). CXR shows left pleural effusion and nodular infiltrates on bilateral lung fields.

Complications

There were no procedure-related adverse effects.

Post-Intervention

CXR post-pleuroscopy revealed a left hilar mass (Fig. **3**). He underwent a CECT thorax post-pleuroscopy for staging purposes and this revealed a left hilar mass with a left pleural effusion (Fig. **4**). There were also multiple lung nodules, mediastinal lymphadenopathy, liver lesions and lytic bone lesions suggestive of metastases.

HPE revealed metastatic adenocarcinoma (Figs. **5a-c**). No EGFR mutation was detected. He was diagnosed with stage IV lung adenocarcinoma and was subsequently referred to the oncologist.

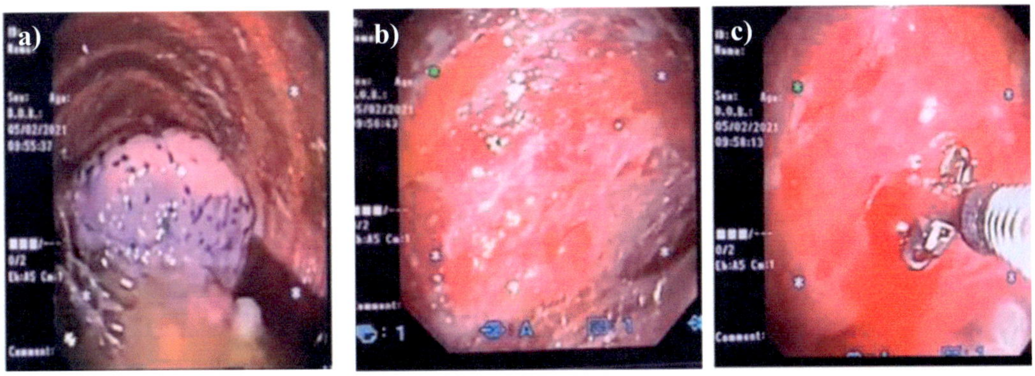

Fig. (2). (a) Upon entering the pleural cavity, atelectatic lung visualized, visceral pleura not thickened. **(b)** Whitish plaques were seen on the parietal pleura. **(c)** Flexible forceps was used to perform biopsies on the parietal pleura.

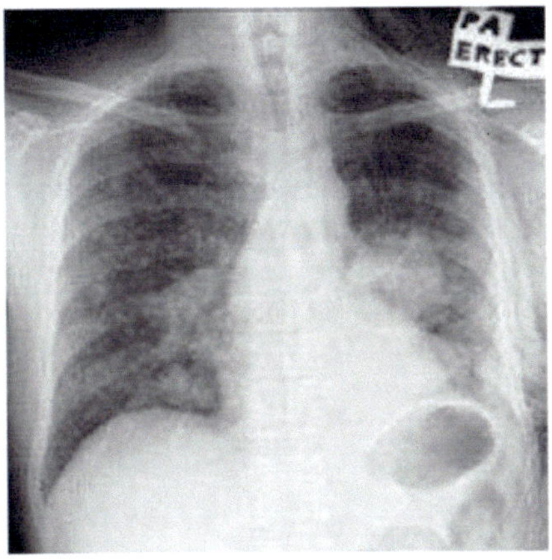

Fig. (3). CXR post-pleuroscopy revealed a left hilar mass.

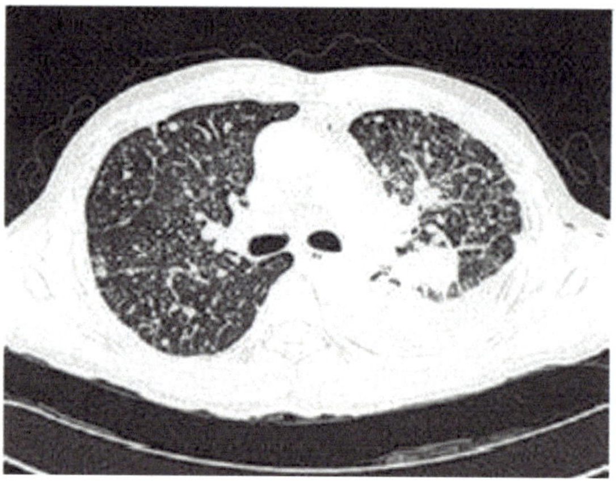

Fig. (4). Axial CT scan shows a left hilar mass, left pleural effusion and bilateral metastatic lung nodules.

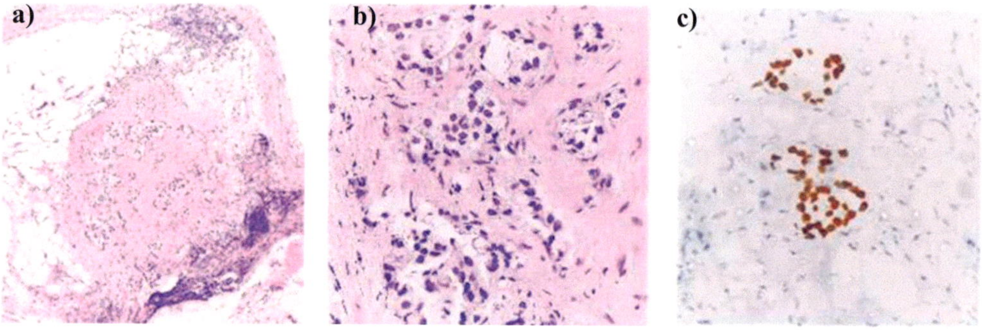

Fig. (5). (a) Histopathological examination (hematoxylin and eosin stain, x10 magnification) shows malignant cells forming irregular glandular pattern associated with desmoplastic stroma. **(b)** Histopathological examination (hematoxylin and eosin stain, x40 magnification) shows malignant cells forming irregular glandular pattern. They display pleomorphic vesicular to hyperchromatic nuclei, some with small conspicuous nucleoli, and moderate amount of cytoplasm. **(c)** The malignant glands are positive for TTF-1 immunohistochemical stain.

Learning Points

- In our patient, pleural fluid cytology showed atypical cells, suspicious of malignancy. However, it was insufficient for further analysis. The diagnostic rate for malignancy from pleural fluid cytology has been reported to have a mean sensitivity of about 60% (range 40–87%) [1]. Although closed pleural biopsy using Abrams needle is an option, the diagnostic rate is 57% for malignancy [1]. Furthermore, malignant deposits are usually seen close to the diaphragm and this area is avoided when a closed pleural biopsy is performed

[1]. Pleuroscopy is a safe procedure, with a 92.6% diagnostic sensitivity for malignant pleural disease [1]. In patients with suspected malignant effusion, pleuroscopy not only allows direct visualization of the parietal and visceral pleurae, but also facilitates drainage of pleural fluid and the performance of biopsies from the parietal pleura. Talc poudrage can also be performed during pleuroscopy to prevent recurrence in selected patients.

Video

The pleural cavity during pleuroscopy and the technique of taking a biopsy from the parietal pleura.

CONSENT FOR PUBLICATION

Not applicable.

CONFLICT OF INTEREST

The author declares no conflict of interest, financial or otherwise.

ACKNOWLEDGEMENTS

The author acknowledges the support received from Dr. Sugunah Sallapan, Department of Pathology, Queen Elizabeth Hospital, Kota Kinabalu, Sabah, Malaysia.

REFERENCE

[1] Hooper C, Lee YCG, Maskell N. Investigation of a unilateral pleural effusion in adults: British Thoracic Society pleural disease guideline 2010. Thorax 2010; 65(Suppl. 2): ii4-ii17. [http://dx.doi.org/10.1136/thx.2010.136978] [PMID: 20696692]

Case 4

'TB or Not TB?'- A Call for Pleuroscopy when Investigations are Not Confirmatory

Hema Yamini Ramarmuty[1,*]

[1] *Respiratory Department, Queen Elizabeth Hospital, Kota Kinabalu, Sabah, Malaysia*

Keywords: Pleuroscopy, Pleural fluid adenosine deaminase, Pleural biopsy, Thoracentesis, Tuberculosis.

Presentation

A 63-year-old gentleman presented with shortness of breath and dry cough for 1-month duration. He did not report any constitutional symptoms. No family history of malignancy.

Comorbidities

Hypertension and dyslipidemia. He is a non-smoker.

Chest Imaging

The CXR on admission showed blunting of bilateral costophrenic angle, with suspected bilateral pleural effusion (Fig. **1a**). Thoracic USG confirmed the presence of bilateral pleural effusion, with a larger effusion seen on the left side (Fig. **1b**). Diaphragm appeared irregular with an ill-defined nodule seen on its surface (Fig. **1c**).

USG-guided thoracentesis revealed a straw-coloured, exudative pleural fluid. Pleural fluid gram stain and cultures were negative. Pleural fluid ADA was 30 U/L and pleural fluid cytology showed lymphocyte predominance.

Intervention

We performed a pleuroscopic examination under conscious sedation (Fentanyl and Midazolam) using an Olympus LTF 160 semirigid pleuroscope. Once adequate

*Corresponding author Hema Yamini Ramarmuty:** Respiratory Department, Queen Elizabeth Hospital, Kota Kinabalu, Sabah, Malaysia; E-mail: yamini8254@hotmail.com

Jamalul Azizi Abdul Rahaman & Tinku Joseph (Eds.)

local anaesthesia was administered (optimal entry site predetermined by USG performed in a lateral decubitus position), a 1-2cm skin incision was made at the middle of the selected intercostal space (parallel to the rib). Blunt dissection using artery forceps was performed till the pleural cavity was reached. A disposable 8mm flexible trocar was then inserted in a corkscrew motion through the tract created by the blunt dissection. The trocar was removed leaving the outer cannula in. The semirigid pleuroscope was then advanced under direct vision through the cannula into the pleural cavity.

Upon entering the pleural cavity, 500ml straw-coloured pleural fluid was drained. The visceral pleura did not appear thickened. The lung was initially collapsed; however upon removing fluid, there was re-expansion of the lung. The parietal pleura was hyperaemic. There were multiple nodules of varying sizes, some of which appeared to be tiny 'sago like' nodules (Fig. **2a**). These nodules were not only seen at the posterior chest wall but also seen on the surface of the diaphragmatic pleura (Fig. **2b**).

Biopsies using flexible biopsy forceps were performed with a 'tearing motion', at the nodules on the parietal pleura (Fig. **2c**). Specimens were sent for histopathological analysis and Mycobacterium tuberculosis (MTB) culture. A 18F chest tube was inserted after the procedure and was connected to underwater seal drainage.

Complications

There were no procedure related adverse effects.

Post-Intervention

HPE revealed multiple granulomas associated with multinucleated giant cells and epithelioid histiocytes (Figs. **3a** and **b**). Caseous necrosis was also present. These findings were compatible with a diagnosis of TB pleuritis. The patient was prescribed anti-TB therapy.

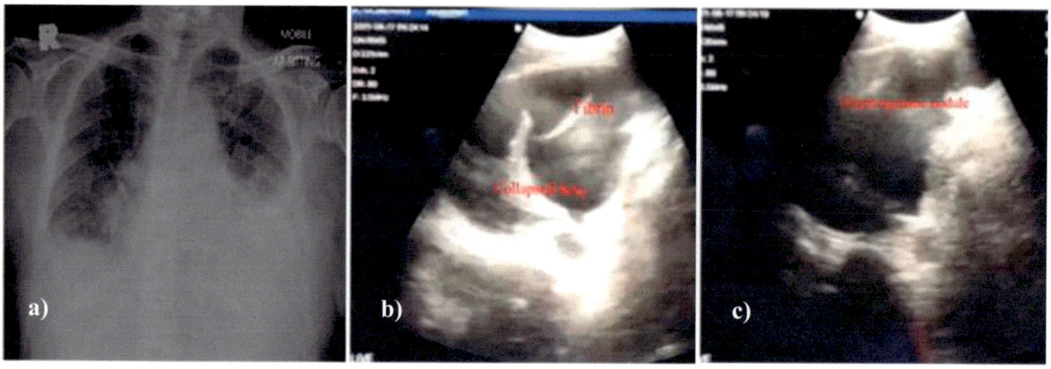

Fig. (1). (a) CXR shows bilateral pleural effusion, more on the left side. **(b)** USG examination of the left hemithorax demonstrates a large pleural effusion causing compressive atelectasis of adjacent lung. **(c)** Diaphragm appears irregular with an ill-defined nodule seen on its surface.

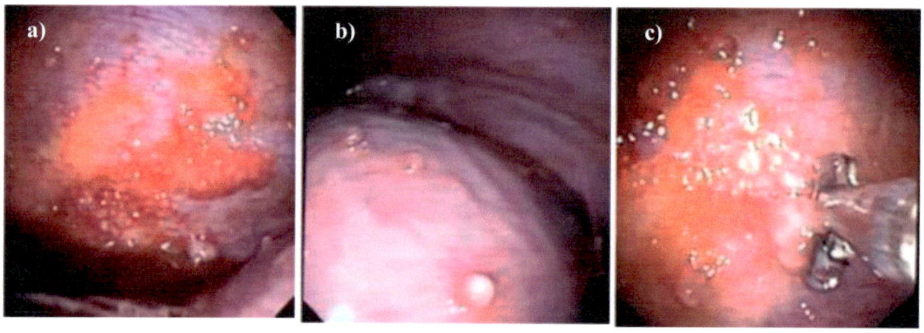

Fig. (2). (a) Multiple nodules seen on the parietal pleura**. (b)** Nodules seen on the diaphragmatic pleura. **(c)** Flexible biopsy forceps used to perform biopsies on the nodular surface of the parietal pleura.

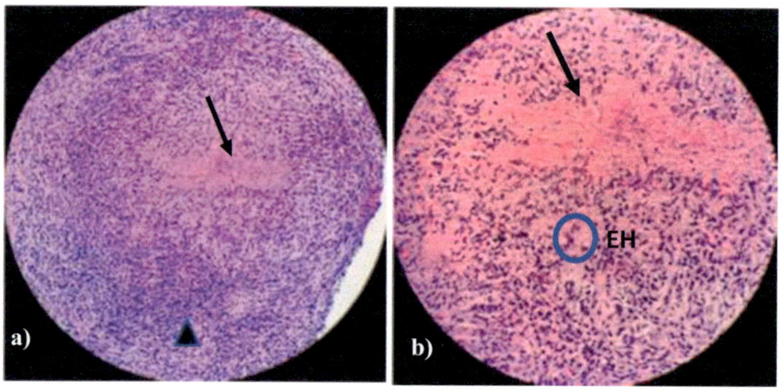

Fig. (3). (a) HPE (haematoxylin and eosin stain, x20 magnification) shows a background of dense lymphoplasmacytic infiltrates (arrowhead) associated with chronic granulomatous inflammation, epithelioid histiocytes and areas of necrosis (arrow). **(b)** HPE (haematoxylin and eosin stain, x40 magnification) demonstrates dense lymphoplasmacytic infiltrates associated with chronic granulomatous inflammation, epithelioid his tiocytes (EH) and areas of necrosis (arrow).

Learning Points

- TB pleuritis occurs due to the presence of TB antigen in the pleural space which results in a delayed hypersensitivity reaction mediated by CD4 cells. Pleural fluid microscopic examination for AFB is positive only in less than 5% of the cases [1]. Mycobacterial culture of pleural fluid has low sensitivity (24-58%) and is limited by a delay of several weeks in obtaining results [1]. This makes diagnosing TB pleuritis challenging.
- Pleural fluid adenosine deaminase (pfADA) is a useful biomarker that can be used as an adjunct in the diagnosis of pleural TB. Although a pfADA cut-off level of 40 U/L has been used to diagnose tuberculous pleural effusion, this value has been derived from overseas data. A single-centre, observational, prospective study of patients with exudative pleural effusion conducted at our centre established a local pfADA cut-off of 29.6 U/L for tuberculous pleural effusion [2].
- As this was an elderly gentleman with bilateral effusion (not typically seen in TB pleuritis) and a borderline pfADA, we decided to confirm the diagnosis by obtaining a pleural biopsy for histopathological analysis and MTB culture. Although closed pleural biopsy using an Abrams needle is an option in TB pleuritis (diagnostic yield 50-60%), we decided to perform a pleuroscopy as malignant effusion was a possible differential diagnosis in this gentleman. Common pleuroscopy findings in TB pleuritis include 'sago like' nodules or micronodules and adhesions.
- Larger and more precise biopsies can be obtained from abnormal areas under direct vision, thus improving the diagnostic yield. Pleuroscopy is an excellent tool to confirm the diagnosis of TB pleuritis in centres where it is available.

Video

Pleural USG demonstrating irregular diaphragm with an ill-defined nodule on its surface and the technique of taking a pleural biopsy of the nodules on the parietal pleura.

CONSENT FOR PUBLICATION

Not applicable.

CONFLICT OF INTEREST

The author declares no conflict of interest, financial or otherwise.

ACKNOWLEDGEMENTS

The author acknowledges the support received from Dr. Khor See Yee, Department of Pathology, Queen Elizabeth Hospital, Kota Kinabalu, Sabah, Malaysia.

REFERENCES

[1] Trajman A, Pai M, Dheda K, *et al.* Novel tests for diagnosing tuberculous pleural effusion: what works and what does not? Eur Respir J 2008; 31(5): 1098-106. [http://dx.doi.org/10.1183/09031936.00147507] [PMID: 18448504]

[2] Huan N-C, Khor IS, Ramarmuty HY, *et al.* Optimising the utility of pleural fluid adenosine deaminase for the diagnosis of tuberculous pleural effusion. Proceed Singapore Healthcare 2020; 30(4): 271-8.

Case 5

Flexi-Rigid Pleuroscope-Guided Cryobiopsy

Kho Sze Shyang[1,2,*], **Larry Ellee Nyanti**[3] and **Tie Siew Teck**[1]

[1] *Division of Respiratory Medicine, Sarawak General Hospital, Kuching, Malaysia*

[2] *Department of Pulmonology, Serdang Hospital, Selangor, Malaysia*

[3] *Medical Department, Faculty of Medicine and Health Sciences, Universiti Malaysia Sabah, Kota Kinabalu, Sabah, Malaysia*

Keywords: Cryobiopsy, Diagnostic pleuroscopy, Medical thoracoscopy, Pleuroscopy, Pleural effusion, Parietal pleura.

Presentation

A 69-year-old gentleman with two-month history of progressive shortness of breath and dry cough associated with loss of weight and appetite. No fever or hemoptysis. He was tachypneic at rest with oxygen saturation of 91% under room air.

Comorbidities

No known chronic medical illness. Previous smoker.

Chest Imaging

Plain CXR revealed right homogeneous opacity with meniscus sign and obliteration of the right heart border suggestive of pleural effusion (Fig. **1**). Transthoracic ultrasound thorax revealed a unilocular right pleural effusion with thickened parietal pleura.

Intervention

USG-guided thoracocentesis confirmed an exudative pleural effusion with atypical cells seen on cytological examination. Under conscious sedation, right pleural cavity was accessed *via* an 11mm metallic trocar after pneumothorax induction. Pleuroscopy was performed using flexi-rigid pleuroscope (LTF- 160, Olympus, Tokyo, Japan). Multiple hard pleural nodules were visualized around the parietal

*Corresponding author Kho Sze Shyang:** Division of Respiratory Medicine, Sarawak General Hospital, Kuching, Malaysia; E-mail: khosze@moh.gov.my pleura and right hemi-diaphragm which were difficult to be grasped with flexible forceps. Pleuroscopic cryobiopsy was then performed using the 950mm 2.4mm flexible cryoprobe (ERBE, Medizintechnik, Tübigen, Germany) through the working channel of the pleuroscope (Fig. **2**). The cryoprobe was activated for 4-5 seconds under direct vision and the specimen was removed by pulling out the cryoprobe and flexi-rigid scope en bloc through the metallic trocar (Fig. **3**).

Complications

No bleeding was observed after a total of 4 cryo activations. The patient did not complain of pain and no bleeding was encountered post-procedure.

Post-Intervention

Post-pleuroscopic cryobiopsy CXR shows adequate lung expansion with parietal pleural thickening (Fig. **4**). Talc pleurodesis was performed post-procedure and the intercostal chest tube was removed after 48 hours uneventfully. Histopathological and immunohistochemical examination confirmed malignant mesothelioma with a biopsy specimen adequately showing malignant cells infiltrating the extrapleural adipose tissue (Fig. **5**). Immunohistochemical staining was positive for calretinin and showed nuclear positivity to BAP- 1 (BRCA-1 associated protein). The patient was subsequently referred to the oncologist for systemic chemotherapy.

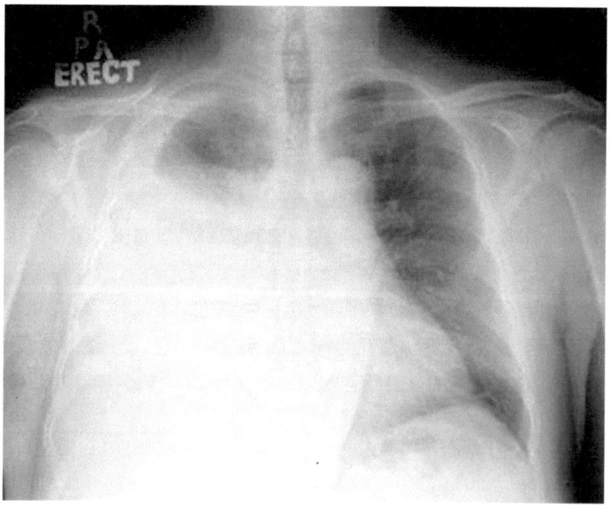

Fig. (1). Massive right pleural effusion with meniscus sign on plain CXR.

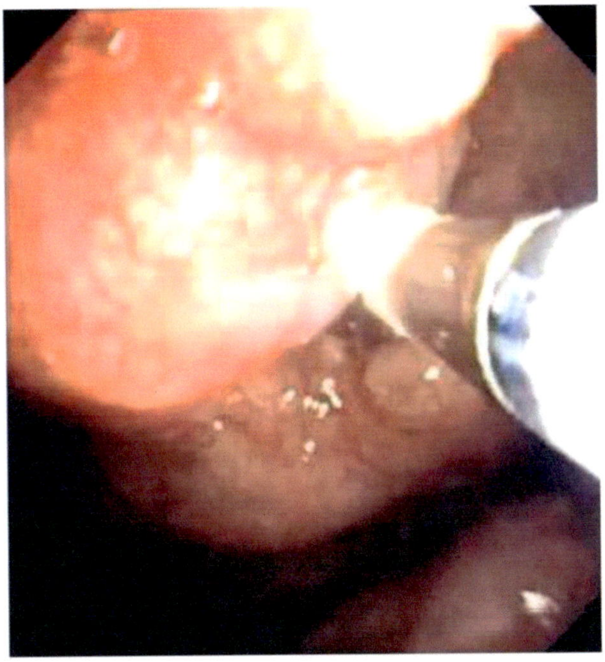

Fig. (2). 950mm 2.4mm flexible cryoprobe activated over the hardened parietal pleural nodule.

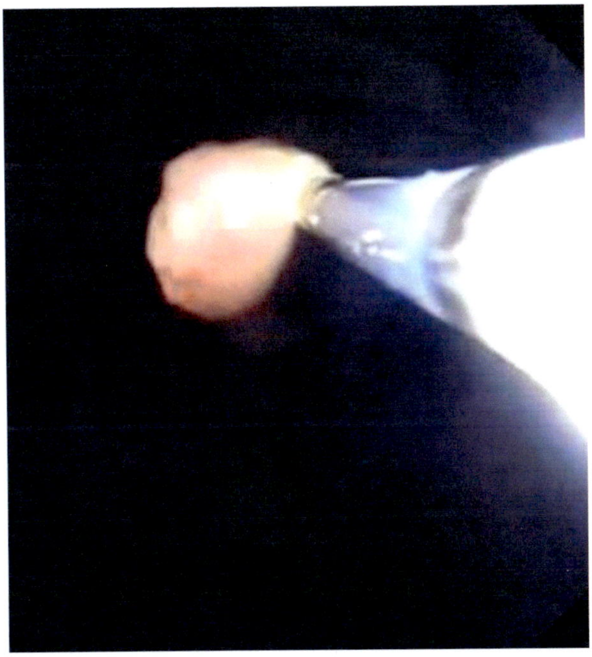

Fig. (3). Biopsy specimen was extracted by pulling out the pleuroscope and cryoprobe en bloc.

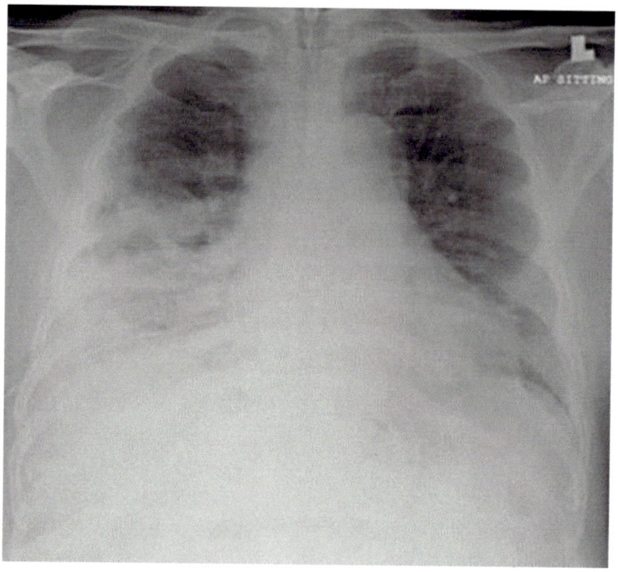

Fig. (4). Post-pleuroscopic cryobiopsy CXR shows adequate lung expansion with parietal pleural thickening.

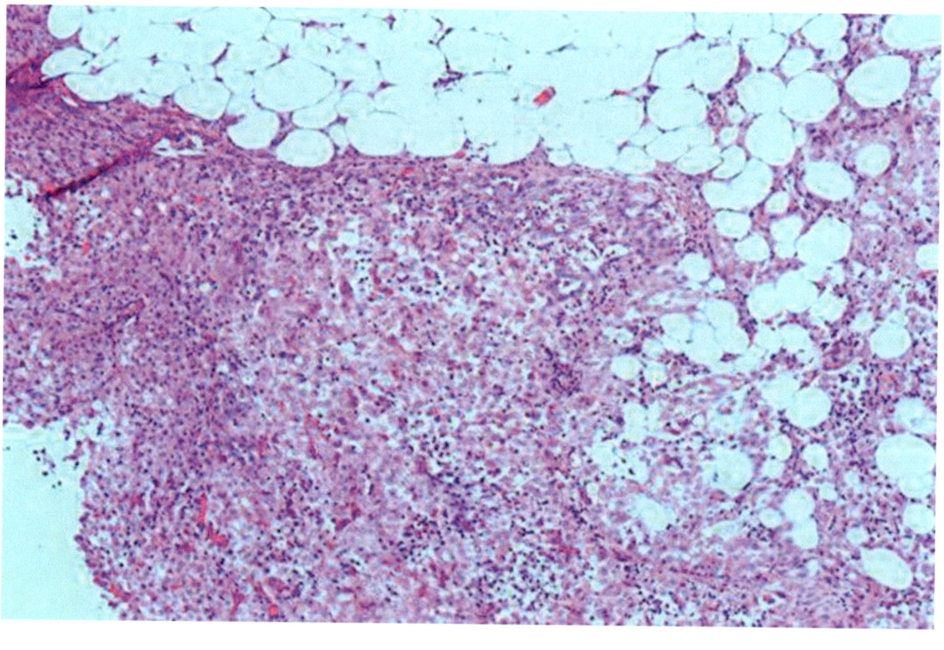

Fig. (5). Atypical mesothelial cells infiltrating through the connective tissue into extrapleural adipose tissue (Hematoxylin and Eosin Stain, x200 magnification).

Learning Points

- Pleuroscopic cryobiopsy is useful in acquiring adequate depth of tissue especially in the diagnosis of malignant mesothelioma. In our early experience, we demonstrated safety and good diagnostic yield of pleuroscopic cryobiopsy in a cohort of six patients with a mean aggregate specimen size of 9.2+/-1.9mm [1]. This technique may serve as an adjunct to conventional forceps biopsy especially when dealing with hard pleural nodules or thickening.

Video

Cryobiopsy of the parietal pleural nodule. Biopsy specimen was extracted by pulling out the pleuroscope and cryoprobe en bloc.

CONSENT FOR PUBLICATION

Not applicable.

CONFLICT OF INTEREST

The author declares no conflict of interest, financial or otherwise.

ACKNOWLEDGEMENTS

The authors acknowledge the support received from Dr. Fatin Izni Nazri, Department of Pathology, Sarawak General Hospital, Sarawak, Malaysia.

REFERENCE

[1] Nyanti L, Kho SS, Chai CS, *et al*. Cryobiopsy in flexi-rigid pleuroscopy in a region with low mesothelioma prevalence. EMJ Respiratory 2020; 8(1): 137-45. [http://dx.doi.org/10.33590/emjrespir/20-00053]

Case 6

Transthoracic Ultrasound and Veress Needle Assisted Pleuroscopy in a Patient with Minimal Pleural Effusion

Kho Sze Shyang[1,2,*] and **Tie Siew Teck**[1]

[1] *Division of Respiratory Medicine, Sarawak General Hospital, Kuching, Malaysia*

[2] *Department of Pulmonology, Serdang Hospital, Selangor, Malaysia*

Keywords: Medical thoracoscopy, Pleuroscopy, Pleural effusion, Pneumothorax induction, Transthoracic ultrasound, Veress needle.

Presentation

A 50-year-old lady was referred for incidental finding of unilateral pleural effusion. She was asymptomatic.

There was no family history of lung malignancy and no recent close TB contact. Pleural fluid analysis confirmed exudative pleural effusion.

Comorbidities

Chronic myeloid leukemia ten years ago and was on oral dasatinib 100mg once daily since then.

Chest Imaging

Right costophrenic angle was blunted on plain CXR suggestive of pleural effusion (Fig. **1**). Transthoracic ultrasound confirmed the presence of minimal, unilocular pleural effusion in the dependent supine position. In the left lateral position, echogenic lung sliding sign was present at the right mid-clavicular line, 6th intercostal rib space with no pleural effusion at the entry point.

*__Corresponding author Kho Sze Shyang:__ Department of Pulmonology, Serdang Hospital, Selangor, Malaysia; E-mail: khosze@moh.gov.my

Jamalul Azizi Abdul Rahaman & Tinku Joseph (Eds.)

Intervention

Under conscious sedation (midazolam and pethidine), local anaesthesia was infiltrated under real-time ultrasound guidance. Veress needle (Figs. **2** and **3**) was then guided towards the pleural line while observing lung sliding on real time ultrasound. Pneumothorax was confirmed once a "give" was felt with concurrent observation of exaggerated A-line with disappearance of B-lines and lung sliding on transthoracic ultrasound (Fig. **4**). Blunt dissection into the pleural cavity was then performed followed by insertion of a 6mm flexible trocar (40120NAL, Karl Storz, Germany).

Rigid pleuroscopy performed using a 0° viewing thoracoscope (26072BA, Hopkins, Karl Storz, Germany) with an optical biopsy forceps (26072A, Karl Storz, Germany) showed diffusely thickened parietal pleura with minimal pleural effusion at the dependent area (Fig. **5**). No pleural adhesion was noted and exploration of pleural cavity was adequate. Pleural biopsy was taken and a 20Fr intercostal chest tube was inserted for drainage of residual fluid.

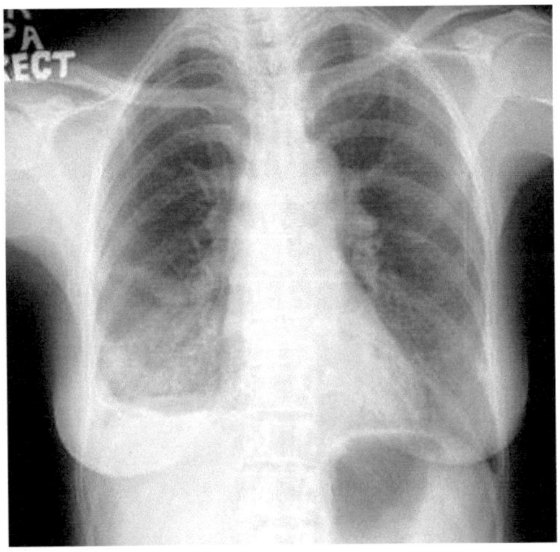

Fig. (1). Plain CXR demonstrated blunted right costophrenic angle with meniscus sign.

Complications

Intercostal chest tube was removed 24 hours later after CXR showed adequate lung expansion with minimal drainage of pleural effusion. No prolonged air leak was encountered.

Post-Intervention

HPE of the pleural biopsy demonstrated chronic inflammatory changes with no evidence of malignancy or TB. Diagnosis of likely dasatinib induced pleural effusion was concluded after discussion with the haematology team. The patient was switched to nilotinib for the management of her chronic myeloid leukemia and the right pleural effusion did not recur on one-month follow-up (Fig. **6**).

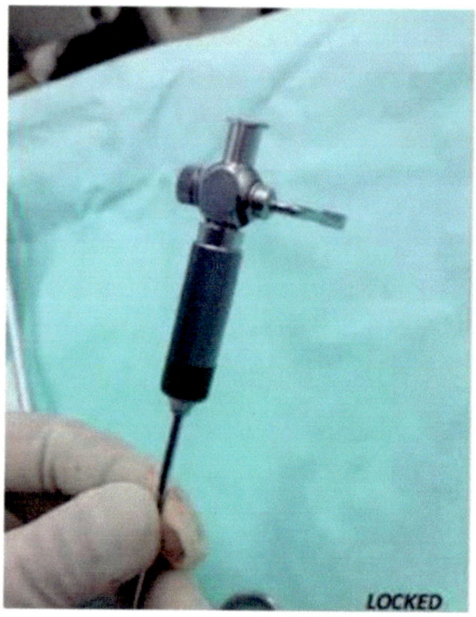

Fig. (2). Veress needle in locked position.

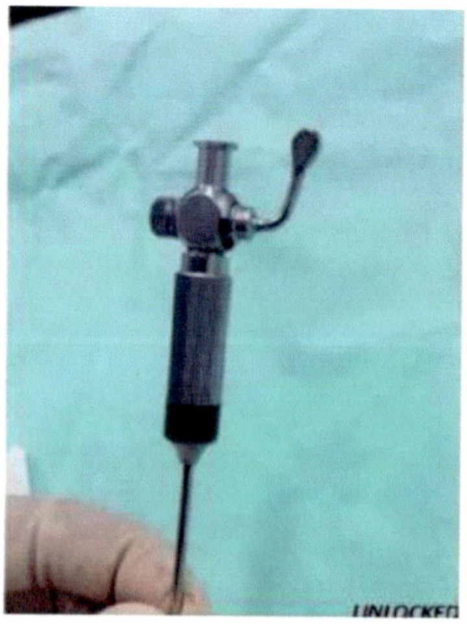

Fig. (3). Veress needle in unlocked position allowing the introduction of air into pleural cavity, thus, inducing pneumothorax for safe access into pleural cavity *via* pleuroscope.

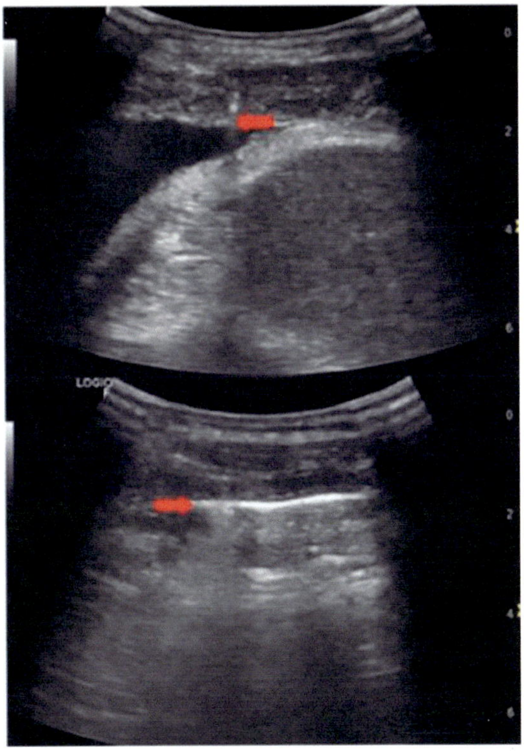

Fig. (4). Minimal pleural effusion on transthoracic ultrasound at right costophrenic angle. Veress needle (red arrow) was inserted under real time ultrasound guidance into pleural cavity. Pneumothorax was confirmed once the tip of Veress needle (red arrow) was guided into the pleural cavity which shows exaggerated A lines, loss of B lines and absence of lung sliding.

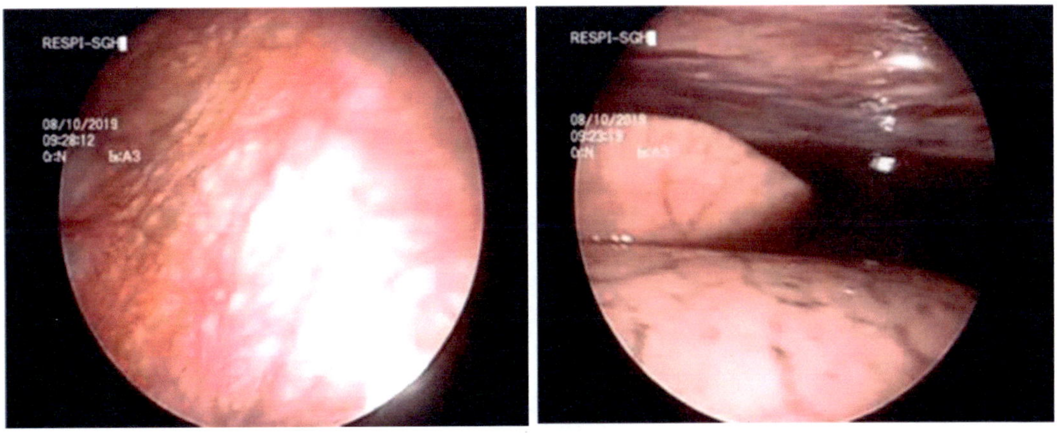

Fig. (5). (Left and Right) Pleural cavity was free from adhesion upon entry with minimal pleural effusion. Diffuse parietal pleural thickening noted during endoscopic examination.

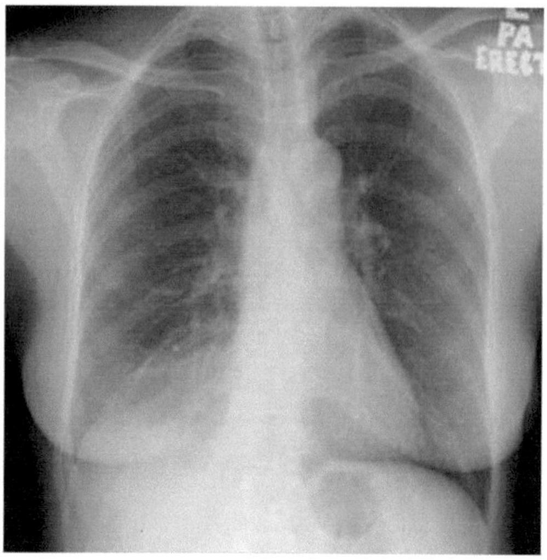

Fig. (6). No recurrence of pleural effusion one month post-procedure.

Learning Points

- Pleuroscopy is an essential tool in the approach to pleural diseases. However, this can be challenging especially in the absence of pleural effusion or even when effusion is minimal. The early study had shown promising safe results in USG-guided pleuroscopy in the absence of pleural effusion [1]. Our case demonstrated that transthoracic ultrasound and Veress needle assisted pleuroscopy in patients with minimal pleural effusion is feasible and safe especially in the presence of echographic lung sliding at the point of entry.

Video

The induction of pneumothorax using the Veress needle before entering the pleural space.

CONSENT FOR PUBLICATION

Not applicable.

CONFLICT OF INTEREST

The author declares no conflict of interest, financial or otherwise.

ACKNOWLEDGEMENT

Declared none.

REFERENCE

[1] Marchetti G, Valsecchi A, Indellicati D, Arondi S, Trigiani M, Pinelli V. Ultrasound-guided medical thoracoscopy in the absence of pleural effusion. Chest 2015; 147(4): 1008-12. [http://dx.doi.org/10.1378/chest.14-0637] [PMID: 25188712]

Case 7

Medical Thoracoscopy with "Induction Pneumothorax"

Soo Chun Ian[1,*]

[1] *Division of Respiratory Medicine, University of Malaya Medical Center, Kuala Lumpur, Malaysia*

Keywords: Lung cancer, Medical thoracoscopy, Pleuroscopy, Pneumothorax, Pleural effusion.

Case Presentation

A 54-year-old lady was admitted for progressive chronic cough for 12 months. Her symptoms did not improve after receiving outpatient treatment from various general practitioners. Her cough was mainly nonproductive, and there was no history of hemoptysis. She also experienced some degree of shortness of breath two weeks before her admission. She denied having fever but had lost 10kg in 4 months despite a regular diet.

On admission, her oxygen saturation was 85% on room air. Clinically, she was afebrile (Temperature of 37.2°C) and breathless (respiratory rate of 36 breaths per minute). She was fully conscious, and she had stable hemodynamics. Clinical examination and CXR confirmed a right-sided pleural effusion. A chest drain (12Fr) was inserted using the Seldinger method. The effusion was exudative and lymphocytic. Repeated cytology examination of the pleural fluid was negative for malignancy. Full septic and Mycobacterium TB screening were negative.

Comorbidities

Anxiety disorder and hypertension.

Chest Imaging

A CT thorax demonstrated the presence of residual right-sided pleural effusion and collapse of the right middle lobe with multiple mediastinal and hilar lymphadenopathy (Figs. **1a-c**).

[*]**Corresponding author Soo Chun Ian:** Division of Respiratory Medicine, University of Malaya Medical Center, Kuala Lumpur, Malaysia; E-mail: scianray@gmail.com

Jamalul Azizi Abdul Rahaman & Tinku Joseph (Eds.)

Intervention

The patient was posted for a medical thoracoscopy with an option to proceed for bronchoscopy under conscious sedation. The instruments used are shown (Figs. **2a-d**). The patient was put in the left lateral position. Guided by a thoracic USG, the entry area was identified, marked, cleaned, draped under sterile technique, and anesthetized with lignocaine 2% infiltrated to the skin and the thoracic wall. Following this, a 3cm incision was made, and the muscle fibers were dissected using artery forceps until the pleural cavity was eached (Fig. **3**). Next, a blunt trocar was introduced through the thoracic wall into the pleural cavity in a corkscrew motion. Subsequently, a semi-rigid thoracoscope was advanced into the pleural cavity under direct vision through the trocar (Fig. **4**).

During the procedure, a concomitant lung expansion occurred as pleural fluid was removed through the thoracoscope to improve visualization of the pleural cavity (Fig. **5**). This had resulted in a diminished pleural space (Fig. **6**). The thoracoscope was then rotated facing the apex of the lung and slowly maneuvered between the expanded lung and the chest wall to an area of a slightly larger pleural cavity. A modified "induction pneumothorax" was performed. The thoracoscope was in position by the operator while the assistant induced repeated pneumothorax by using a 20cc syringe plunger through the working channel of the thoracoscope until a reasonable pleural space was achieved (Fig. **7**). The vital signs of the patient were closely monitored throughout the entire procedure. The parietal pleura was biopsied under direct visualization (Fig. **8**). After the thoracoscope was withdrawn, a chest drain (22Fg) was inserted into the pleural cavity and connected to an underwater seal drainage system.

A bronchoscopy was also performed immediately after the medical thoracoscopy, given the 'normal looking' parietal pleura. Endobronchial biopsy confirmed primary lung adenocarcinoma. Pleural fluid collected during pleuroscopy detected the presence of malignant cells but was not enough for IHC.

Complications

Nil.

Post-Intervention

Diagnosis: Stage IV lung adenocarcinoma.Talc pleurodesis was carried out once diagnosis was confirmed.

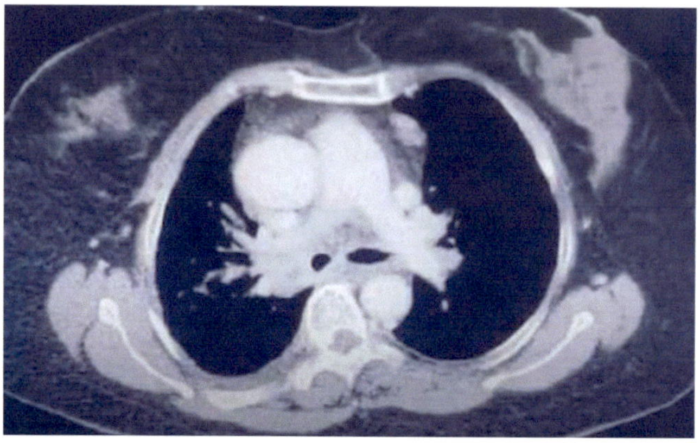

Fig. (1a). Mediastinal and hilar lymphadenopathy.

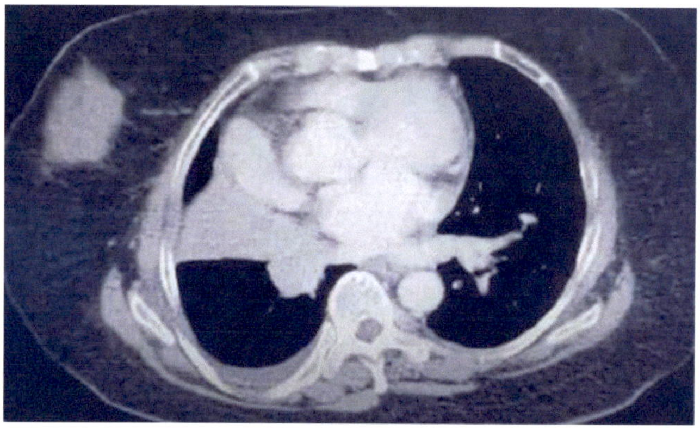

Fig. (1b). Collapse of the right middle lobe.

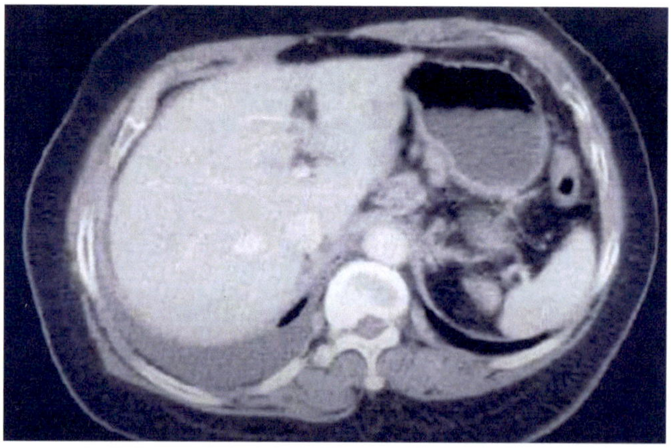

Fig. (1c). Moderate amount of right pleural effusion.

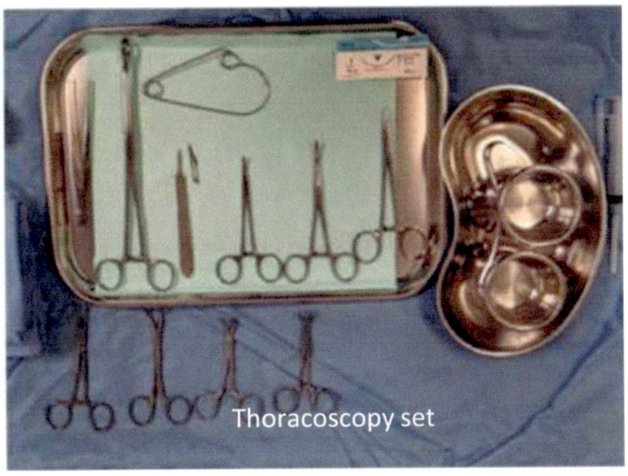

(a)

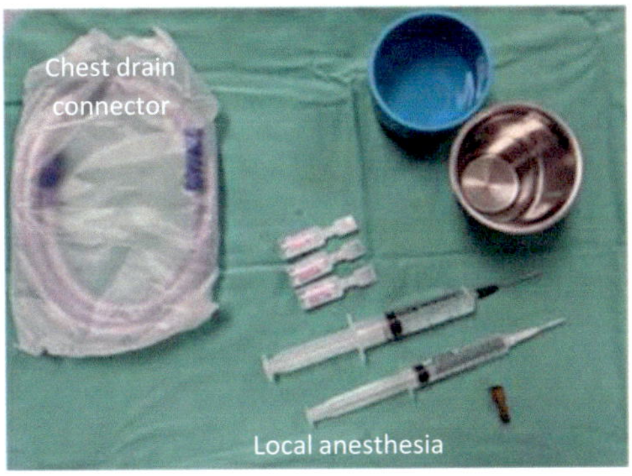

(b)

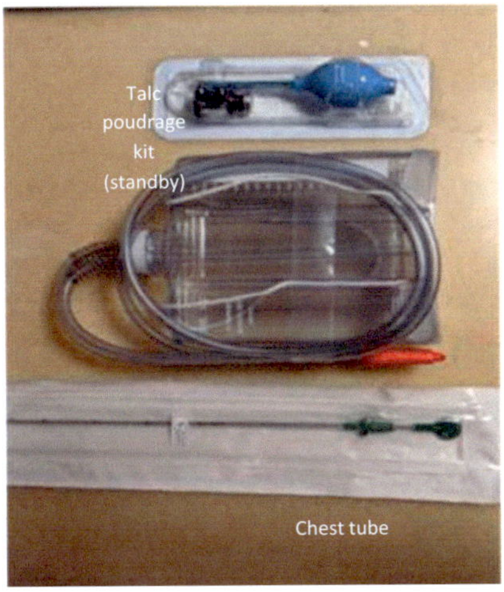

(c)

(Fig. 2) contd.....

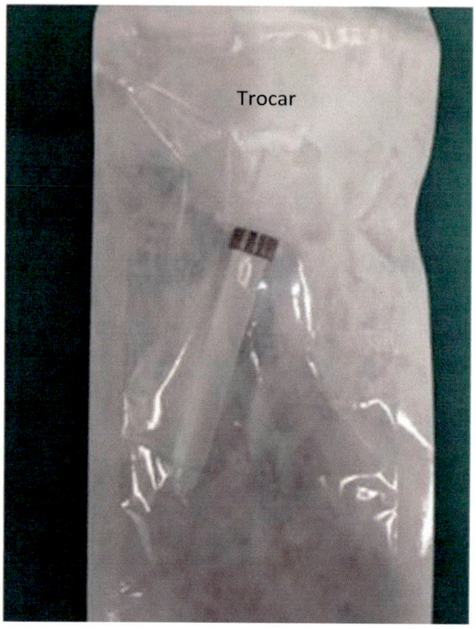

(d)

Fig. (2). (a-d) Instruments for medical thoracoscopy.

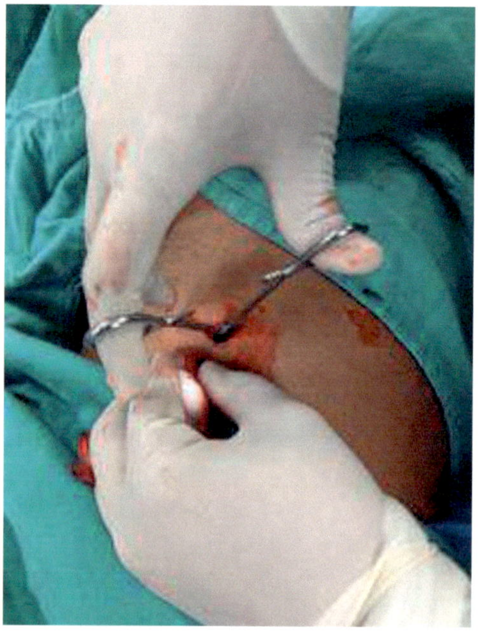

Fig. (3). Dissection of muscle fibers using artery forceps.

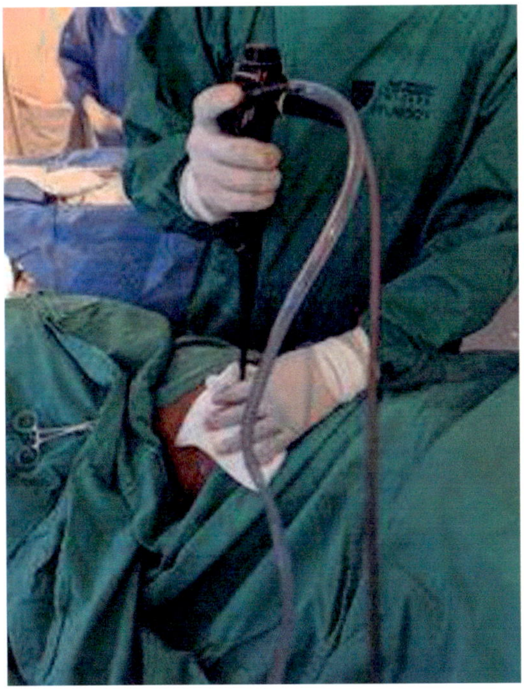

Fig. (4). Semi-rigid thoracoscope inserted into the pleural cavity *via* the trocar.

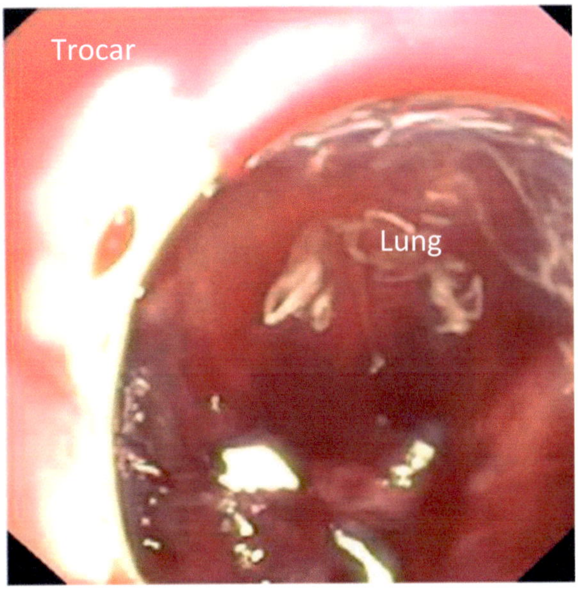

Fig. (5). Lung expansion following evacuation of pleural fluid (viewed *via* thoracoscopy).

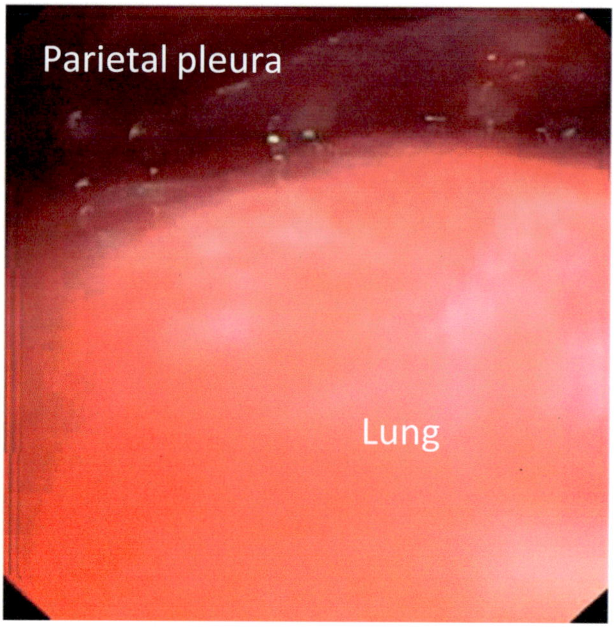

Fig. (6). Small pleural space.

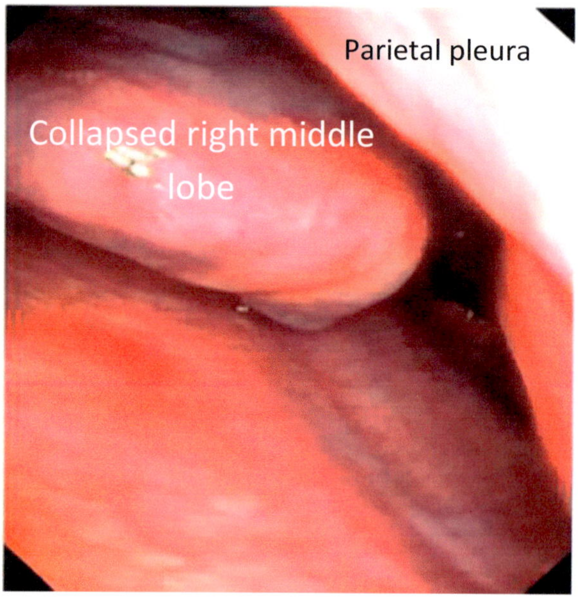

Fig. (7). Larger pleural space (after inducing pneumothorax).

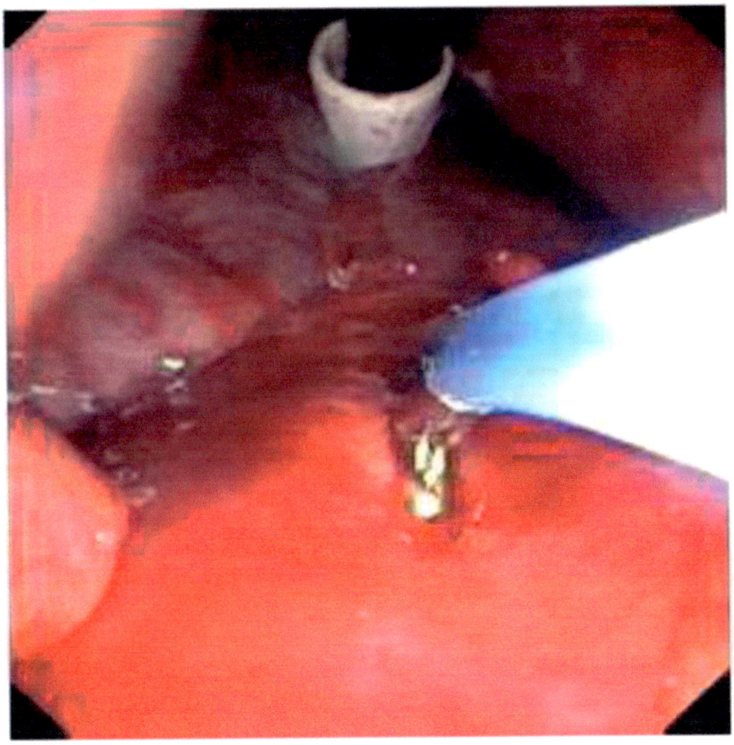

Fig. (8). Biopsy of parietal pleura.

Learning Points

- Induction pneumothorax was previously described nearly two decades ago [1]. Over the years, based on the original concept described, various methods have been improvised for medical thoracoscopy especially in cases with limited pleural space. The Boutin needle is a standard device used for the induction of pneumothorax. The success of pneumothorax induction can be confirmed through the "hissing" sound heard when the parietal pleura is punctured [2]. The current case highlights a few essential points for medical thoracoscopy. First, evacuation of pleural fluid (for small to moderate pleural effusion) may lead to rapid lung expansion and limit the available space safe for medical thoracoscopy. Second, the flexi-rigid thoracoscope can be safely guided to a larger pleural space to allow a modified induction pneumothorax to be carried out. Finally, induction pneumothorax should only be carried out by an experienced proceduralist with close monitoring of the patient's vital signs.

CONSENT FOR PUBLICATION

Not applicable.

CONFLICT OF INTEREST

The author declares no conflict of interest, financial or otherwise.

ACKNOWLEDGEMENT

Declared none.

REFERENCES

[1] Tchertkoff IG, Selikoff IJ, Robitzek EH. The role of trauma in initial pneumothorax. Dis Chest 1948; 14(4): 475-90.
[http://dx.doi.org/10.1378/chest.14.4.475] [PMID: 18873012]

[2] Alraiyes AH, Dhillon SS, Harris K, Kaphle U, Kheir F. Medical Thoracoscopy. Pleura (Thousand Oaks) 2016; 3.
[http://dx.doi.org/10.1177/2373997516632752]

Case 8

Rigid Thoracoscopy

Rigid Thoracoscopy in Undiagnosed Exudative Pleural Effusion

Tinku Joseph[1,*] and **Sathish C. Reddy**[1]

[1] *Division of Interventional Pulmonology, Amrita Institute of Medical Sciences, Kochi, Kerala, India*

Keywords: Exudative effusion, Pleural effusion, Pleural tuberculosis, Rigid thoracoscopy, Thoracoscopy.

Presentation

A 35-year-old gentleman presented with non-productive cough and breathlessness on exertion of 2 weeks duration. No fever, chest pain or weight loss.

Comorbidities

Systemic hypertension, Post-COVID-19 status.

Chest Imaging

CXR showed a right-sided moderate pleural effusion (Fig. **1**).

Plain CT Thorax Findings:

- Moderate right-sided pleural effusion measuring 7cm in depth in supine position.
- Small loculations noted in the fluid in right upper pleural cavity.
- No obvious nodular pleural thickening or masses.
- Passive collapse of posterior aspect of the right upper lobe and medial segment of right middle lobe.
- Few sub-centimetric right paratracheal and subcarinal lymph nodes, the largest measuring 8mm.

He was initially evaluated on an outpatient basis and ultrasound-guided diagnostic pleural fluid aspiration was done. Pleural fluid analysis revealed exudative effusion with ADA of 38.5 U/L.

*__Corresponding author Tinku Joseph:__ Division of Interventional Pulmonology, Amrita Institute of Medical Sciences, Kochi, Kerala, India; E-mail: tinkujoseph2010@gmail.com

Pleural fluid cytology was suggestive of lymphocyte-rich pleural effusion. Pleural fluid for AFB smear and GeneXpert were negative. In view of inconclusive pleural fluid analysis reports, a plan was made to do rigid thoracoscopy and pleural biopsy.

Intervention

Under general anesthesia, the patient was intubated with double lumen endotracheal tube. Then patient's position was changed to left lateral position with the affected side (right lung) up. The site of trocar puncture (6th inter- costal space in mid axillary line) was marked under ultrasound guidance. Trocar site was then infiltrated with 4% lignocaine injection. The skin, subcutaneous tissue, the upper border of the lower rib and its periosteum were anesthetized. A 5cm wide skin incision was made parallel to the ribs in midaxillary line and dissection was performed through the subcutaneous planes to the intercostal muscles (muscles should always be split with forceps, avoid cutting it since it delays the healing process and increases the chances of fistula formation). The trocar was later introduced into the pleural cavity and subsequently rigid thoracoscope with suction tube attached was inserted.

The next step was to suction out 80 percent of the pleural fluid to visualize both costal and diaphragmatic pleurae clearly. Rapid clearance of the pleural fluid can predispose to re-expansion pulmonary edema. Thoracoscopy showed multiple sago grain nodules over costal and diaphragmatic pleurae with minimal adhesions and septations within the pleural cavity (Fig. **2**). Multiple biopsies (Pleural peels) were taken subsequently from the visualized pleural nodules with rigid biopsy forceps. Adequate haemostasis was achieved after pleural biopsy.

After obtaining adequate pleural biopsies and breaking the adhesions with the rigid forceps a 24F chest tube was inserted into the pleural cavity through the trocar site and subsequently connected to the underwater seal drain. The incision site was closed with 1 zero silk mattress suture and a tight sterile bandage was applied around the chest tube. The patient tolerated the procedure well, there was no evidence of air leak post-procedure and the patient was extubated on the table.

Complications

No immediate post-procedure complications were noted.

Post-Intervention

Post-procedure CXR showed adequate lung expansion with a chest tube *in situ* (Fig. **3**). Histopathological examination of the pleural biopsy specimen was suggestive of necrotizing granulomatous inflammation. Pleural tissue GeneXpert for mycobacterium tuberculosis was also positive. He was subsequently initiated on anti-tubercular medications and the chest drain was removed once the drain was less than 100ml in 24 hours.

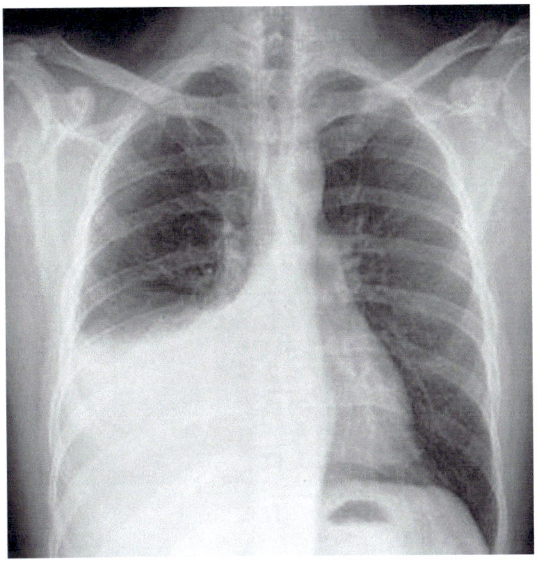

Fig. (1). Pre-procedure CXR: Right-sided moderate pleural effusion.

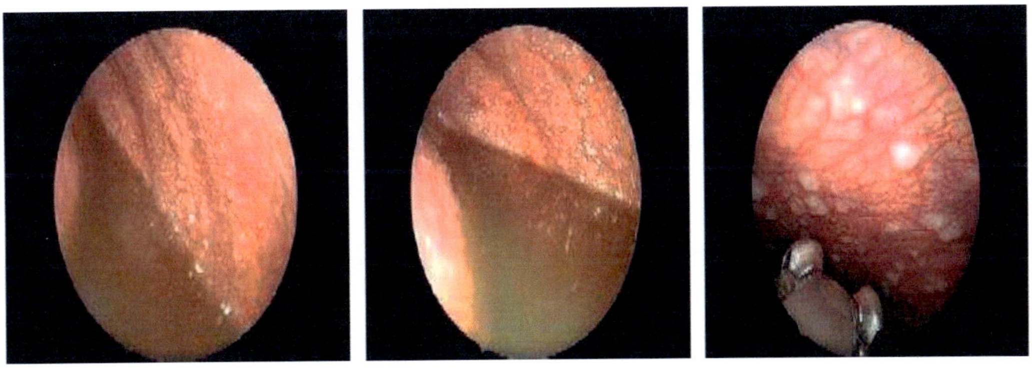

Fig. (2). Thoracoscopic view: Sago grain nodules over parietal pleura.

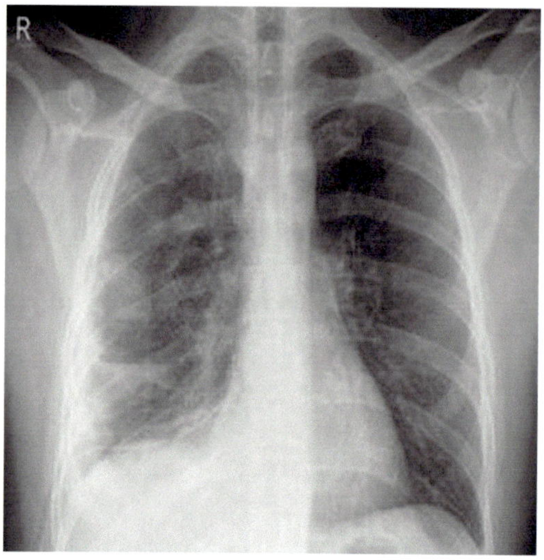

Fig. (3). Post-procedure CXR: Lung expansion with ICD *in situ*.

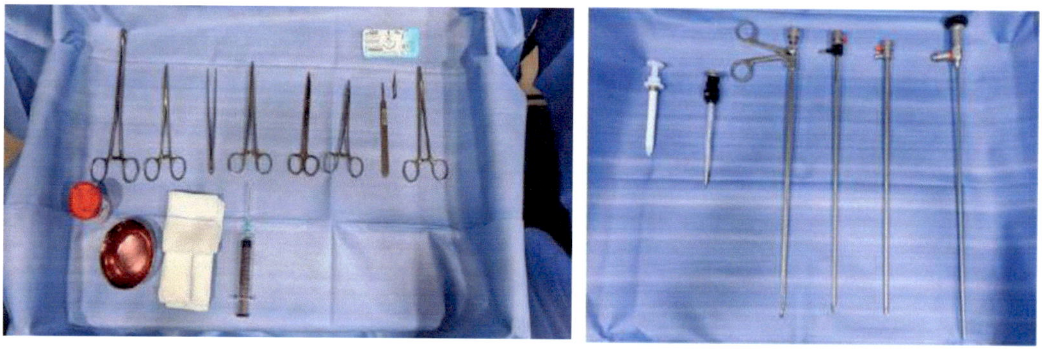

Fig. (4). Instruments required to perform rigid thoracoscopy.

Learning Points

- Rigid thoracoscopy and flexi-rigid pleuroscopy instruments present different advantages and,
- Disadvantages.
- Rigid thoracoscopy has marginally increased diagnostic yield compared to flexi-rigid pleuroscope.
- Advantages of rigid thoracoscopy (Fig. **4**).
- Provides larger biopsy specimens with minimal crush artifact.
- A useful tool in breakage of pleural septations/ adhesions using rigid optical forceps and L cautery.

- Helps in talc pleurodesis in same sitting (Talc poudrage).
- Cost-effective compared to flexi-rigid thoracoscope.
- Disadvantages of rigid thoracoscopy.
- Should be handled by an experienced interventional pulmonologist – Instrument tip is sharp compared to flexi-rigid pleuroscope and this can cause injury to the lung parenchyma [1].

The ideal pleural service should be equipped with rigid thoracoscope, mini-thoracoscope and a flexi-rigid pleuroscope to tailor for individual patients' pleural conditions.

CONSENT FOR PUBLICATION

Not applicable.

CONFLICT OF INTEREST

The author declares no conflict of interest, financial or otherwise.

ACKNOWLEDGEMENT

Declared none.

REFERENCE

[1] Dhooria S, Singh N, Aggarwal. AN, Gupta D. A randomized trial comparing the diagnostic yield of rigid and semirigid thoracoscopy in undiagnosed pleural effusions. Respir Care 2014; 59(5): 756-64.

Case 9

Grains of Sago in the Chest: Rigid Thoracoscopy for TB Pleural Effusion

Harikishan Gonuguntla[1,*] and **Belgundi Preeti Vidyasagar**[1]

[1] *Division of Interventional Pulmonology, Yashoda Hospital, Secunderabad, India*

Keywords: Biopsy, Lymphocytes, Pleural effusion, Thoracoscopy, Sago grains, Ultrasound.

Presentation

A 60-year gentleman was referred to our center with a request for medical thoracoscopy-guided pleural biopsy after an initial inconclusive thoracentesis and pleural fluid analysis. His medical history revealed loss of weight and appetite over the last 30 days.

Comorbidities

None.

Chest Imaging

CXR and CT thorax revealed moderate left pleural effusion with slight mediastinal shift and lung collapse (Figs. **1a** and **b**). Chest ultrasound confirmed the presence of pleural effusion with no septations.

Pleural fluid analysis - Straw coloured, exudative, lymphocyte predominance, with borderline ADA. Cytology showed predominantly lymphocytes admixed with histiocytes and neutrophils, negative for atypical cells– Inconclusive analysis.

Intervention

Medical thoracoscopy was performed under conscious sedation (Fentanyl + Dexmedetomidine) using a 6mm rigid thoracoscope (HEINE optical 6mm set, Karl Storz, Germany). The pleural inspection was performed using a 4mm 30-degree Hopkins telescope. Both visceral and parietal pleural surfaces were studded with

*__Corresponding author Harikishan Gonuguntla:__ Division of Interventional Pulmonology, Yashoda Hospital, Secunderabad, India; E-mail: harikishang@gmail.com

Jamalul Azizi Abdul Rahaman & Tinku Joseph (Eds.)

small nodules resembling sago grains (Figs. **2** and **3**). Using the optical biopsy forceps, 4-5 biopsies were obtained from the parietal pleural surface. Following the biopsy, a 28F intercostal drain was inserted into the pleural cavity.

Complications

None.

Post-Intervention

Post-procedure CXR showed an expanded left lung with ICD *in situ* (Fig. **4**). HPE of the pleural biopsy showed granulomatous inflammation with epithelioid histiocytes, lymphocytes, plasma cells and Langhans type of giant cell favoring Mycobacterial etiology (Fig. **5**). Mycobacterium tuberculosis was detected through polymerase chain reaction (PCR) assay from the pleural biopsy spec imen. Rifampicin resistance was not detected. The patient was initiated on standard anti-TB therapy.

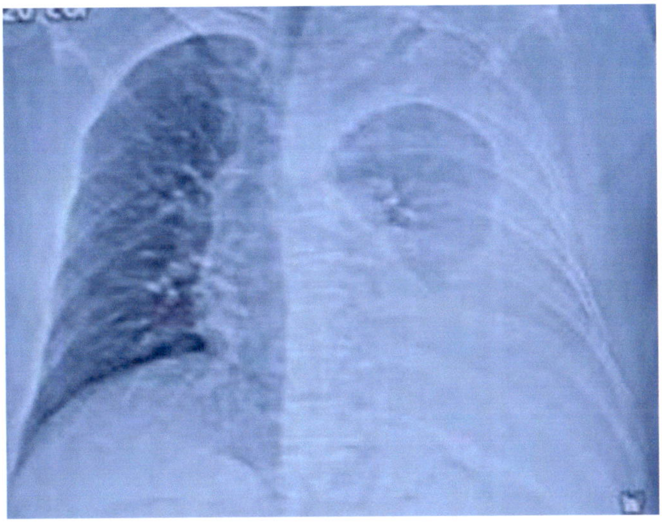

Fig. (1). (a) CXR shows left pleural effusion.

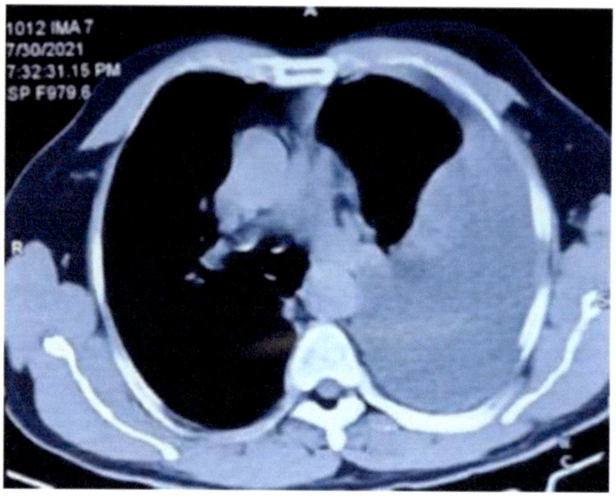

Fig. (1). (b) Axial CT Thorax showing left moderate pleural effusion with slight mediastinal shift and underlying lung collapse.

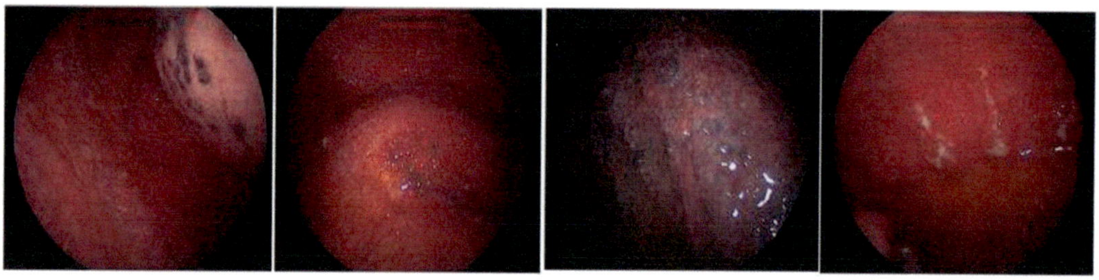

Fig. (2). Rigid thoracoscopic images demonstrating sago grain appearance from left to right: Anterior parietal pleura, diaphragm, visceral pleura and whitish cheesy material on the posterior parietal pleura.

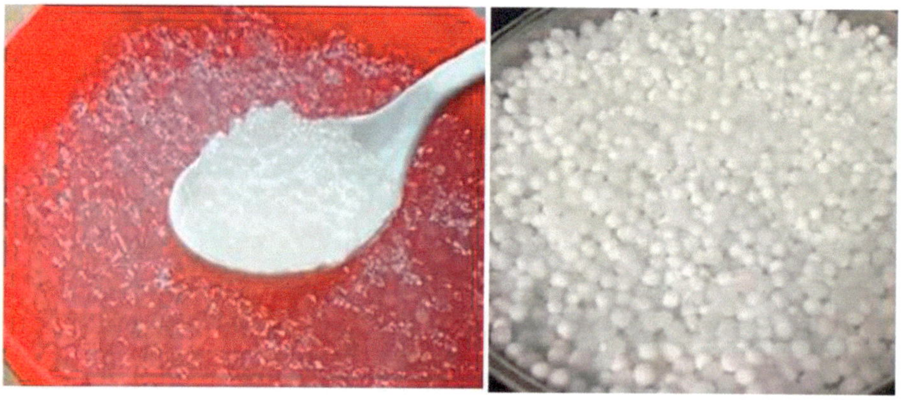

Fig. (3). (Left and Right images) Sago grains.

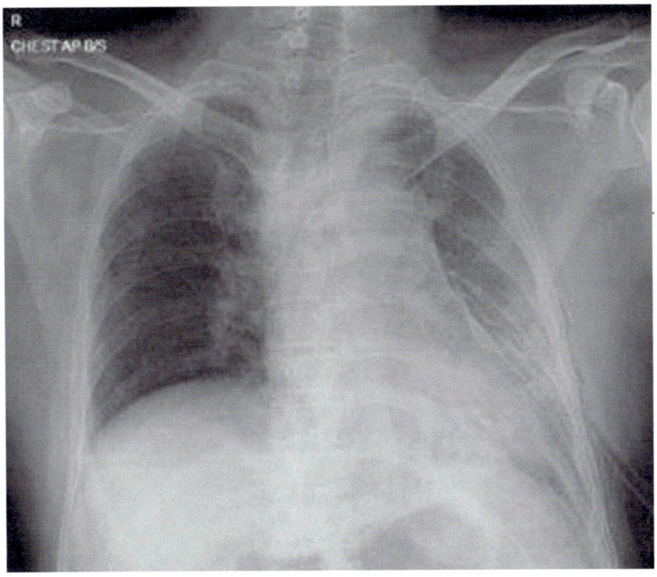

Fig. (4). Post-procedure CXR shows expanded left lung with ICD *in situ.*

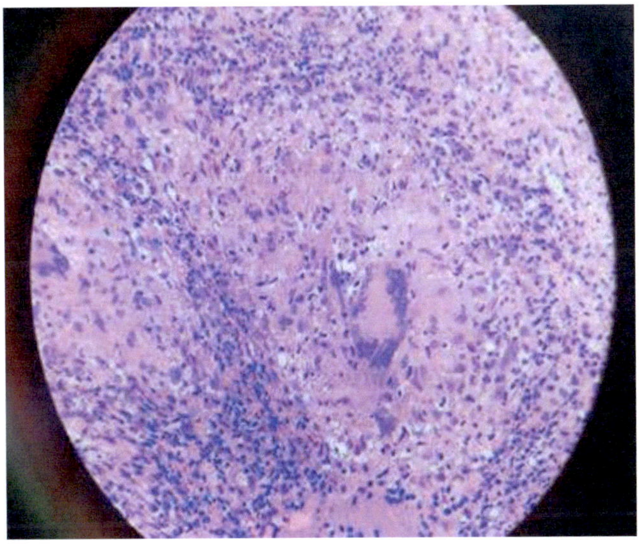

Fig. (5). HPE (hematoxylin and eosin stain, x40 magnification) revealed granulomatous inflammation with Langhans giant cells.

Learning Points

- Thoracoscopic pleural biopsy for demonstration of granulomatous inflammation and/or detection of Mycobacterium with GeneXpert is essential, especially if pleural fluid reports are inconclusive, more so in elderly patients who fail to mount fever response and in whom there is a clinical suspicion of malignancy.

- Tuberculous pleural effusions, on thoracoscopy demonstrate classical features of disseminated, small, solid or caseous, sago-type nodules over the parietal pleura [1]. The yield for diagnosing tuberculous pleural effusion with thoracoscopy is nearly 100% [2]. A point to highlight is the importance of microbiological investigations of the pleural biopsy specimen as demonstrated in our case.

Video

Rigid thoracoscopy procedure in this patient.

CONSENT FOR PUBLICATION

Not applicable.

CONFLICT OF INTEREST

The author declares no conflict of interest, financial or otherwise.

ACKNOWLEDGEMENTS

The authors acknowledge the support received from Dr. Milap Shah, Department of Pathology, Yashoda Hospital, Secunderabad, India.

REFERENCES

[1] Astoul P. Thoracoscopy for Pulmonologists: A Didactic Approach. Springer 2014. [http://dx.doi.org/10.1007/978-3-642-38351-9]

[2] Loddenkemper R. Thoracoscopy: results in non cancerous and idiopathic pleural effusions. Poumon Coeur 1981; 37(4): 261-4. [PMID: 7312756]

Case 10

Indwelling Pleural Catheter

Indwelling Pleural Catheter for Benign Pleural Effusion: A Patient with Lupus Pleurisy

Mohamed Faisal Abdul Hamid[1,*], **Ng Boon Hau**[1], **Nik Nuratiqah Nik Abeed**[1] and **Andrea Ban Yu-Lin**[1]

[1]*Respiratory Unit, Faculty of Medicine, National University of Malaysia, Selangor, Malaysia*

Keywords: Anti-nuclear antibody, Benign, Effusion, Indwelling pleural catheter, Pleurodesis, Systemic lupus erythematosus.

Presentation

A 52-year-old lady, a non-smoker presented with a 2-week history of progressive dyspnea, with preceding arthralgia for one month. Physical examination revealed her oxygen saturation was 97% on room air. Chest examination revealed reduced breath sounds over the left mid-lower zone with reduced vocal resonance and stony dullness on percussion.

Comorbidities

None.

Chest Imaging

Initial CXR revealed a moderate left pleural effusion (Fig. **1**).

Intervention

Thoracentesis was performed. Pleural fluid adenosine deaminase (ADA) was 2.8 U/L, and the Xpert MTB/RIF Ultra (Cepheid, USA) was not detected. Pleuroscopy revealed inflamed pleura and HPE revealed predominantly lymphocytic infiltrates.

Serum ANA subsequently was positive with a titre of 1:640 and anti-double stranded DNA was elevated at 81.10 IU/mL (positive is >75) with reduced complement levels (C3: 35 mg/dL and C4:3.9mg/dL). A diagnosis of systemic lupus erythematosus (SLE) with lupus pleurisy was made.

[*]**Corresponding author Mohamed Faisal Abdul Hamid:** Respiratory Unit, Faculty of Medicine, National University of Malaysia, Selangor, Malaysia; E-mail: faisal.hamid@ppukm.ukm.edu.my

Jamalul Azizi Abdul Rahaman & Tinku Joseph (Eds.)

Despite aggressive treatment with pulse methylprednisolone, cyclophosphamide and tapering doses of oral prednisolone of 1mg/kg/day, the effusion recurred twice in a space of one month. Hence, we decided for indwelling pleural catheter (IPC).

Complications

None.

Post-Intervention

She performed regular IPC drainage of 300–400mL per session, three times per week at home. There were no complications such as infection, symptomatic loculation or IPC blockage. After 3 months post-insertion, she achieved spontaneous pleurodesis, as there was no more drainage from the IPC (Fig. **2**). The IPC was flushed to ensure no blockage before it was removed (Fig. **3**). There were no complications during the removal and the IPC was intact.

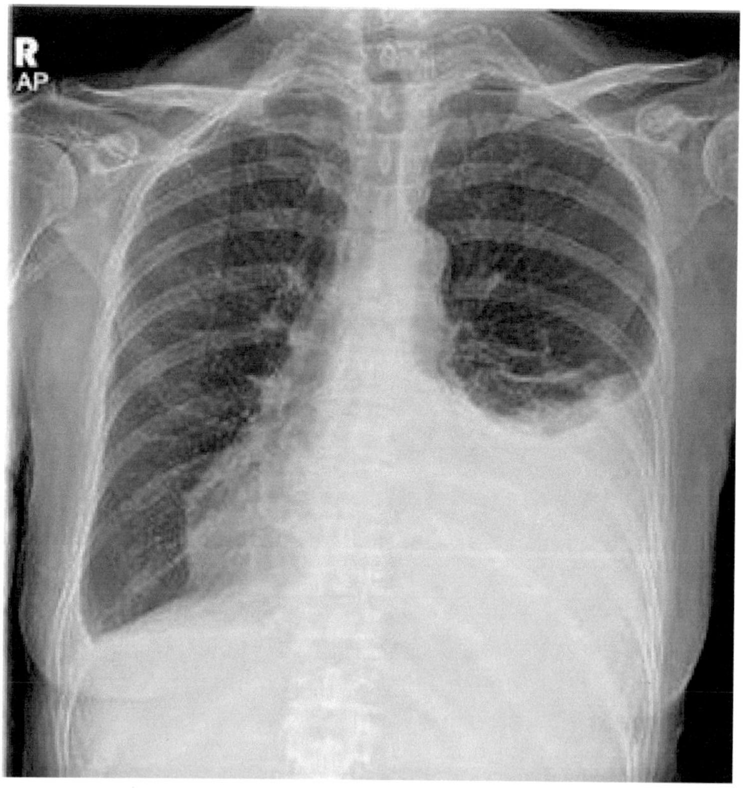

Fig. (1). CXR revealed a moderate left pleural effusion.

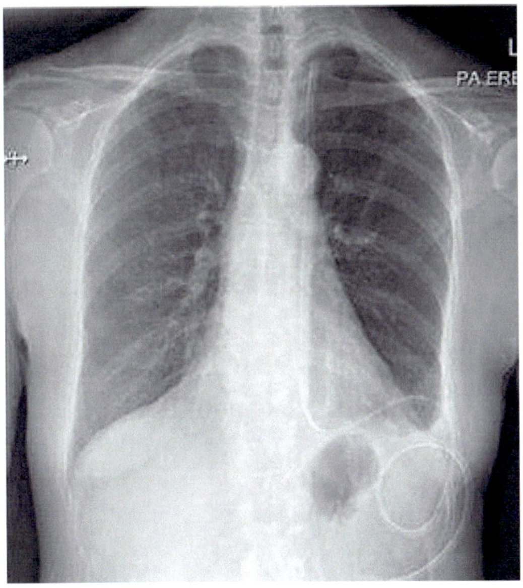

Fig. (2). CXR after 3 months post-IPC insertion revealed mild left pleural thickening.

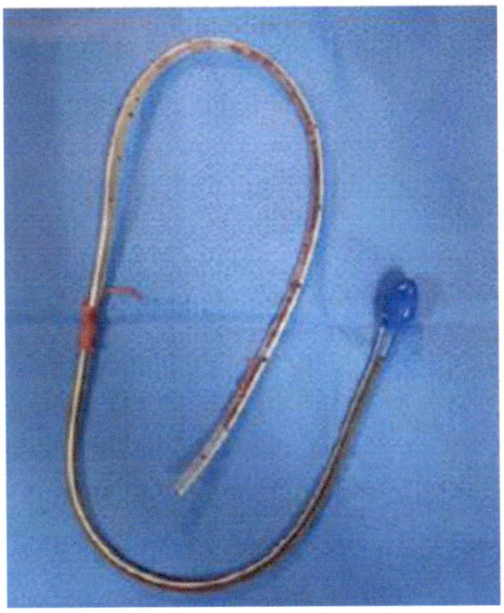

Fig. (3). Intact IPC post-removal.

Learning Points

- IPC may be an alternative treatment to relieve dyspnoea in a refractory benign pleural effusion after optimizing medical treatment; especially when dealing with high output chest drainage. It can be removed once spontaneous pleurodesis is achieved. Spontaneous pleurodesis is generally defined as the finding of minimal IPC drainage (50mL or less) on three consecutive attempts without evidence of symptomatic re-accumulation of fluid [1]. In a multicentre study, spontaneous pleurodesis was achieved at a median time of 71 days in cases with non-malignant pleural effusion [2]. This was similar to our patient.

Video

The technique of IPC removal.

CONSENT FOR PUBLICATION

Not applicable.

CONFLICT OF INTEREST

The author declares no conflict of interest, financial or otherwise.

ACKNOWLEDGEMENT

Declared none.

REFERENCES

[1] Maceachern P, Tremblay A. Pleural controversy: Pleurodesis versus indwelling pleural catheters for malignant effusions. Respirology 2011; 16(5): 747-54. [http://dx.doi.org/10.1111/j.1440-1843.2011.01986.x] [PMID: 21545373]

[2] Bhatnagar R, Reid ED, Corcoran JP, *et al.* Indwelling pleural catheters for non-malignant effusions: a multicentre review of practice: Table 1. Thorax 2014; 69(10): 959-61. [http://dx.doi.org/10.1136/thoraxjnl-2013-204563] [PMID: 24343783]

Case 11

Indwelling Pleural Catheter for Malignant Pleural Effusion. Managing Symptomatic Loculations

Mohamed Faisal Abdul Hamid[1,*]

[1] *Respiratory Unit, Faculty of Medicine, National University of Malaysia, Selangor, Malaysia*

Keywords: Alteplase, DNase, Dornase-alfa, Indwelling pleural catheter, Fibrinolytics, Malignant effusion.

Presentation

A 53-year-old lady, a non-smoker presented with a massive right pleural effusion (Fig. **1**). She was diagnosed with Stage IV lung adenocarcinoma following pleuroscopy. Her tumor driver mutation was negative for EGFR, ALK and ROS-1 mutation. Her lungs failed to re-expand following evacuation of pleural effusion. Her oxygen saturation was 92% on room air.

Comorbidities

None.

Chest Imaging

CXR revealed a non-expandable right lung (Fig. **2**).

Intervention

Indwelling pleural catheter (IPC) was inserted as a treatment modality for recurrent malignant pleural effusion. She continued draining 2-3 times per week. She received 6 cycles of chemotherapy. However, 1 month after IPC insertion, she became more breathless and that there was right pleural loculation which failed to drain *via* the existing IPC (Fig. **3**). Intrapleural alteplase 10mg (diluted in 50mls 0.9% normal saline) was instilled *via* the IPC adaptor and allowed to dwell for 45 minutes before allowing drainage. The cycle was repeated 5 times (12 hourly) which drained a total of 1.45L of hemoserous effusion. Repeat CXR showed resolution of the effusion with non-expandable right lung and pleural thickening (Fig. **4**).

[*] **Corresponding author Mohamed Faisal Abdul Hamid:** Respiratory Unit, Faculty of Medicine, National University of Malaysia, Selangor, Malaysia; E-mail: faisal.hamid@ppukm.ukm.edu.my

Complications

Mild pleuritic pain after draining the fluids which improved with regular analgesia.

Post-Intervention

She continued draining pleural fluid thrice weekly, and her dyspnoea improved. She succumbed 7 months later due to disease progression.

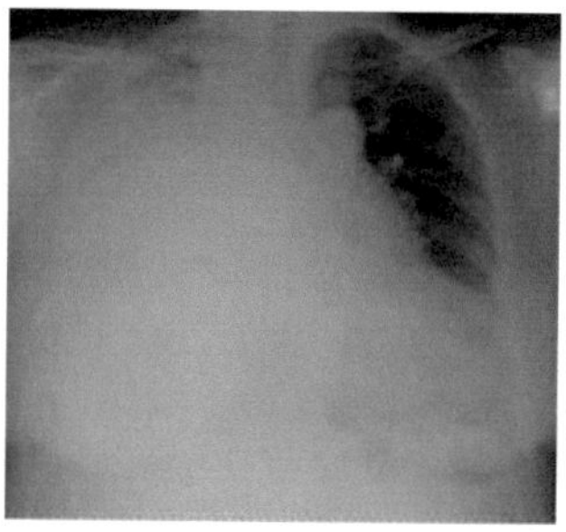

Fig. (1). CXR revealed a massive right pleural effusion.

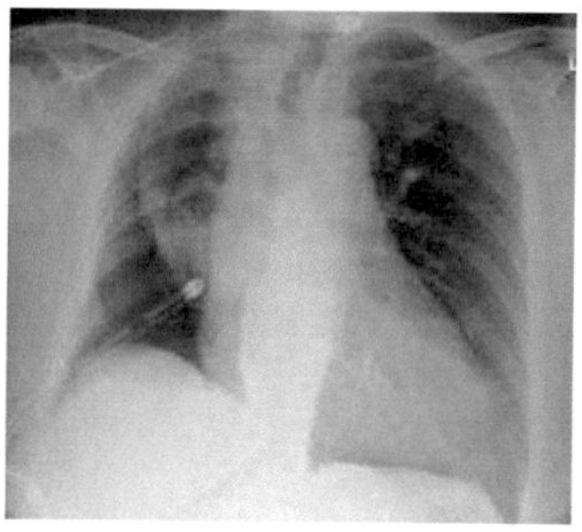

Fig. (2). CXR revealed a non-expandable lung with a 24-Fr chest tube *in situ*.

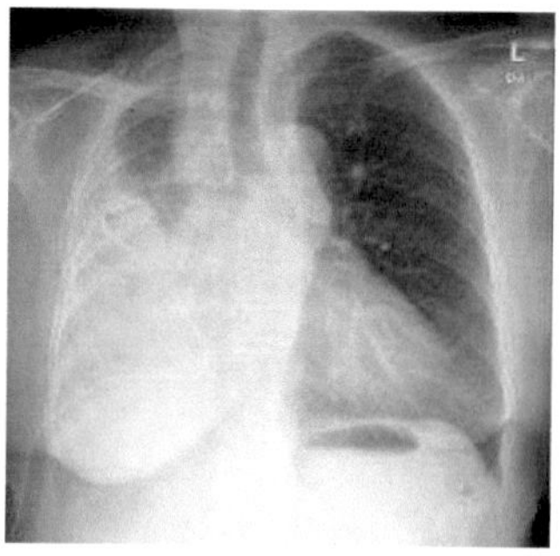

Fig. (3). CXR one month after IPC insertion revealed right pleural loculation which failed to drain *via* IPC.

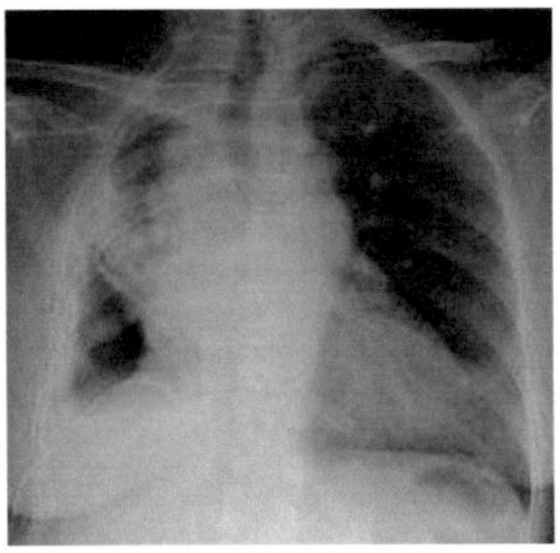

Fig. (4). CXR after 5 doses of intrapleural alteplase which showed resolution of effusion with pleural thickening and a right non-expandable lung.

Learning Points

- Symptomatic loculation is reported to be present in 5-14% of IPC-treated patients.
- It typically occurs at about two months after IPC insertion [1].
- Catheter blockage develops due to the formation of dense fibrinous tissue around and within the IPC.
- Intrapleural fibrinolytics are feasible and safe treatment options to restore patency in a blocked IPC [2].

CONSENT FOR PUBLICATION

Not applicable.

CONFLICT OF INTEREST

The author declares no conflict of interest, financial or otherwise.

ACKNOWLEDGEMENT

Declared none.

REFERENCES

[1] Lui MMS, Thomas R, Lee YCG. Complications of indwelling pleural catheter use and their management. BMJ Open Respir Res 2016; 3(1): e000123.
[http://dx.doi.org/10.1136/bmjresp-2015-000123] [PMID: 26870384]

[2] Faisal M, Nurhanis S, Nik Abeed NN, Ng BH, Ban AYL. Re-establishing indwelling pleural catheter patency with alteplase after failure of streptokinase. Respirol Case Rep 2020; 8 (7): e00639.
[http://dx.doi.org/10.1002/rcr2.639] [PMID: 32774860]

Case 12

Indwelling Pleural Catheter for Malignant Pleural Effusion with Spontaneous Pleurodesis

Mohamed Faisal Abdul Hamid[1,*]

[1]*Respiratory Unit, Faculty of Medicine, National University of Malaysia, Selangor, Malaysia*

Keywords: Adenocarcinoma, Indwelling pleural catheter, Malignant effusion, Non-expandable lung, Pleurodesis, Recurrent effusion.

Presentation

A 52-year-old lady, a non-smoker diagnosed with Stage IV lung adenocarcinoma. Her tumor driver mutation was negative for EGFR, ALK and ROS-1 mutation. She presented with recurrent right malignant pleural effusion which accumulated rapidly within one week. Her oxygen saturation was 93% on room air.

Comorbidities

None.

Chest Imaging

CXR revealed a moderate right pleural effusion (Fig. **1a**).

Intervention

After counselling, she agreed for indwelling pleural catheter (IPC) insertion. IPC is a catheter with multiple fenestrations that is tunneled in the subcutaneous tissue. She also received 5 cycles of permetrexed and cisplatin-based chemotherapy. Following IPC insertion, she continued draining the pleural fluid thrice per week. The CXR showed significant reduction of pleural effusion (Fig. **1b**). Her dyspnoea and quality of life improved and she was able to continue with her activities of daily living.

Complications

None.

[*]**Corresponding author Mohamed Faisal Abdul Hamid:** Respiratory Unit, Faculty of Medicine, National University of Malaysia, Selangor, Malaysia; E-mail: faisal.hamid@ppukm.ukm.edu.my

Jamalul Azizi Abdul Rahaman & Tinku Joseph (Eds.)

Post-Intervention

Four months later, she achieved spontaneous pleurodesis (Fig. **1c**). This was evidenced by pleural drainage amounting to less than 50 mls for 3 consecutive days as well as lung re-expansion seen on CXR. IPC was then removed and there was no recurrence of the malignant pleural effusion.

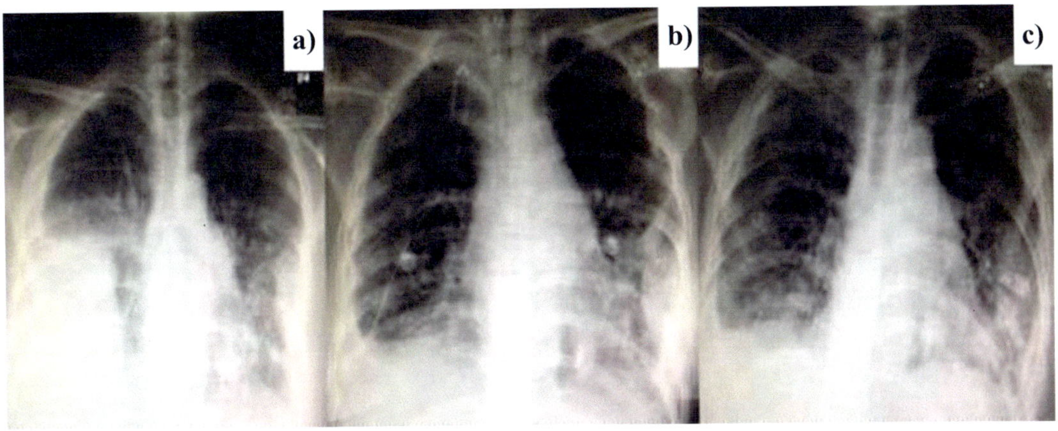

Fig. (1). (a) CXR before IPC insertion showed a moderate right pleural effusion. **(b)** CXR showed IPC *in situ* with significant reduction of pleural effusion. **(c)** CXR showed no recurrence of pleural effusion following the removal of IPC after spontaneous pleurodesis.

Indwelling Pleural Catheter: A Step by Step Approach (Figs. 2-8)

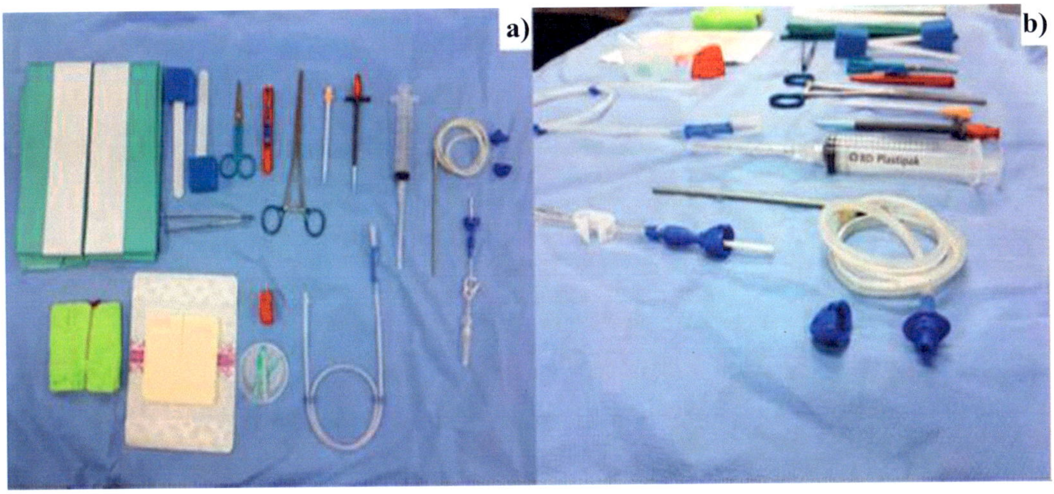

Fig. (2). (**a** and **b**) IPC set.

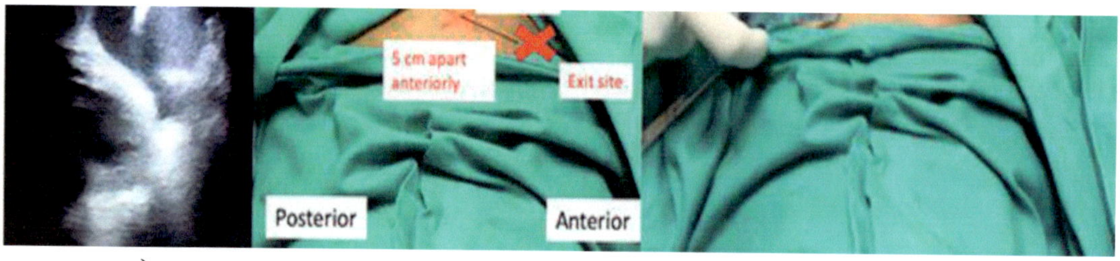

a) b) c)

Fig. (3). (a) After positioning the patient in the lateral position, ultrasound is used to locate the entry site. **(b)** Once entry site is located, mark the exit site about 5 cm anteriorly. **(c)** Under sterile technique, infiltrate lignocaine at the skin of the entry site as well as the periosteum of the rib, and parietal pleura.

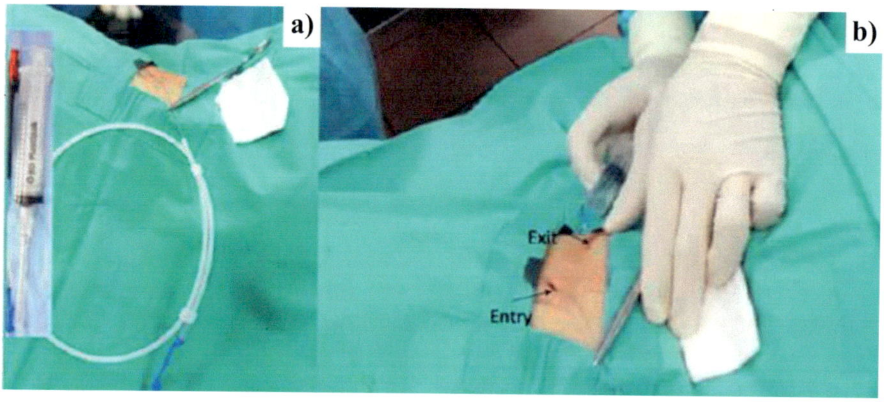

Fig. (4). (a) After locating the pleural cavity, insert the guide wire and remove the needle. Clamp the guide wire to the drape to avoid it getting dislodged. **(b)** Infiltrate lignocaine from the exit site to the entry site.

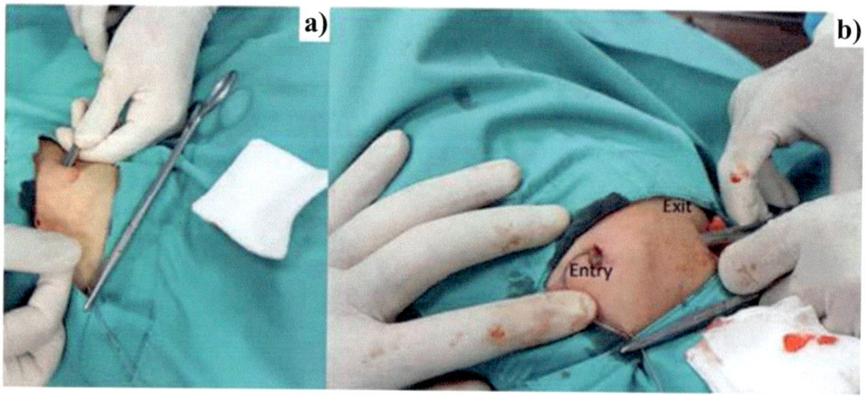

Fig. (5). (a) Create a subcutaneous tunnel starting from exit site to the entry site **(b)**.

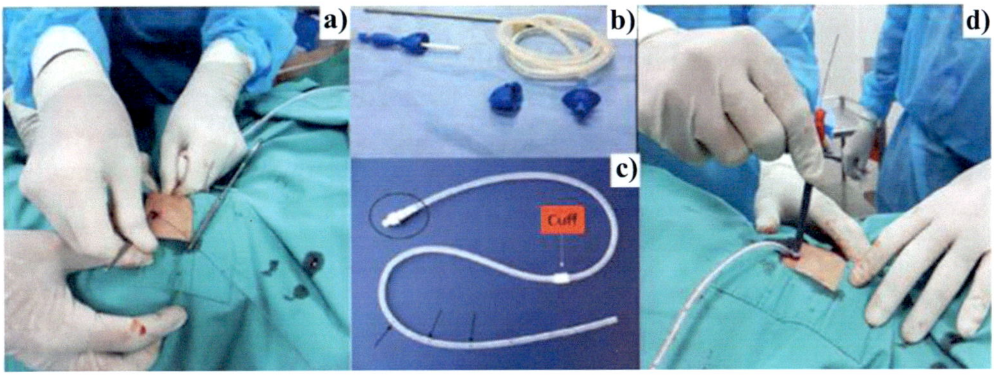

Fig. (6). (a) Insert the trocar attached to the distal end of IPC through the subcutaneous tract. The IPC is shown in **(b)**. The cuff **(c)** needs to be placed between the entry and exit site. **(d)** Dilator with a peel-away sheath being placed over the guide wire.

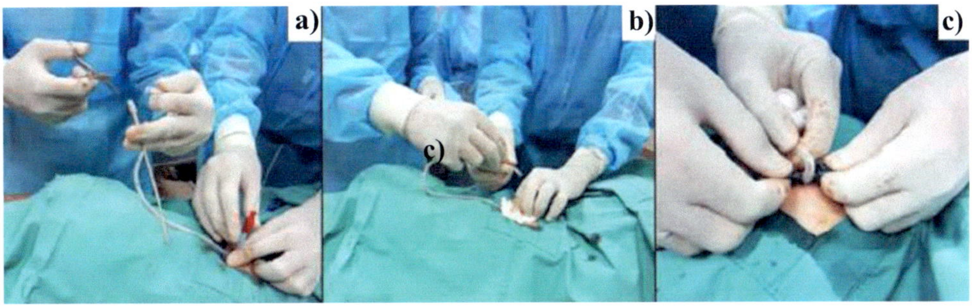

Fig. (7). (a) Use a scissors and cut the end of IPC to remove the trocar. **(b)** Remove the guide wire and dilator. **(c)** Insert the IPC through the sheath before peeling away the sheath.

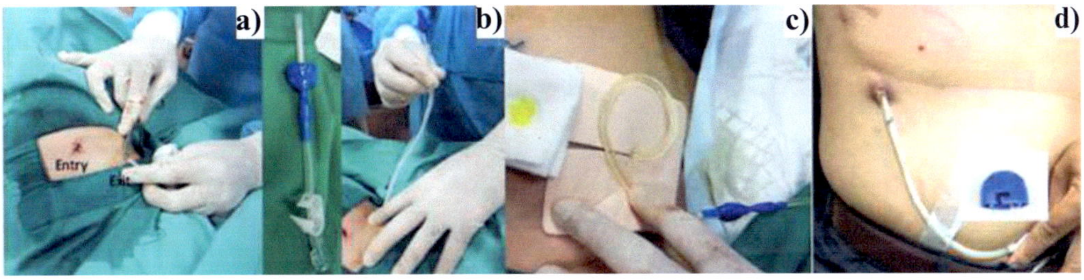

Fig. (8). (a) Suture the entry and exit site. **(b and c)** Connect the IPC adaptor to the catheter. **(d)** Once drained, connect the IPC cap to the catheter.

Learning Points

- IPC has become an accepted practice in the management of malignant pleural effusion especially in patients with non-expandable lung. Infection rate in specialised centres is low and most cases can be treated with antibiotics alone [1]. Spontaneous pleurodesis rate with IPC is about 50%; and there is a growing evidence of combining talc with IPC in selected cases. Chemotherapy should not be viewed as a contraindication for indwelling pleural catheter insertion and similarly chemotherapy should probably not be withheld from patients who have an IPC in place [2].

Video

The technique of IPC insertion (from patient positioning to connection of IPC adaptor).

CONSENT FOR PUBLICATION

Not applicable.

CONFLICT OF INTEREST

The author declares no conflict of interest, financial or otherwise.

ACKNOWLEDGEMENT

Declared none.

REFERENCES

[1] Fysh ETH, Tremblay A, Feller-Kopman D, *et al.* Clinical outcomes of indwelling pleural catheter-related pleural infections: an international multicenter study. Chest 2013; 144(5): 1597-602.
[http://dx.doi.org/10.1378/chest.12-3103] [PMID: 23828305]

[2] Chan Wah Hak C, Sivakumar P, Ahmed L. Safety of indwelling pleural catheter use in patients undergoing chemotherapy: a five-year retrospective evaluation. BMC Pulm Med 2016; 16(1): 41.
[http://dx.doi.org/10.1186/s12890-016-0203-7] [PMID: 26968653]

Case 13

Complication of Indwelling Pleural Catheter in a Patient with Advanced Breast Cancer

Aisya Natasya Musa[1], **Muhammad Amin Ibrahim**[1] and **Mohd Arif Mohd Zim**[1,*]

[1] *Respiratory Unit, Faculty of Medicine, Universiti Teknologi MARA (UiTM), Selangor, Malaysia*

Keywords: Breast cancer, Blocked indwelling pleural catheter, Intrapleural, Multiloculated, Streptokinase, Pleural effusion.

Presentation

A 62-year-old woman presented with progressive breathlessness over 2 weeks. There was no fever. She had a fungating skin lesion on her left breast extending to the left axilla that was biopsied which revealed infiltrating ductal carcinoma (Fig. **1**). Respiratory examination revealed a massive left sided pleural effusion.

Comorbidities

Left breast cancer in 2001 and completed chemotherapy but was subsequently lost to follow up.

Chest Imaging

CT thorax, abdomen and pelvis (CTTAP) confirmed local recurrence of left breast cancer with extensive local infiltration, metastases to bilateral pleurae with massive left pleural effusion, mediastinal and right hilar lymphadenopathies, abdominal lymphadenopathy and multiple lytic sclerotic metastatic bone lesions to T5, T6, T10, left-sided ribs, left humerus, bilateral iliac bones, sacral alae, right acetabulum and bilateral proximal femurs.

Intervention

Indwelling pleural catheter (IPC) was inserted under sedation (IV midazolam 1.5mg and IV Fentanyl 25 mcg). Due to the extensive skin metastases, the IPC was inserted posteriorly to reduce the risk of catheter tract seeding or metastases and pain (Fig. **2**). IPC insertion site location was confirmed with an ultrasound scan.

*****Corresponding author Mohd Arif Mohd Zim:** Respiratory Unit, Faculty of Medicine, Universiti Teknologi MARA (UiTM), Selangor, Malaysia; E-mail: firadhom@yahoo.com

Jamalul Azizi Abdul Rahaman & Tinku Joseph (Eds.)

Complications

3 weeks later, the patient presented with blocked IPC with minimal output for 3 days (Fig. **3**). Bedside USG showed a multiloculated effusion. Despite flushing, the drainage remained poor. Subsequently, 1,500,000 IU intrapleural streptokinase was instilled in 3 divided doses of 500,000 IU at 0,12 and 24 hours.

Post-Intervention

Despite the posterior position of the IPC, it was not associated with pain or discomfort to the patient. Following intrapleural streptokinase instillation, the IPC drainage improved to 3L over 2 days. A repeat CXR showed improvement of the loculated effusion (Fig. **4**). The case was referred to an oncologist and the patient received hormonal chemotherapy (Estrogen Receptor positive). 4 months later, there was a complete resolution of the effusion.

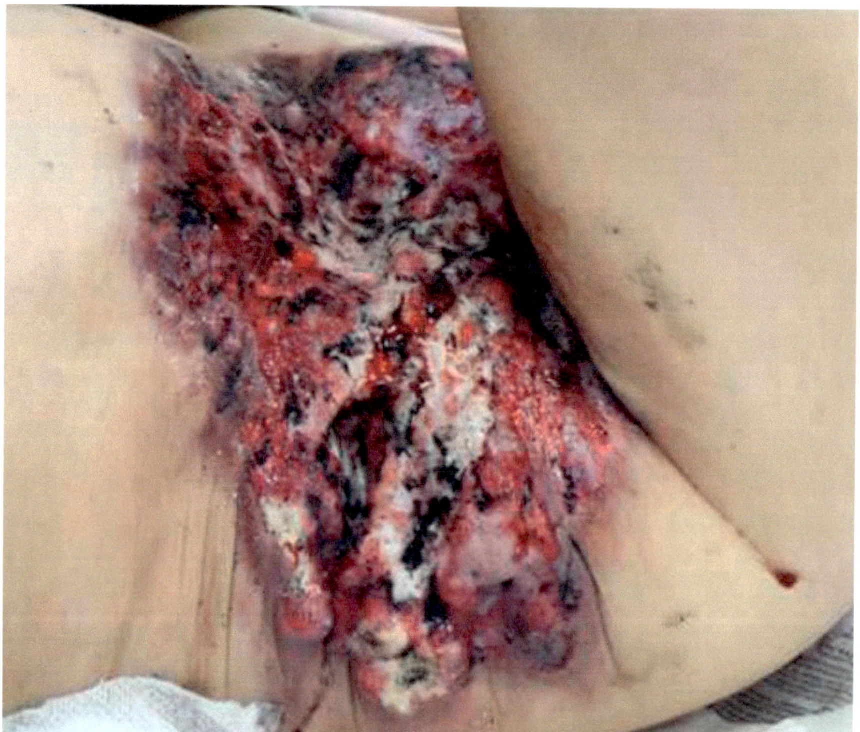

Fig. (1). Extensive skin lesion around the left breast and left axilla which was confirmed to be infiltrating ductal carcinoma.

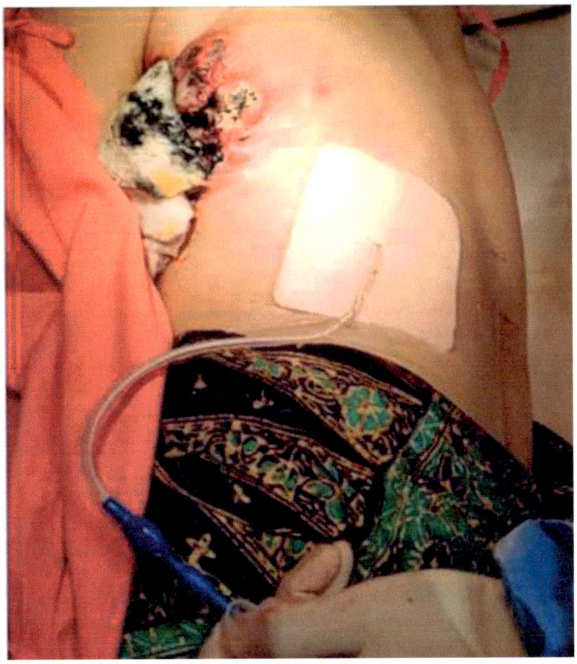

Fig. (2). Post IPC insertion showing its posterior location.

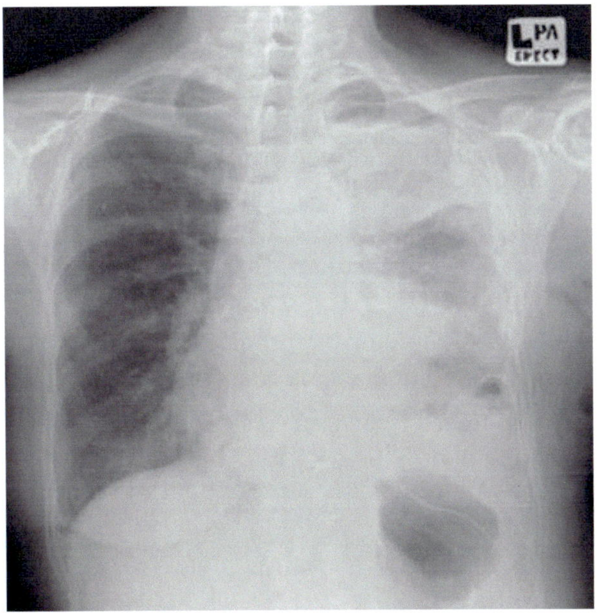

Fig. (3). CXR 3 weeks after IPC insertion when the patient presented with blocked IPC with reduced output showing multiloculated left sided pleural effusion.

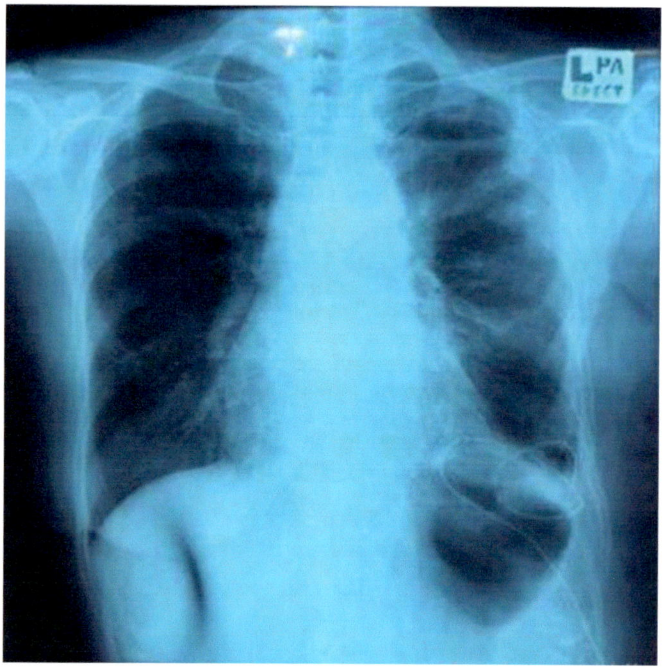

Fig. (4). CXR after intrapleural streptokinase instillation.

Learning Points

- Posterior insertion of IPC is possible in cases where insertion in the safety triangle is not possible. In this patient, it was not associated with discomfort or pain.
- Blocked IPC is uncommon and occurs in less than 5% in malignant pleural effusion which results from accumulation of fibrinous exudates within and surrounding the catheter lumen [1]. It is normally managed by flushing the tube or by instilling fibrinolytic agent; commonly alteplase. Our case highlights the fact that intrapleural streptokinase can be used as a cheaper alternative.
- Malignant pleural effusion responds to systemic chemotherapy [2]. This case also highlights the resolution of effusion after hormonal chemotherapy in a patient with metastatic pleural effusion secondary to breast cancer.

CONSENT FOR PUBLICATION

Not applicable.

CONFLICT OF INTEREST

The author declares no conflict of interest, financial or otherwise.

ACKNOWLEDGEMENT

Declared none.

REFERENCES

[1] Chalhoub M, Saqib A, Castellano M. Indwelling pleural catheters: complications and management strategies. J Thorac Dis 2018; 10(7): 4659-66.
[http://dx.doi.org/10.21037/jtd.2018.04.160] [PMID: 30174919]

[2] Dixit R, Agarwal KC, Gokhroo A, *et al*. Diagnosis and management options in malignant pleural effusions. Lung India 2017; 34(2): 160-6.
[http://dx.doi.org/10.4103/0970-2113.201305] [PMID: 28360465]

Case 14

Removal of Indwelling Pleural Catheter for Complicated Pleural Infection

Aisya Natasya Musa[1], **Muhammad Amin Ibrahim**[1] and **Mohd Arif Mohd Zim**[1,*]

[1] *Respiratory Unit, Faculty of Medicine, Universiti Teknologi MARA (UiTM), Selangor, Malaysia*

Keywords: EGFR positive, Indwelling pleural catheter, Lung adenocarcinoma, Purulent, Pleural effusion, Pseudomonas.

Presentation

A 41-year-old woman presented with recurrent right-sided pleural effusion. A lung biopsy confirmed adenocarcinoma of the lung with positive EGFR mutation. A pigtail was initially inserted to drain the effusion. However, due to persistent drainage, an indwelling pleural catheter (IPC) was inserted and the patient was discharged well (Fig. **1**). 2 weeks post-IPC insertion, the patient presented again with purulent pleural fluid and fever (Fig. **2**). Culture from the pleural fluid grew pseudomonas which was sensitive to amikacin, gentamicin and cefepime but resistant to Augmentin. The patient was subsequently treated with intravenous cefepime.

Comorbidities

Asthma, old pulmonary TB and hepatitis B carrier.

Chest Imaging

CT Thorax showed a multiloculated effusion with a split pleural sign suggestive of empyema (Fig. **3**).

Intervention

As the temperature continued to spike despite antibiotic, a decision was made to remove the IPC.

Complications

There were no complications following removal of the IPC (Fig. **4**).

***Corresponding author Mohd Arif Mohd Zim:** Respiratory Unit, Faculty of Medicine, Universiti Teknologi MARA (UiTM), Selangor, Malaysia; E-mail: firadhom@yahoo.com

Post-Intervention

The temperature settled and the patient was discharged well with oral antibiotics. She was commenced on gefitinib (TKI) by the oncologist and had no recurrence of the pleural effusion (Fig. **5**).

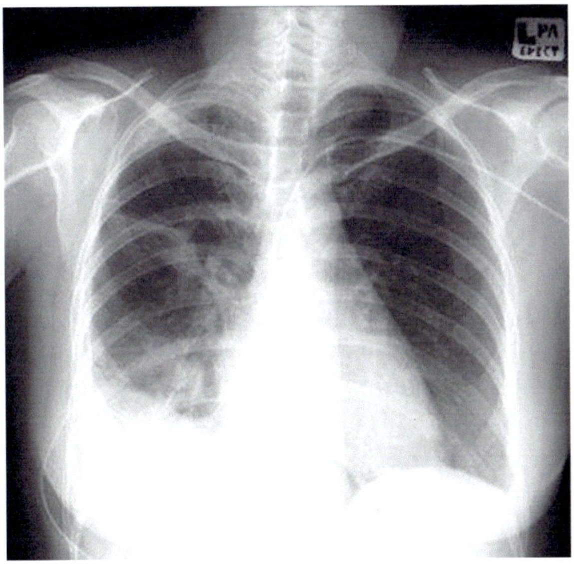

Fig. (1). CXR post-IPC insertion.

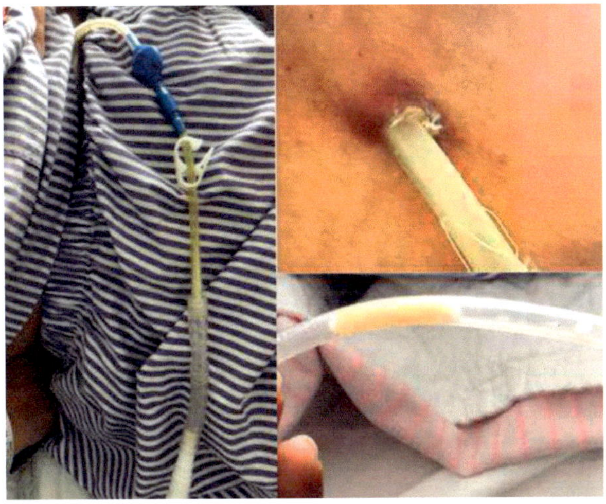

Fig. (2). Purulent pleural effusion from the IPC with a clean exit.

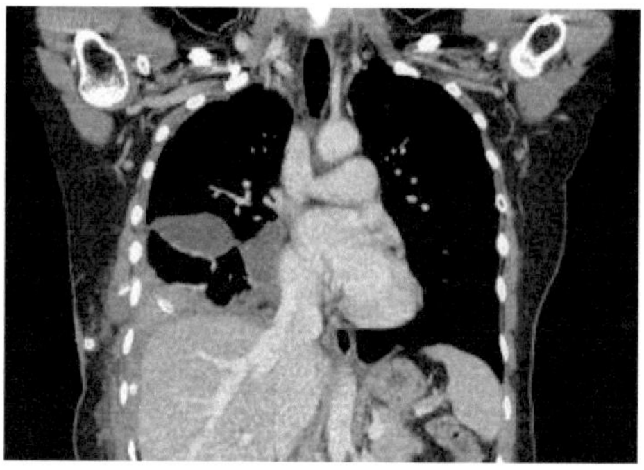

Fig. (3). Coronal CT Thorax shows the IPC position and the empyema.

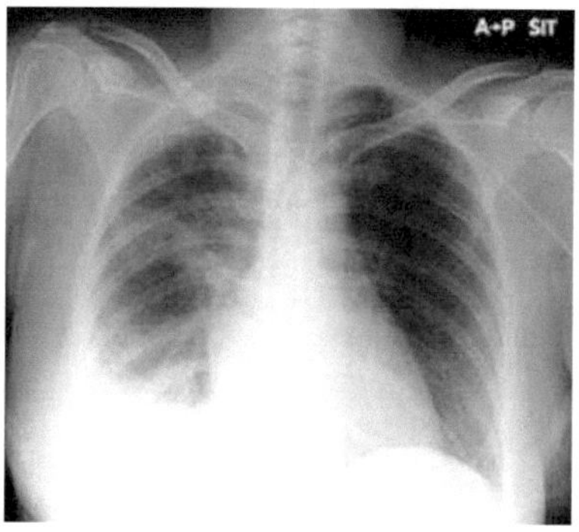

Fig. (4). CXR post-IPC removal.

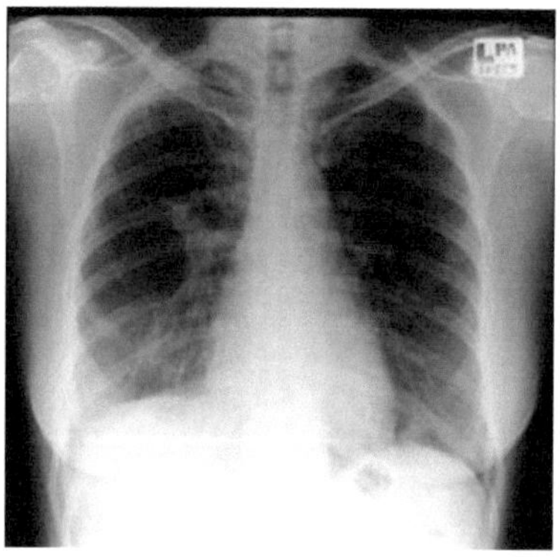

Fig. (5). CXR after 2 months on gefitinib.

Learning Points

- Catheter related empyema is normally managed with antibiotics [1]. Removal of IPC is only necessary if the infection is not responding to antibiotics as in this case [2]. Malignant pleural effusion (MPE) in an EGFR positive lung adenocarcinoma typically responds to TKI [3]. Therefore, in this group of patients, it is possible to look for resolution of the MPE after commencement of TKI before performing an invasive procedure such as IPC.

Video

The technique of IPC removal.

CONSENT FOR PUBLICATION

Not applicable.

CONFLICT OF INTEREST

The author declares no conflict of interest, financial or otherwise.

ACKNOWLEDGEMENT

Declared none.

REFERENCES

[1] Chalhoub M, Saqib A, Castellano M. Indwelling pleural catheters: complications and management strategies. J Thorac Dis 2018; 10(7): 4659-66. [http://dx.doi.org/10.21037/jtd.2018.04.160] [PMID: 30174919]

[2] Lui MMS, Thomas R, Lee YCG. Complications of indwelling pleural catheter use and their management. BMJ Open Respir Res 2016; 3(1): e000123. [http://dx.doi.org/10.1136/bmjresp-2015-000123] [PMID: 26870384]

[3] Dunscombe AO, Maskell NA. Common iatrogenic pleural complications. Curr Respir Care Rep 2012; 1(2): 82-90. [http://dx.doi.org/10.1007/s13665-012-0009-x]

Case 15

Malposition of Indwelling Pleural Catheter into the Liver

Aisya Natasya Musa[1], **Muhammad Amin Ibrahim**[1] and **Mohd Arif Mohd Zim**[1,*]

[1] *Respiratory Unit, Faculty of Medicine, Universiti Teknologi MARA (UiTM), Selangor, Malaysia*

Keywords: Indwelling pleural catheter, Lung adenocarcinoma, Malposition, Liver, Pleural effusion, Trapped lung.

Presentation

A 68-year-old woman was referred to our centre for pleuroscopy. She presented with a 2-week history of cough, loss of weight and loss of appetite. Clinical examination revealed a massive right sided pleural effusion. There was no cervical lymphadenopathy and breast examination was unremarkable. She had recurrent episodes of right sided pleural effusion and was treated as parapneumonic effusion. A conventional chest tube was inserted at the referring hospital to drain the pleural fluid (Fig. **1**).

Comorbidities

Hypertension.

Chest Imaging

CT Thorax showed a massive right sided pleural effusion with thickened pleura suggestive of empyema. There were multiple left lung nodules.

Intervention

Pleuroscopy under sedation showed chronic inflamed pleura with poor rib to rib differentiation throughout the anterior, posterior, diaphragmatic and apical pleurae. There were multiple nodules throughout (Fig. **2**). The lung was trapped and not expanding. Biopsy of the nodules from the anterior pleura confirmed metastatic lung adenocarcinoma (EGFR positive).

[*]**Corresponding author Mohd Arif Mohd Zim:** Respiratory Unit, Faculty of Medicine, Universiti Teknologi MARA (UiTM), Selangor, Malaysia; E-mail: firadhom@yahoo.com

Jamalul Azizi Abdul Rahaman & Tinku Joseph (Eds.)

As the pleural effusion did not resolve, an indwelling pleural catheter (IPC) was inserted 2 weeks later. This was done under sedation and ultrasound guidance to confirm the position without any immediate complications (Fig. **3**). Post IPC, a total of 2L of fluid was removed and she was discharged well and referred to the oncologist who prescribed gefitinib (TKI).

Complications

1 week post IPC insertion, there was leaking at the IPC site, skin breakdown with slough surrounding the exit site. This was managed with de-sloughing, re-suturing the exit site and she was treated as exit-site infection and remained well. She was managed as an outpatient till 2 months later when she had fever and greenish discharge from the IPC. Her IPC was not draining, and aspirate yielded a small amount of pus. She was admitted and was treated as nosocomial pneumonia and empyema with intravenous Tazosin.

CXR and CT thorax showed malposition of the IPC in the liver (Figs. **4** and **5**). The decision was made to remove the IPC with cardiothoracic and surgical backup. The IPC was removed without any complications and the patient remained stable throughout.

Post-Intervention

The patient continued to improve on gefitinib with no recurrence of the effusion till her disease progressed one year later.

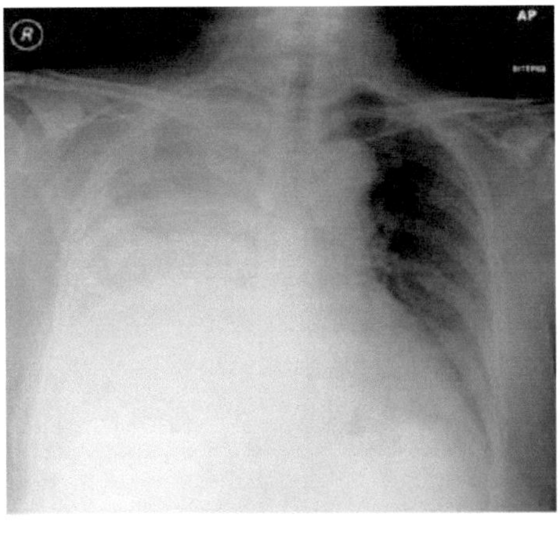

Fig. (1). CXR prior to conventional chest drain insertion by the referring hospital.

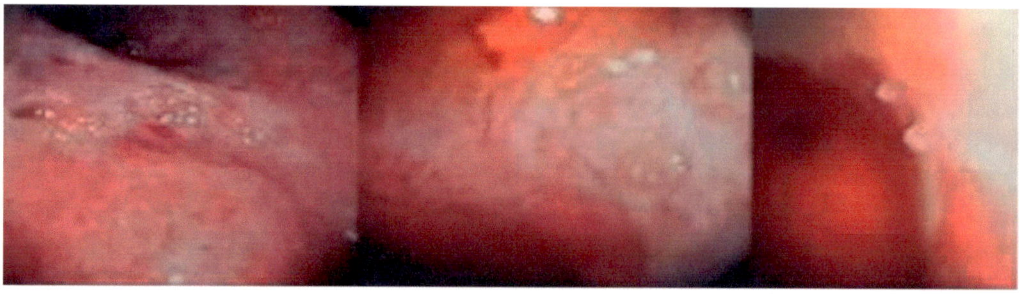

Fig. (2). Pleuroscopy findings showing chronic inflamed parietal pleura with multiple nodules.

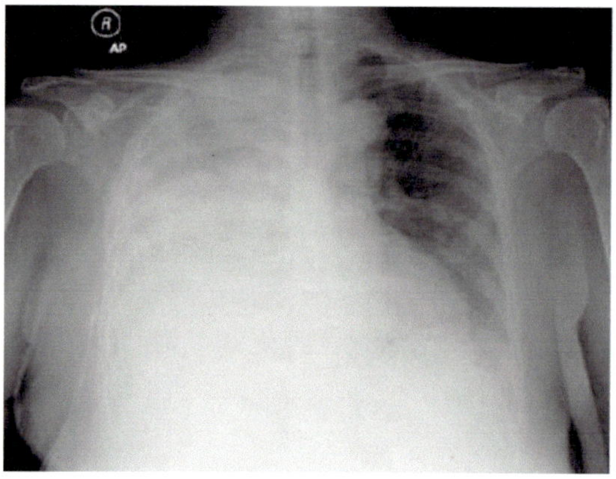

Fig. (3). CXR post-IPC insertion.

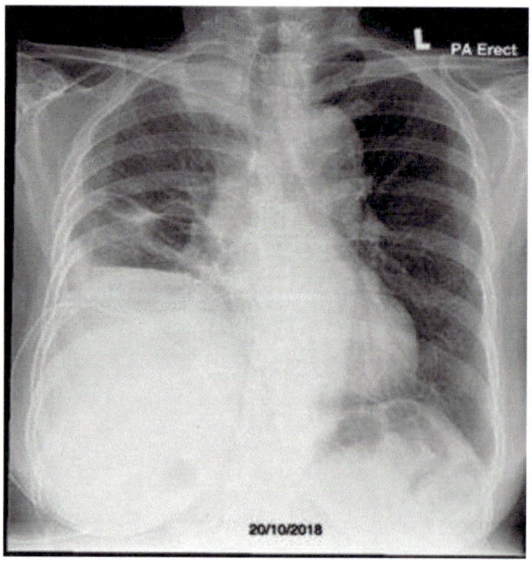

Fig. (4). Location of the IPC traversing the pleural space and through the diaphragm and liver.

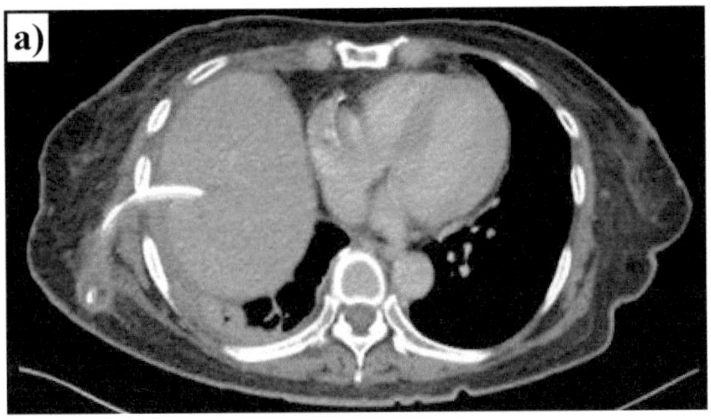

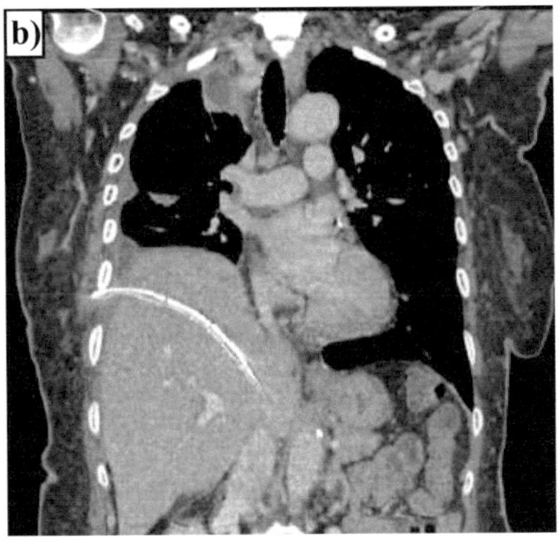

Fig. (5). (a and **b)** Axial and coronal CT thorax showing the IPC traversing the pleural space and through the diaphragm and liver.

Learning Points

- Drain malposition can occur in 2.4% of cases and is commoner in the conventional chest tube with trocar [1]. In order to avoid this, pleural USG should be done prior to chest tube insertion. As IPC insertion is a blunt technique, it is not possible for the pleural catheter to pierce the diaphragm and the liver. It is likely that the previous chest tube insertion had created a tract which the pleural catheter followed. This case highlights the importance of imaging when performing procedures in the pleural space to avoid injuries to other organs such as the liver and diaphragm.

CONSENT FOR PUBLICATION

Not applicable.

CONFLICT OF INTEREST

The author declares no conflict of interest, financial or otherwise.

ACKNOWLEDGEMENT

Declared none.

REFERENCE

[1] Dunscombe AO, Maskell NA. Common iatrogenic pleural complications. Curr Respir Care Rep 2012; 1(2): 82-90.
[http://dx.doi.org/10.1007/s13665-012-0009-x]

Case 16

Intrapleural Fibrinolytics

Alternative Regimen of Intrapleural Fibrinolytics with Alteplase and Pulmozyme for Complex Effusion in a Post-Surgery Patient

Mas Fazlin Mohamad Jailaini[1] and **Mohamed Faisal Abdul Hamid**[1,*]

[1] *Respiratory Unit, Faculty of Medicine, National University of Malaysia, Selangor, Malaysia*

Keywords: Alteplase, Complex effusion, DNase, Dornase-alfa, Fibrinolytic, Pulmozyme.

Presentation

A 68-year-old woman, presented with haematuria was diagnosed with bilateral staghorn renal calculi and bilateral hydronephrosis. Bilateral ureteric stenting followed by a right percutaneous nephrolithotomy (PCNL) was performed. However, 48 hours post-operatively, she developed high grade fever with right pleuritic chest pain.

Post-operatively, she developed nosocomial pneumonia which progressed into a right parapneumonic effusion requiring non-invasive ventilation. She was febrile with temperature 38.40 C, pulse rate 120/min, blood pressure 105/70 mmHg, oxygen saturation 90% on room air. Chest examination revealed reduced breath sounds over the right hemithorax with reduced vocal resonance and stony dullness on percussion.

She was prescribed Tazobactam/Piperacillin. She desaturated and required non-invasive ventilation. Bedside thoracic sonography revealed multi-septated effusion. A 12 Fr intercostal chest catheter (ICC) was inserted under ultrasound guidance, and pleural fluid analysis revealed exudative effusion with LDH of 1100 IU/L, with pleural to serum creatinine ratio <1 indicating no evidence of nephro-pleural fistula. The pleural fluid culture revealed no growth.

Comorbidities

None.

[*] **Corresponding author Mohamed Faisal Abdul Hamid:** Respiratory Unit, Faculty of Medicine, National University of Malaysia, Selangor, Malaysia; E-mail: faisal.hamid@ppukm.ukm.edu.my

Chest Imaging

CXR revealed right moderate pleural effusion (Fig. **1**).

Intervention

Intrapleural fibrinolysis in view of minimal chest drainage following ICC insertion. This had to be done with caution as the patient had surgery 48 hours earlier. We used a lower dose of intrapleural alteplase 2.5mg and pulmozyme 5mg which were administered sequentially 12 hours apart. The chest catheter was flushed with saline to ensure its patency prior to the procedure and oral tramadol 50mg was given. Fifteen minutes later, alteplase at 2.5mg diluted in 50mL of 0.9% sodium chloride was instilled intrapleurally *via* ICC, which was then allowed to dwell for 45 minutes and then unclamped to allow free drainage for 45 minutes. The same procedure was then repeated for Pulmozyme 5mg (diluted in 50mL of 0.9% sodium chloride). The remainder of the diluted medication was kept in the fridge. Therapy was given 12 hours apart.

Complications

None.

Post-Intervention

After 3 doses of intrapleural alteplase and pulmozyme, a total of 2.1L of hemoserous fluid was drained. Serial CXR and bedside thoracic sonography revealed minimal effusion (Figs. **2-4**). Her clinical condition improved gradually, and she was discharged well after completing 1 week of intravenous antibiotics.

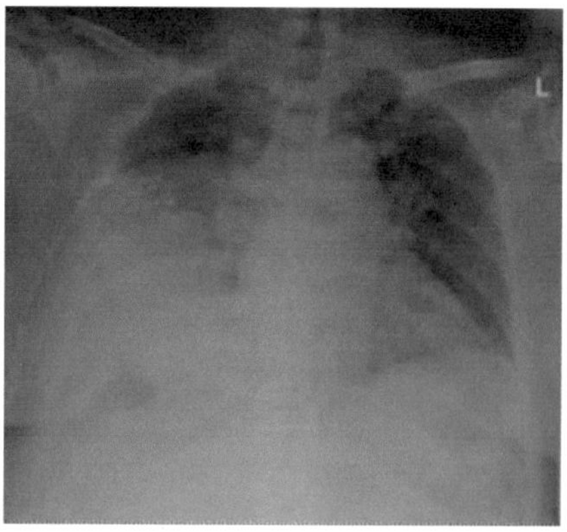

Fig. (1). CXR on initial presentation showed moderate right pleural effusion with ICC *in situ*.

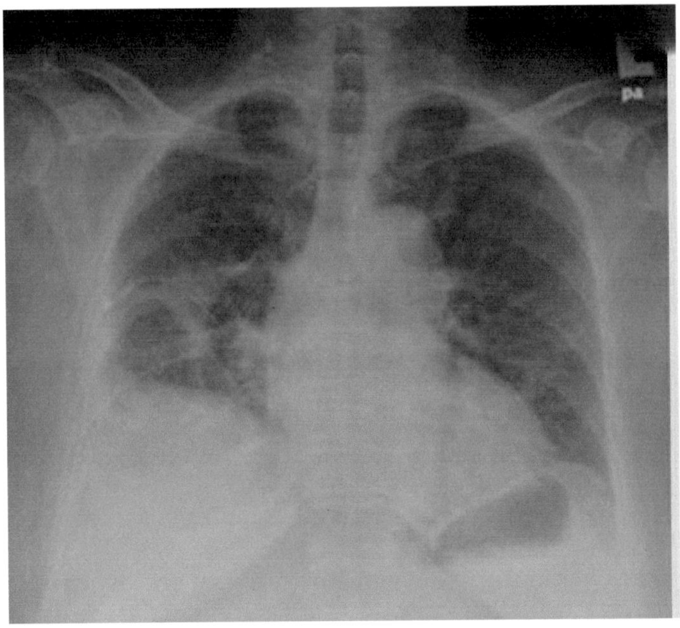

Fig. (2). CXR 3 days post intrapleural alteplase and pulmozyme showed significant reduction of right pleural effusion.

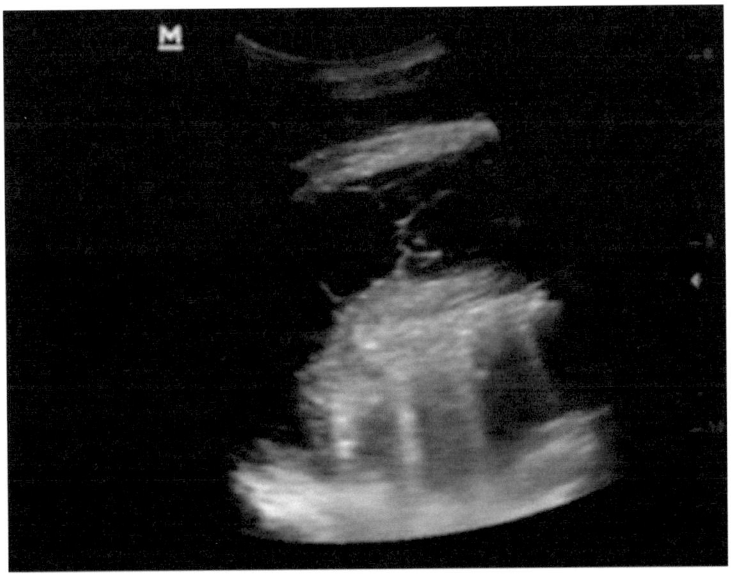

Fig. (3). Thoracic sonography pre-intrapleural fibrinolysis showed septated effusion.

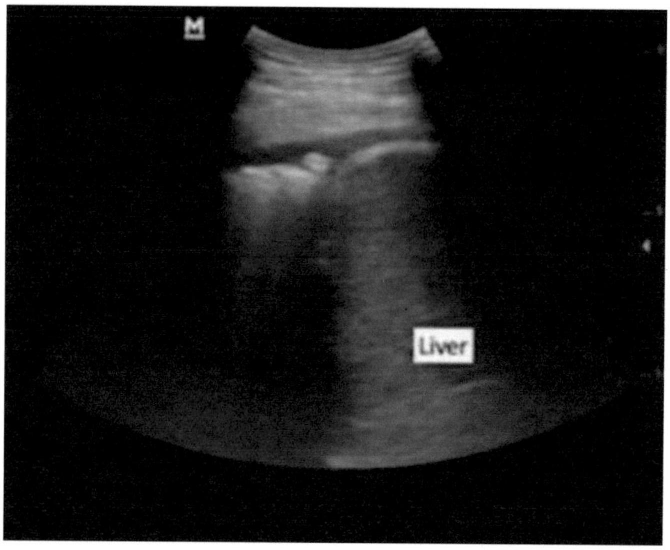

Fig. (4). Thoracic sonography 24 hours post-fibrinolysis showed minimal effusion.

Learning Points

- There is no standardized regimen for intrapleural alteplase and pulmozyme and the dosing needs to be individualized. Studies looking at lower doses of alteplase (2.5mg-5mg) showed similar efficacy compared with 10mg alteplase in combination with 5mg Pulmozyme [1, 2]. We opted to use 2.5 mg alteplase in our patient to minimize the risk of bleeding as the patient had a recent surgery; although the systemic bleeding rate from the use of intrapleural alteplase was reported to be low.

CONSENT FOR PUBLICATION

Not applicable.

CONFLICT OF INTEREST

The author declares no conflict of interest, financial or otherwise.

ACKNOWLEDGEMENT

Declared none.

REFERENCES

[1] Ip H, West A, Wallace D, Noorzad F, Ahmed L. Safety and efficacy of reduced dose intrapleural alteplase and DNAase for pleural infection. Eur Respir J 2018; 52(Suppl. 62): PA4712.

[2] Popowicz N, Bintcliffe O, De Fonseka D, *et al.* Dose de-escalation of intrapleural tissue plasminogen activator therapy for pleural infection. The alteplase dose assessment for pleural infection therapy project. Ann Am Thorac Soc 2017; 14(6): 929-36. [http://dx.doi.org/10.1513/AnnalsATS.201609-673OC] [PMID: 28324671]

Case 17

Intrapleural Fibrinolytics with Alteplase and Pulmozyme for Complex Tuberculous Effusion

Mohamed Faisal Abdul Hamid[1,*]

[1] *Respiratory Unit, Faculty of Medicine, National University of Malaysia, Selangor, Malaysia*

Keywords: Alteplase, DNase, Dornase-alfa, Fibrinolytic, Pulmozyme, Tuberculous effusion.

Presentation

A 35-year-old gentleman, a chronic smoker presented with fever for 1 week associated with chronic cough for the past 6 months. He was febrile with temperature 39.40 C, pulse rate 110/min, blood pressure 130/90 mmHg, and oxygen saturation 94% on room air. Chest examination revealed reduced breath sounds over right mid-lower zone with reduced vocal resonance and stony dullness on percussion.

He was prescribed Tazobactam/Piperacillin, however, he had a persistent spike of temperature. CXR revealed right moderate pleural effusion (Fig. **1a**). CT Thorax revealed loculated right pleural effusion with collapse consolidation of the anterior segment of right upper, middle and lower lobes with the presence of lytic bone lesion at the right posterior 8th rib and 10th ribs (Figs. **2a** and **b**). Thoracentesis revealed exudative effusion and pleuroscopy revealed hyperemic inflamed costal pleura with minimal septations at the apex. CXR post-pleuroscopy revealed persistent right pleural effusion (Fig. **3**).

Further investigations revealed pleural fluid adenosine deaminase of 57 U/L, and parietal pleural biopsy revealed chronic granulomatous inflammation suggestive of tuberculosis. He was treated as tuberculous pleural effusion with bone (rib) involvement.

Comorbidities

None.

[*]**Corresponding author Mohamed Faisal Abdul Hamid:** Respiratory Unit, Faculty of Medicine, National University of Malaysia, Selangor, Malaysia; E-mail: faisal.hamid@ppukm.ukm.edu.my

Chest Imaging

CXR revealed right moderate pleural effusion.

Intervention

As chest tube was not draining and CT showed loculated effusion, intrapleural fibrinolytics were administered. Prior to the procedure, the chest tube was flushed to ensure its patency. Oral tramadol 50mg was given 15 minutes before the procedure. Sequential alteplase at 16mg and Pulmozyme 5mg were instilled intrapleurally. Both medications were diluted in 50mL of 0.9% sodium chloride solution. Alteplase 16mg was instilled first intrapleurally *via* the chest tube, which was then allowed to dwell for 45 minutes and then unclamped to allow free drainage for 45 minutes. The same procedure was then repeated for Pulmozyme 5mg. Therapy was given 12 hours apart for a maximum of 3 doses. However, our patient only required 2 doses as there was significant drainage of pleural fluid following the intervention.

Complications

None.

Post-Intervention

After 2 doses of intrapleural alteplase and Pulmozyme, a total of 2.3L of hemoserous fluid was drained. Bedside thoracic sonography revealed minimal effusion (Figs. **4a** and **b**) and a repeat CT Thorax showed significant radiological improvement (Fig. **5**). Patient's temperature subsided, the chest tube was removed, and he was discharged well.

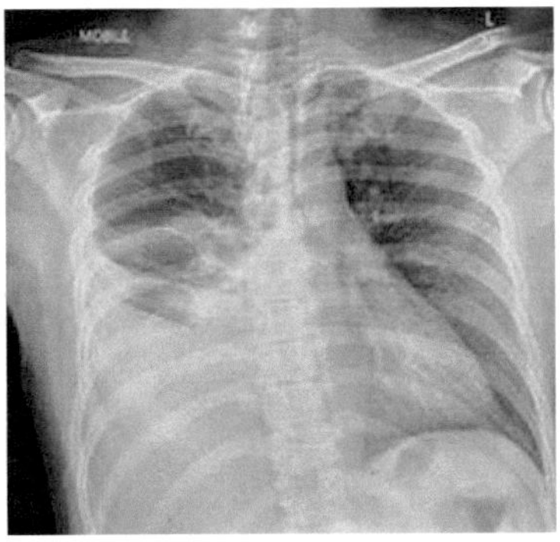

Fig. (1). CXR on initial presentation showed moderate right pleural effusion.

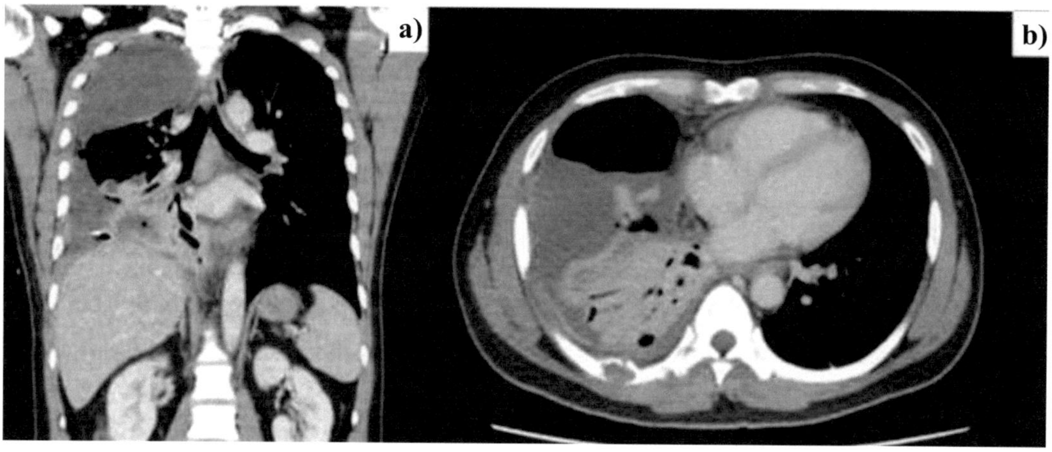

Fig. (2). **(a)** Coronal CT Thorax showed right loculated pleural effusion. **(b)** Axial CT Thorax showed loculated right pleural effusion with collapse consolidation of the right lower lobe and lytic lesion at right posterior 8th and 10th ribs.

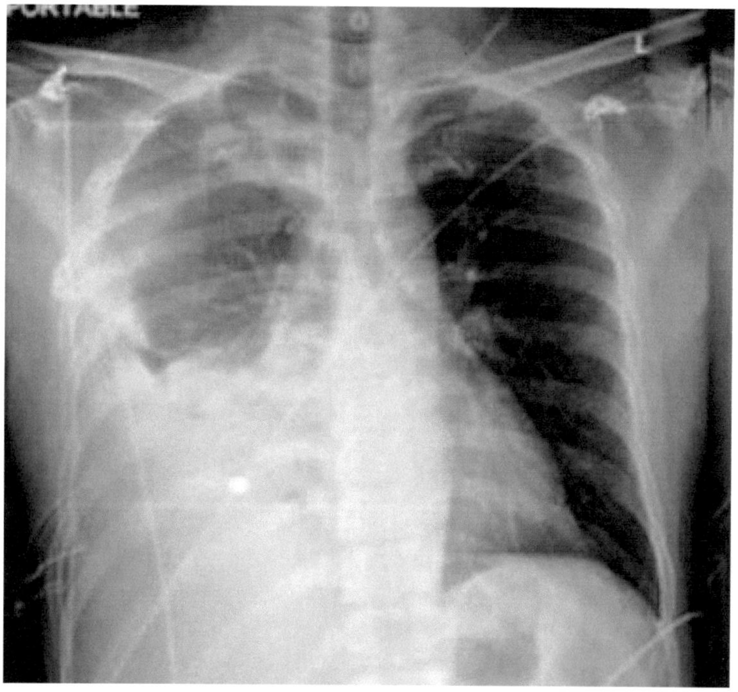

Fig. (3). CXR post-pleuroscopy revealed persistent right pleural effusion.

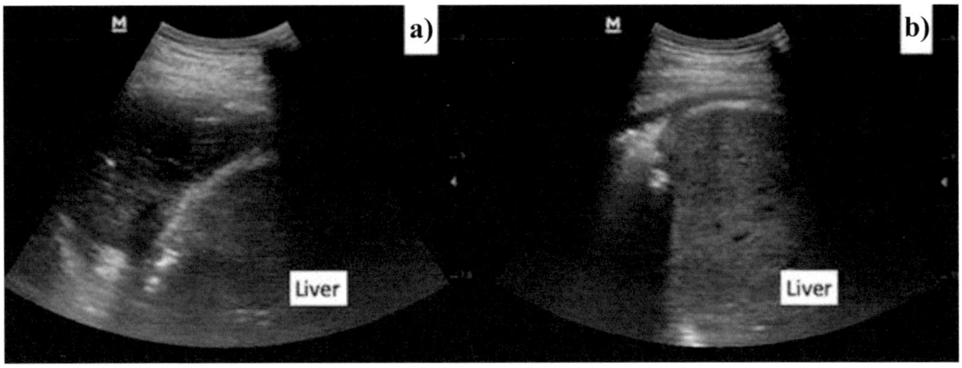

Fig. (4). (a) Thoracic sonography pre-intrapleural fibrinolysis showed septated effusion which resolved 48 hours post-intrapleural fibrinolysis **(b)**.

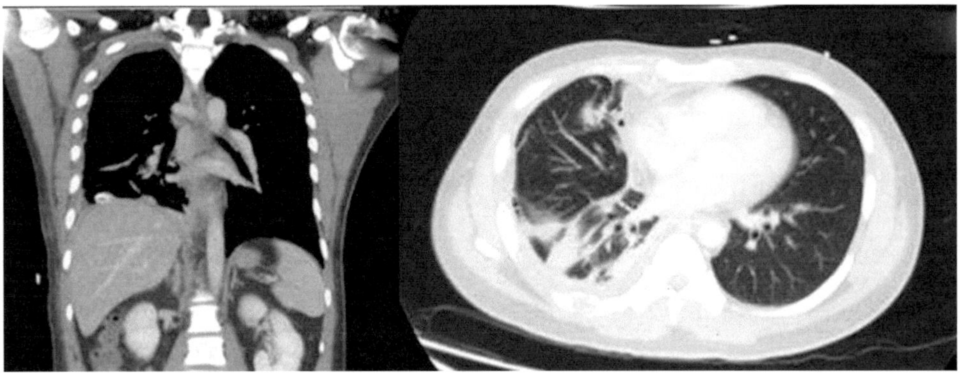

Fig. (5). (Left) Coronal CT Thorax and (Right) axial CT thorax 48 hours after 2 doses of intrapleural alteplase and pulmozyme revealed minimal right pleural effusion with minimal consolidation of the right lower lobe.

Learning Points

- Combination of alteplase and pulmozyme improves pleural drainage and reduces the rate of surgical referral as demonstrated by Multi-center Intra-pleural Sepsis Trial (MIST-2) using alteplase 10mg and pulmozyme 5mg [1]. Our regimen of 16mg alteplase and 5mg pulmozyme can be an alternative regimen in centers with different alteplase formulations, as it is effective with an acceptable safety profile [2]. However, the dosage of intrapleural alteplase needs to be individualized depending on bleeding risk (*e.g.*, post-surgical, thrombocytopenia/coagulopathy), nature of effusion (*e.g.*, empyema *vs* hemothorax) and patient's general condition.

CONSENT FOR PUBLICATION

Not applicable.

CONFLICT OF INTEREST

The author declares no conflict of interest, financial or otherwise.

ACKNOWLEDGEMENT

Declared none.

REFERENCES

[1] Rahman NM, Maskell NA, West A, *et al.* Intrapleural use of tissue plasminogen activator and DNase in pleural infection. N Engl J Med 2011; 365(6): 518-26. [http://dx.doi.org/10.1056/NEJMoa1012740] [PMID: 21830966]

[2] Cheong XK, Yu-Lin Ban A, Abdul Hamid MF. Short-course intrapleural alteplase and DNase in complex effusion with bleeding risk. Respirol Case Rep 2020; 8(7): e00648. [http://dx.doi.org/10.1002/rcr2.648] [PMID: 32864139]

Case 18

Chest Ultrasonography

Parapneumonic Effusion with Collapsed Consolidated Lung

Muhammad Redzwan S. Rashid Ali[1,*]

[1] *KPJ Johor Specialist Hospital, Johor Bahru, Malaysia*

Keywords: Consolidation, Loculation, Pleural effusion, Septations, Thoracic, Ultrasonography (USG).

Presentation

A 28-year-old patient, non-smoker presented with cough, fever, dyspnoea and pleuritic pain of 4 days duration.

Comorbidities

Nil.

Chest Imaging

Gross consolidation of the left lung on CXR (Fig. **1**).

CT Thorax showed bilateral diffuse consolidation more on the left lung with mild loculation and septa tion suggestive of exudative pleural effusion (Fig. **2**).

Thoracic USG showed echogenic pleural effusion with antecedent dense consolidation of the left lung (Fig. **3**).

Intervention

Broad spectrum intravenous antibiotics, pleural aspiration, drainage and oxygen.

Complications

None.

*Corresponding author Muhammad Redzwan S. Rashid Ali:** KPJ Johor Specialist Hospital, Johor Bahru, Malaysia; E-mail: redzwanrashid@gmail.com

Post-Intervention

Improvement after intravenous antibiotics, oxygen support, pleural aspiration and drainage.

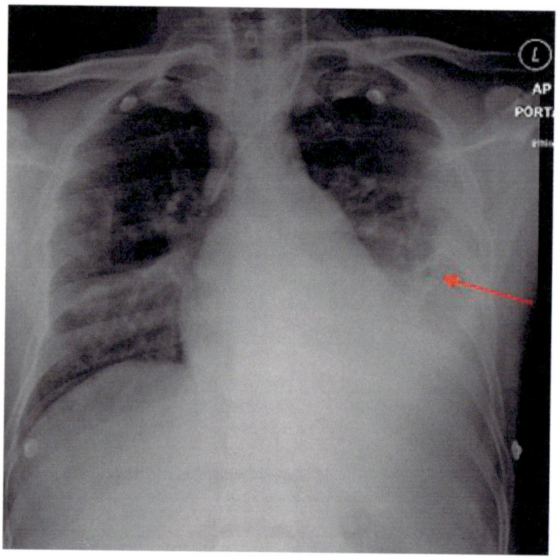

Fig. (1). CXR showing left lobar consolidation with early evidence of pleural effusion (red arrow).

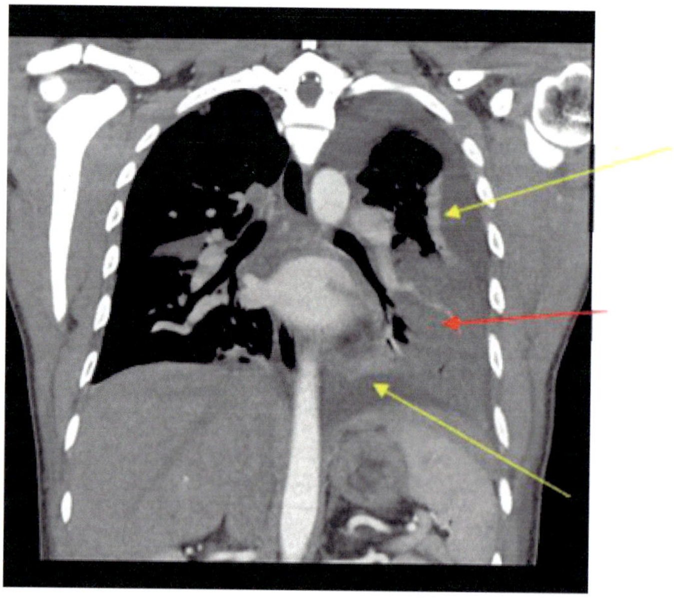

Fig. (2). Coronal CT Thorax showing a dense left lobar consolidation (red arrow) with adjacent pleural effusion (yellow arrows).

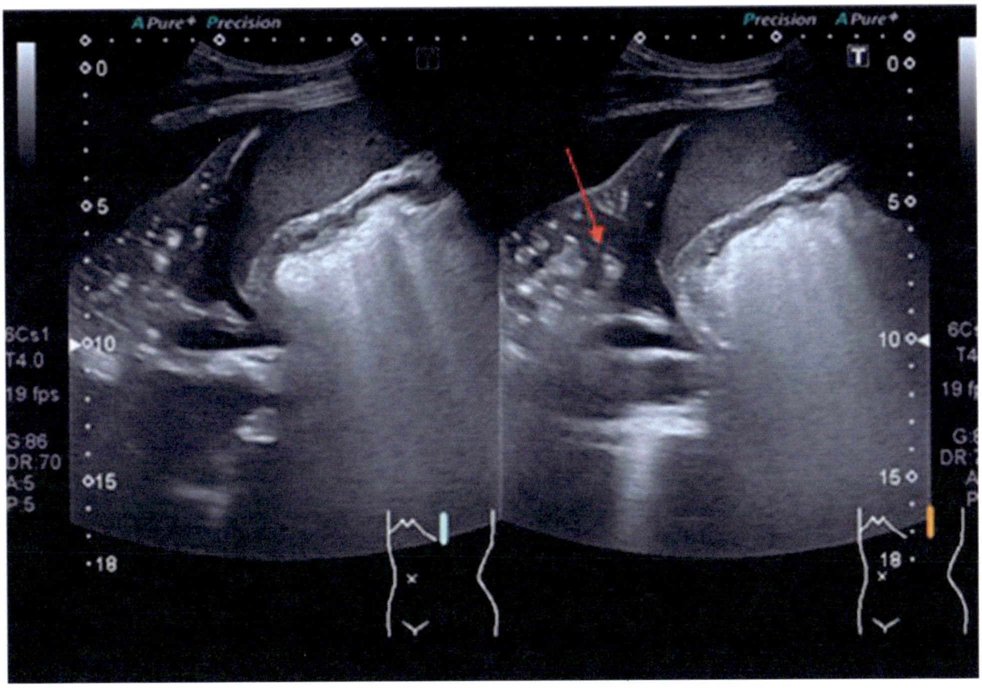

Fig. (3). Thoracic USG revealed a dense echogenic consolidated left lung (sonographic air bronchograms) (red arrow) with adjacent pleural effusion which was aspirated twice.

Learning Points

- Early institution of antibiotics and pleural aspiration prevents progression to complicated parapneumonic effusion and empyema. Transthoracic USG can be a useful bedside tool to differentiate worsening consolidation or presence of parapneumonic effusion to alter antibiotic therapy, for drainage of the infected pleural fluid and to monitor clinical progression of patient together with biochemical parameters [1].

CONSENT FOR PUBLICATION

Not applicable.

CONFLICT OF INTEREST

The author declares no conflict of interest, financial or otherwise.

ACKNOWLEDGEMENT

Declared none.

REFERENCE

[1] Koegelenberg CFN, von Groote-Bidlingmaier F, Bolliger CT. Transthoracic ultrasonography for the respiratory physician. Respiration 2012; 84(4): 337-50. [http://dx.doi.org/10.1159/000339997] [PMID: 22832423]

Case 19

Rapid Detection of Pneumothorax by Thoracic Sonography

Mohamed Faisal Abdul Hamid[1,*]

[1]Respiratory Unit, Faculty of Medicine, National University of Malaysia, Selangor, Malaysia

Keywords: Barcode sign, Lung point, Pneumothorax, Stratosphere sign, Sliding sign, Seashore sign.

Presentation

A 16-year-old boy presented to our center complaining of sudden onset of left sided pleuritic chest pain. There was no preceding trauma or respiratory tract infections.

On presentation, he was slightly tachypnoeic with a respiratory rate of 22/minute, blood pressure was 110/70mm Hg and heart rate of 100/minute. Examination of the respiratory system revealed reduced breath sound over the left hemithorax with hyper-resonance on percussion.

Comorbidities

None.

Chest Imaging

A quick bedside thoracic sonography on the left hemithorax revealed loss of sliding sign and absence of B lines, while on M mode revealed stratosphere sign (barcode sign) (Fig. **1a**) as opposed to seashore sign demonstrated on the normal lung (Fig. **1b**). There was presence of "lung point" postero-laterally indicating the boundary of pneumothorax (Fig. **2a**). These findings were confirmed with CXR that revealed left-sided pneumothorax mea suring >2cm at the hilar level (Fig. **2b**).

Intervention

We performed needle thoracentesis at the left 2nd intercostal space in the midclavicular line. Following local anaesthetic with lignocaine 2%, a 16G cannula was inserted and 750mls of air aspirated. Bedside ultrasound was done which

*Corresponding author Mohamed Faisal Abdul Hamid:** Respiratory Unit, Faculty of Medicine, National University of Malaysia, Selangor, Malaysia; E-mail: faisal.hamid@ppukm.ukm.edu.my

Jamalul Azizi Abdul Rahaman & Tinku Joseph (Eds.)

revealed the presence of a sliding sign with a seashore sign indicating resolved pneumothorax.

Complications

Nil.

Post-Intervention

The patient was discharged the following day as there was complete re-expansion of the lung. There was no recurrence of pneumothorax upon clinic review.

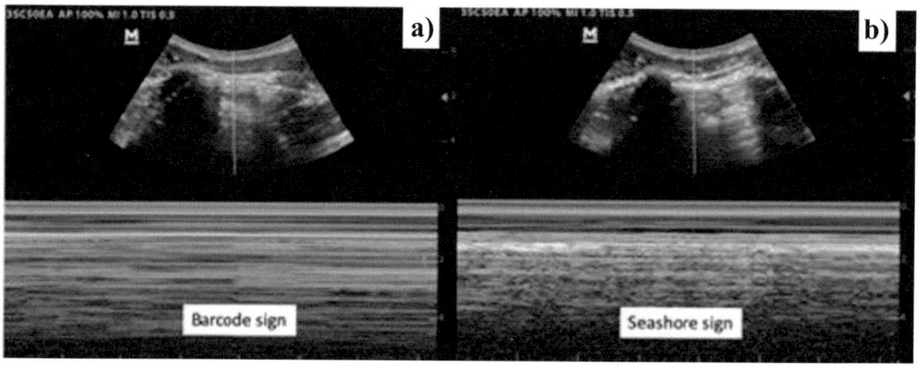

Fig. (1). (a) Ultrasound of the left hemothorax revealed Barcode sign (Stratosphere sign) indicating presence of pneumothorax. **(b)** Ultrasound on the right hemithorax (normal lung) revealed seashore sign indicating normal lung sliding.

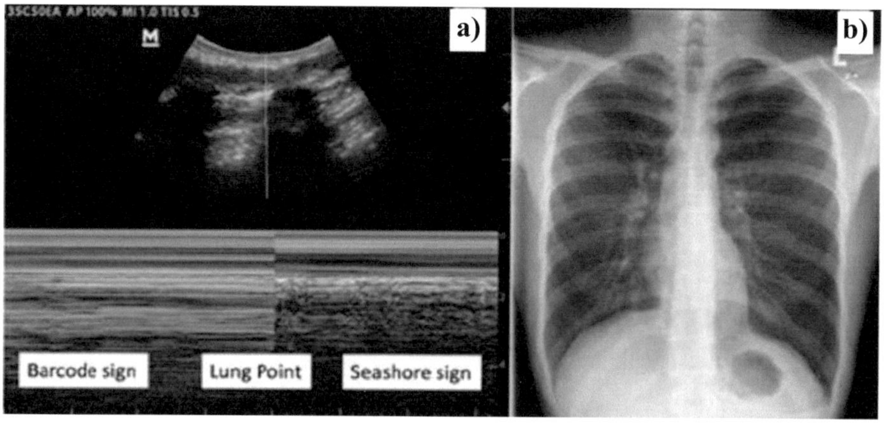

Fig. (2). (a) Ultrasound of the left hemithorax indicating lung point which is the boundary of the pneumothorax. **(b)** CXR revealed left-sided pneumothorax.

Learning Points

- Thoracic sonography is useful to diagnose pneumothorax especially when there is delay in performing CXR. Signs of pneumothorax on ultrasound include loss of sliding sign, absence of B lines (comet-tail sign), stratosphere sign (barcode sign), lung point as well as lung pulse. The presence of lung sliding with comet tail artifacts excludes pneumothorax (high negative predictive value) but the reverse is not true [1]. Identification of lung point is 100% specific for pneumothorax [2].

Video

Sonographic signs of pneumothorax in the above patient.

CONSENT FOR PUBLICATION

Not applicable.

CONFLICT OF INTEREST

The author declares no conflict of interest, financial or otherwise.

ACKNOWLEDGEMENT

Declared none.

REFERENCES

[1] Husain L, Hagopian L, Wayman D, Baker W, Carmody K. Sonographic diagnosis of pneumothorax. J Emerg Trauma Shock 2012; 5(1): 76-81. [http://dx.doi.org/10.4103/0974-2700.93116] [PMID: 22416161]

[2] Lichtenstein D, Mezière G, Biderman P, Gepner A. The "lung point": an ultrasound sign specific to pneumothorax. Intensive Care Med 2000; 26(10): 1434-40. [http://dx.doi.org/10.1007/s001340000627] [PMID: 11126253]

Case 20

Point of Care Thoracic Ultrasound (Diaphragm) in a Post-COVID-19 Patient

Soo Chun Ian[1,*]

[1] *University of Malaya Medical Center, Kuala Lumpur, Malaysia*

Keywords: Thoracic ultrasound, Diaphragm ultrasound, COVID-19, Pulmonary rehabilitation, Respiratory infection.

Presentation

A 68-year-old man with a 50-pack year smoking history was admitted for fever and lethargy for three days associated with progressive dyspnea and non-resolving cough. He had a COVID-19 (category 4) infection and was recently discharged a week ago. Premorbid, he was independent and able to self-care (modified medical research council: mMRC dyspnea scale of 2). On his readmission, his oxygen saturation was 70% on room air. Clinically, he was febrile (Temperature of 38.5°C) and had a 40 breaths per minute respiratory rate. However, he was fully conscious, and he had stable hemodynamics. There was no bronchospasm, but lung auscultation revealed a generalized prolonged expiratory phase and scattered fine and coarse crepitations at both lung bases. His arterial blood gas on a non-rebreather mask (two flaps removed) with 15L oxygen showed type I hypoxemic respiratory failure (HRF) with an alveolar-arterial gradient of 408mmHg. He had an elevated white cell count 15.1x109/L, C-reactive protein 115mg/L. The other blood parameters were grossly insignificant. His infective workup was negative. He was treated for nosocomial infection with post- COVID-19 interstitial lung disease with a background of severe emphysema complicated with hospital- acquired pneumonia.

Comorbidities

Hypertension and gout.

Chest Imaging

His CXR is shown (Fig. **1**). A CTPA showed lung changes consistent with post-COVID-19 infection with fibrotic changes, minimal right-sided pleural effusion,

*Corresponding author Soo Chun Ian:** University of Malaya Medical Center, Kuala Lumpur, Malaysia; E-mail: scianray@gmail.com and generalized emphysematous changes (Figs. **2a** and **b**).

Intervention

He required non-invasive ventilation support for two days. Following that, he required High flow nasal cannula oxygen therapy (Flow 60L/min/ FiO_2 60%). On completion of antibiotics, he had no fever, and there was an improvement in the laboratory and inflammatory parameters. However, the patient had difficulty weaning off ventilation with persistent HRF.

A pulmonary rehabilitation assessment concluded the patient had pulmonary insufficiency secondary to the underlying lung parenchymal disease and reduced pulmonary capacity complicated with severe deconditioning secondary to reduced mobility and prolonged hospital stay.

Landmarks for sonography examination of the diaphragm (Figs. **3a** and **b**).

A sonography examination of the diaphragm assessment was also performed (Figs. **4a-c** and **5a-b**).

Diaphragm excursion in normal adult individuals (Fig. **6**).

Complications

None.

Post-Intervention

Patient achieved good recovery after intervention and was able to self-ambulate with a walking stick (Figs. **7** and **8**).

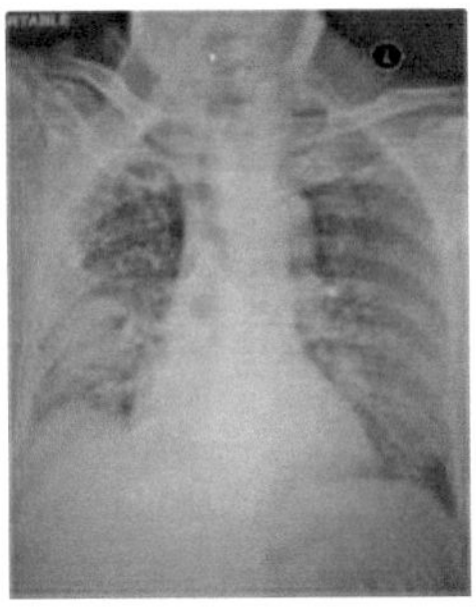

Fig. (1). CXR (portable) on admission demonstrating bilateral lung infiltrates of COVID-19 infection.

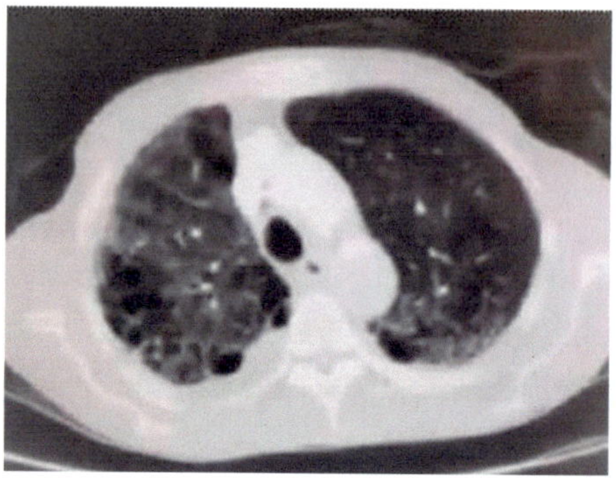

(a)

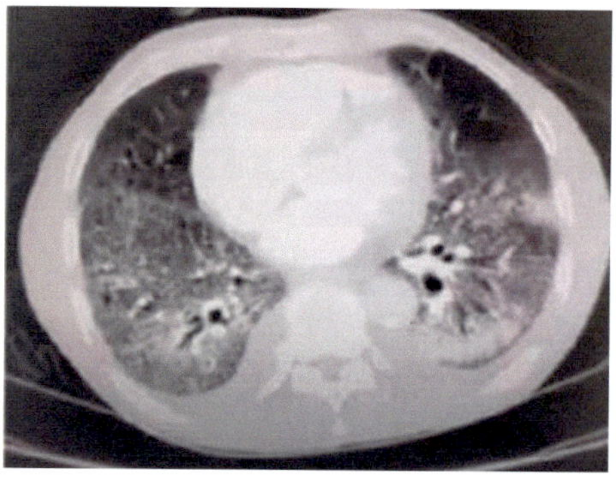

(b)

Fig. (2). (a) CT thorax: Axial images of upper zone showing extensive emphysematous lung changes. **(b)** Axial images of lower zone showing extensive inflammatory interstitial lung changes secondary to COVID-19 infection.

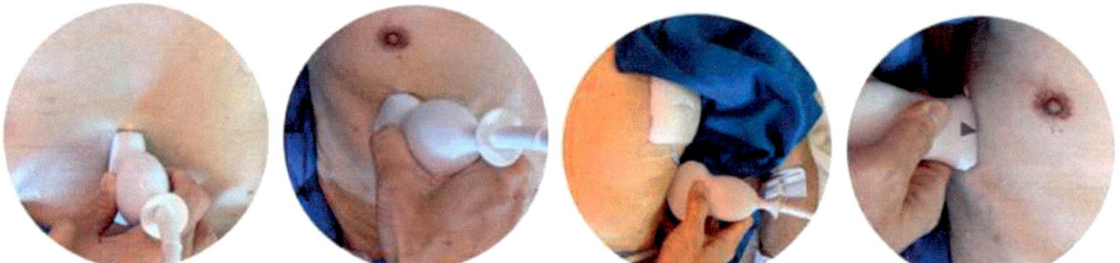

Fig. (3). (a) A: Starting Point: inferior to xiphisternum. Slide the US probe in the lateral direction (Approximately 5-6cm) until the liver and the dome of the diaphragm are visualized. **B:** Right Subcostal: Assessment of the right diaphragm excursion. **C:** Left Subcostal: Assessment of the left diaphragm excursion. **D:** Inferior Intercostal: 8th-9th intercostal space, mid-axillary line (Zone of apposition of pleura and diaphragm).

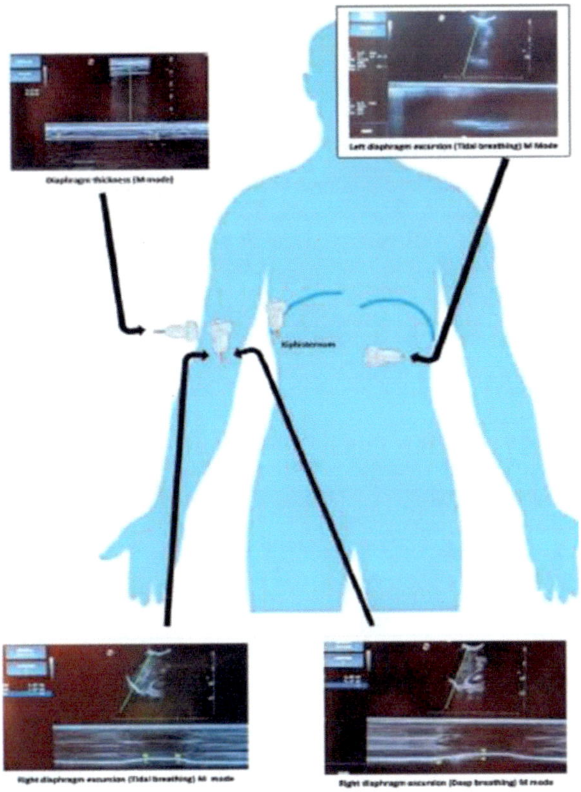

Fig. (3). (b) Landmarks for sonography examination of the diaphragm.

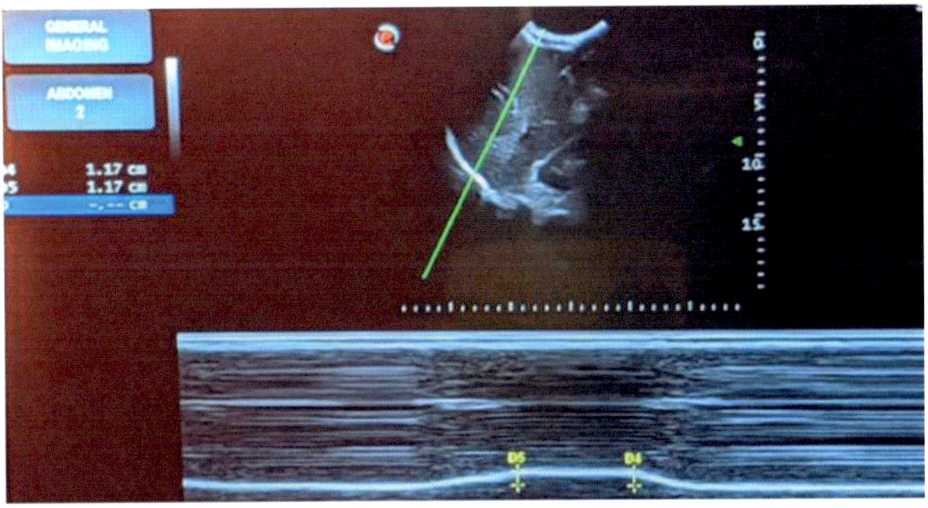

Fig. (4). (a) Right diaphragm excursion on tidal breathing (1.17cm).

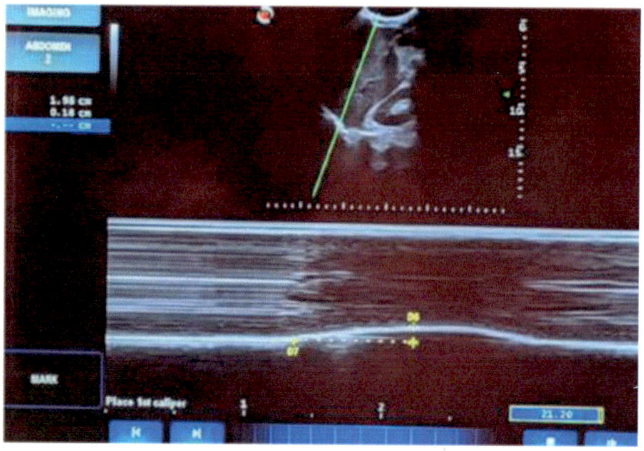

Fig. (4). (b) Right diaphragm excursion on deep breathing (1.98cm).

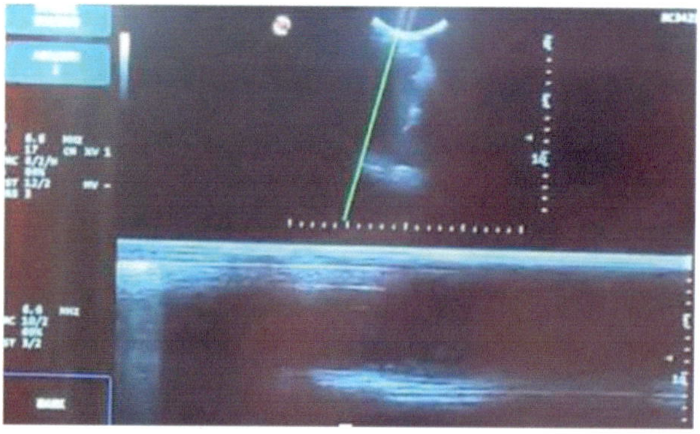

Fig. (4). (c) Left diaphragm excursion (Frequently not well visualized and obliterated by the lung and occasionally bowel shadow).

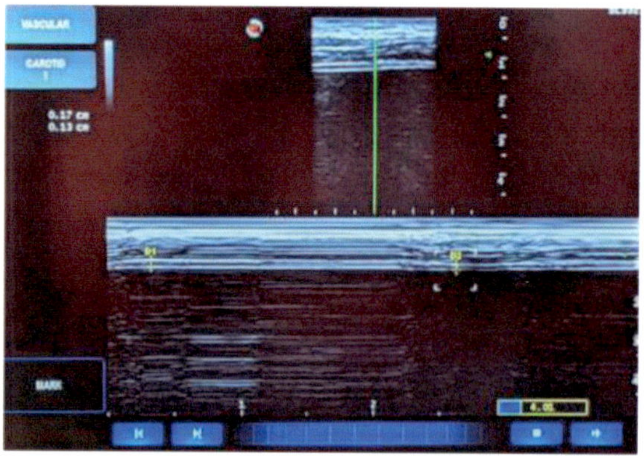

Fig. (5). (a) Measurement of diaphragm thickness (Total lung capacity 0.17cm, end expiratory 0.13cm) M mode.

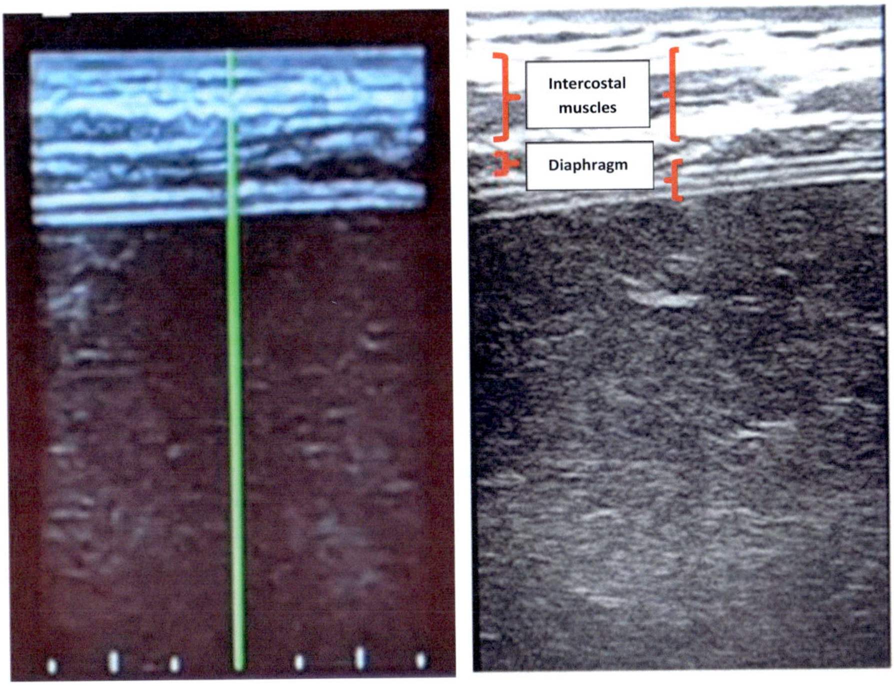

Fig. (5). (b) Measurement of diaphragm thickness.

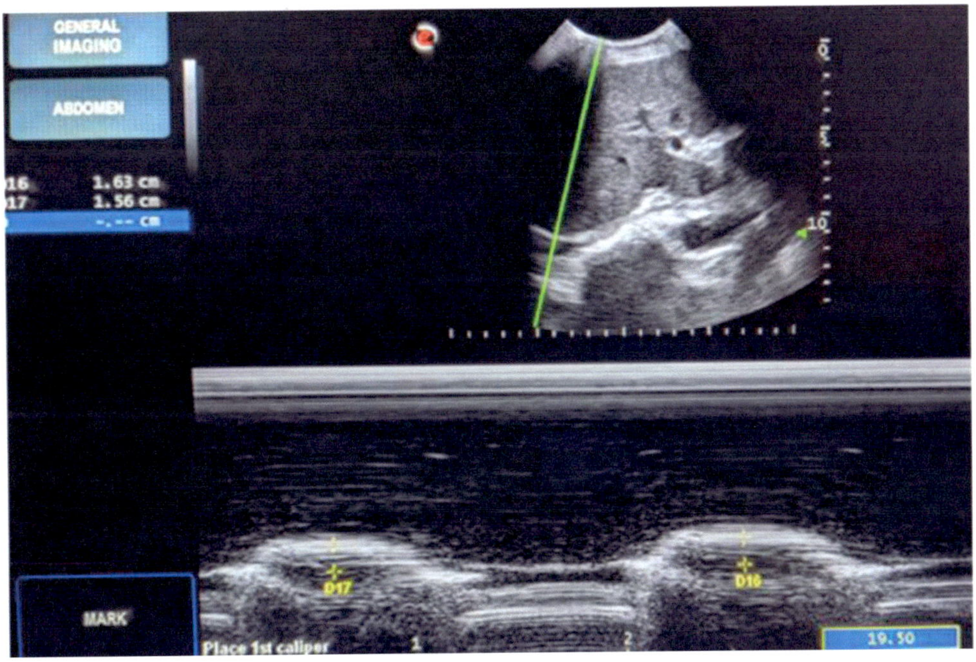

Fig. (6). Diaphragm excursion in normal adult individuals.

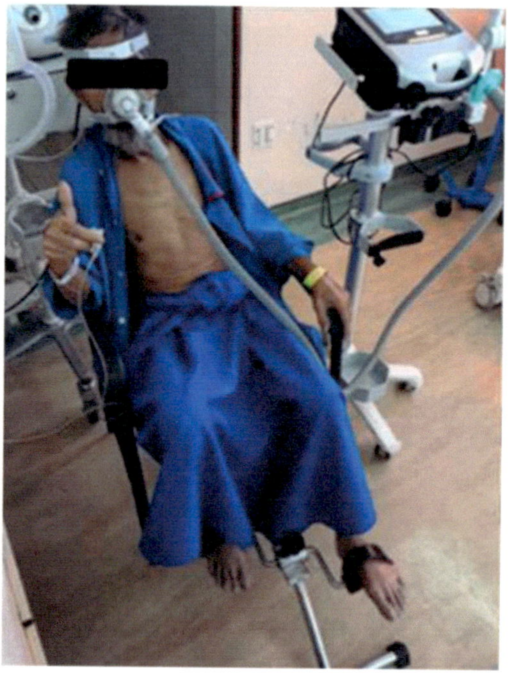

Fig. (7). (a) Cycle ergometer exercise supported by non-invasive ventilator.

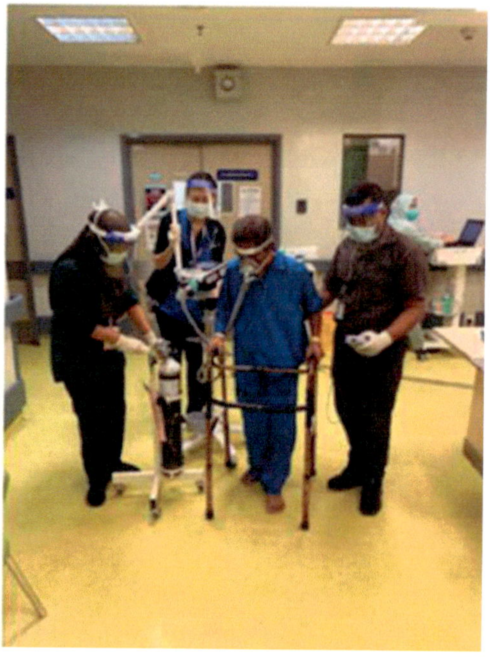

Fig. (7). (b) Ambulation with non-invasive ventilator.

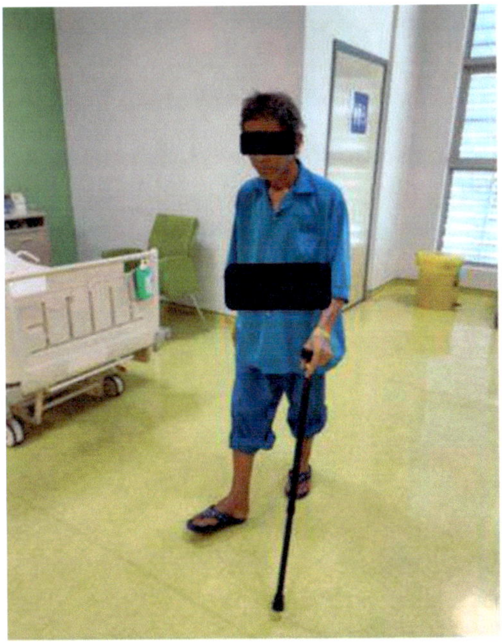

Fig. (8). Patient achieved good recovery and was able to self-ambulate with a walking stick.

Learning Points

- The diaphragm is made up of fatigue-resistant slow-twitch type I and fast twist type II amyofibres. It is innervated by the phrenic nerve from cervical 3, 4 and 5. The movement of the diaphragm can result in a 75% increase in lung volume during quiet breathing, and therefore the diaphragm is a major respiratory muscle for ventilation.
- Numerous neurological conditions are commonly known to affect diaphragm excursion. In addition, underlying hyperinflation with a recent severe lung infection (COVID-19), glucocorticoid usage, and disuse atrophy can further aggravate the diaphragm.
- During the sonographic examination of this patient's diaphragm as part of his assessment during the pulmonary rehabilitation (Figs. **4a-c**), the patient's diaphragm excursion is at the lower margin of the normal range for healthy males (Quiet breathing: 1.1-2.5cm (Fig. **6**) and markedly reduced (Deep breathing: 4.7-9.2cm) [1].
- The reported average thickness of the diaphragm in healthy volunteers ranges from 0.22 - 0.28cm. At the end of expiration, a thickness of < 0.2cm suggests diaphragm atrophy [2]. The diaphragm thickness of this patient ranges from 0.13 - 0.17cm (Fig. **5**). The thickening fraction of the diaphragm is 31% ((0.17-

0.13)/0.13). A thickening fraction below 20% has been reported to be consistent with the diagnosis of diaphragm paralysis [3]. The overall sonographic evidence in this patient could suggest he has some degree of diaphragm atrophy. In addition, a prolonged hospital stay, reduced mobility, and poor nutrition could also have contributed to the deconditioning of the patient.

- The patient was incorporated into an aggressive pulmonary rehabilitation (Figs. **7a** and **b**) supported by non-invasive ventilation, and two weeks later, he was successfully weaned off ventilation support. He was discharged home after three weeks of pulmonary rehabilitation (Fig. **8**).
- In summary, sonography examination of the diaphragm is a useful ancillary tool for weaning off ventilation support and pulmonary rehabilitation for patients with chronic respiratory disorders.

CONSENT FOR PUBLICATION

Not applicable.

CONFLICT OF INTEREST

The author declares no conflict of interest, financial or otherwise.

ACKNOWLEDGEMENT

Declared none.

REFERENCES

[1] Boussuges A, Gole Y, Blanc P. Diaphragmatic motion studied by m-mode ultrasonography: methods, reproducibility, and normal values. Chest 2009; 135(2): 391-400. [http://dx.doi.org/10.1378/chest.08-1541] [PMID: 19017880]

[2] Justin Hale, Hugh Dowlen, Michael Cartwright, and Aarti Sarwal Neuromuscular Ultrasound for Evaluation of the Normal and Abnormal Diaphragm. Neurology 2013; 12: 80-5.

[3] Summerhill EM, El-Sameed YA, Glidden TJ, McCool FD. Monitoring recovery from diaphragm paralysis with ultrasound. Chest 2008; 133(3): 737-43. [http://dx.doi.org/10.1378/chest.07-2200] [PMID: 18198248]

Section D

Paediatric Interventional Pulmonology

Case 1

Foreign Body Removal (Different Techniques)

Peanut in the Airway- A Hard Nut to Crack?

Harikishan Gonuguntla[1,*] and **Belgundi Preeti Vidyasagar**[1]

[1] *Department of Interventional Pulmonology, Yashoda Hospital, Secunderabad, India*

Keywords: Bronchoscope, Basket, Emergency, Foreign body, Stridor.

Presentation

A 2-year-old child was rushed to the emergency room with complaints of sudden onset of cough after a witnessed episode of peanut ingestion. No stridor or cyanosis was noted at presentation. His resting room air oxygen saturation was 98%. Clinical examination showed bilateral conducted sounds on auscultation.

Comorbidities

None.

Chest Imaging

Plain CXR demonstrated bilateral parenchymal infiltration (Fig. **1**).

Intervention

Diagnostic bronchoscopy (BF 190, Olympus Medical, Tokyo, Japan) was performed under general anaesthesia using a supraglottic device. The foreign body was localised to RB10 (Postero-basal segment of the right lower lobe) (Figs. **2a** and **b**).

A 4mm Fogarty embolectomy catheter (Edward Lifesciences, USA) (Fig. **3**) was passed through the working channel of the bronchoscope and was placed distal to the foreign body and inflated (Fig. **4**). Pus was noted oozing from the side of the

*Corresponding author Harikishan Gonuguntla: Department of Interventional Pulmonology, Yashoda Hospital, Secunderabad, India; E-mail: harikishang@gmail.com

Jamalul Azizi Abdul Rahaman & Tinku Joseph (Eds.)

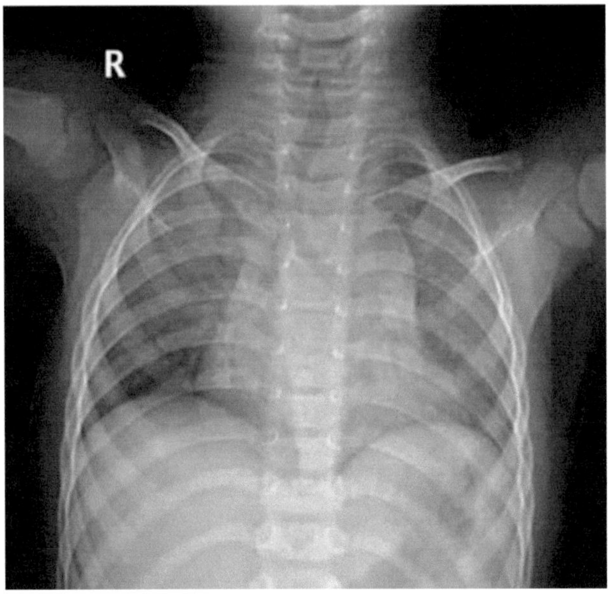

Fig. (1). Plain CXR demonstrated bilateral non-specific parenchymal infiltrates.

foreign body (Figs. **5a** and **b**). With the balloon inflated, the foreign body was dislodged into the lower lobe bronchus by pulling the inflated balloon proximally (Fig. **6**).

Using a 4Fr nitinol urology stone retrieval basket [1] (INDOVASIVE, Biorad medisys, India) (Fig. **7**), the foreign body was grasped and safely secured in the basket and removed en bloc with the bronchoscope. It was held in the basket firmly, pulled proximally through the right main bronchus, trachea, and removed out through the I-Gel successfully (Figs. **8a-c** and **9**).

Complications

The procedure was uneventful with no documented complications.

Post-Intervention

The child was extubated immediately post-procedure and was discharged home after parent counselling about feeding patterns in children.

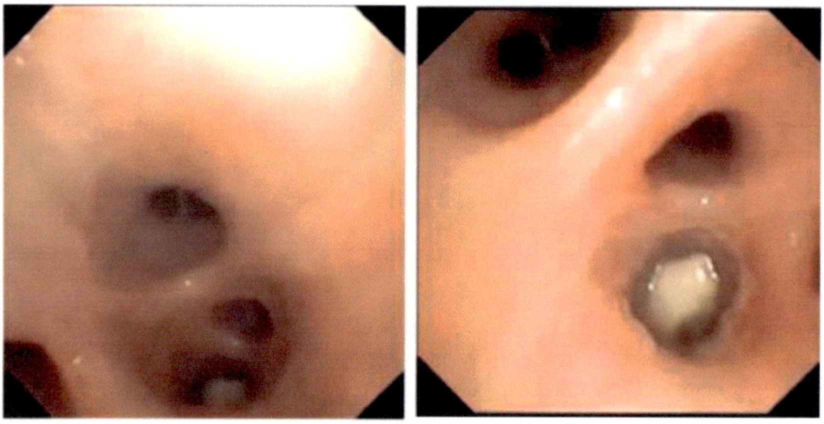

a) b)

Fig. (2). (a and **b)** Foreign body visualised in the postero-basal segment of the right lower lobe.

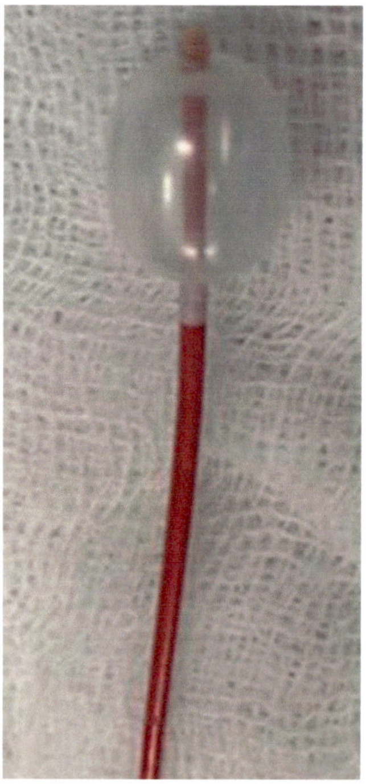

Fig. (3). 4mm Fogarty embolectomy catheter.

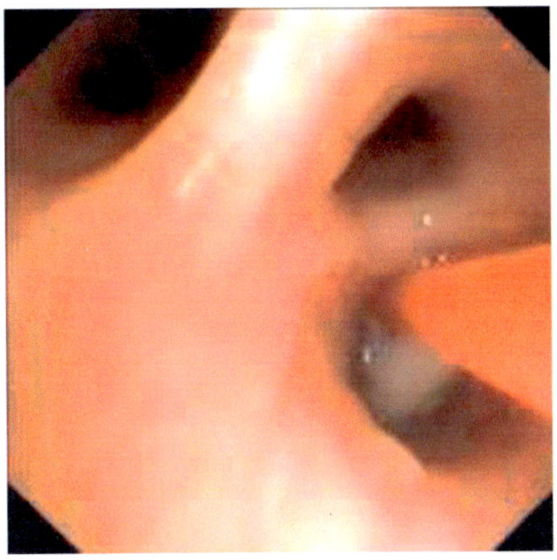

Fig. (4). 4mm Fogarty balloon passed distal to the foreign body and inflated.

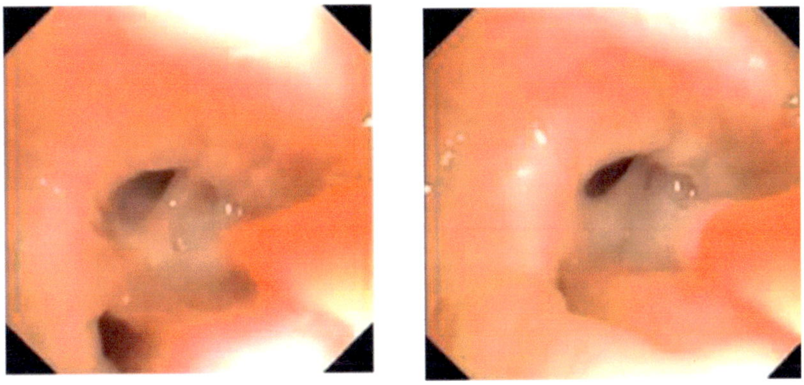

a) b)

Fig. (5). (a and **b)** Pus oozing from the side of the foreign body.

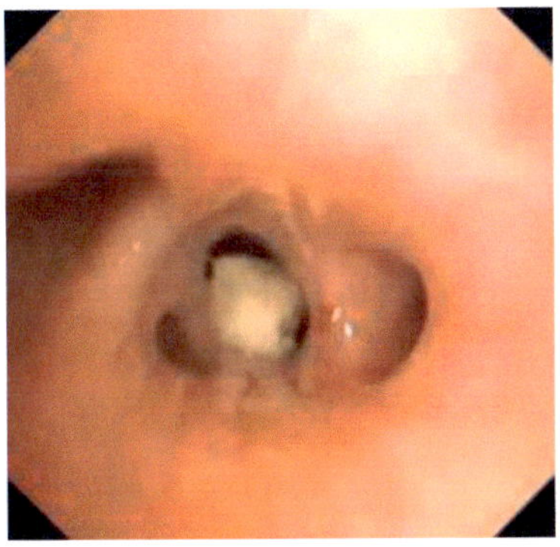

Fig. (6). Foreign body dislodged proximally.

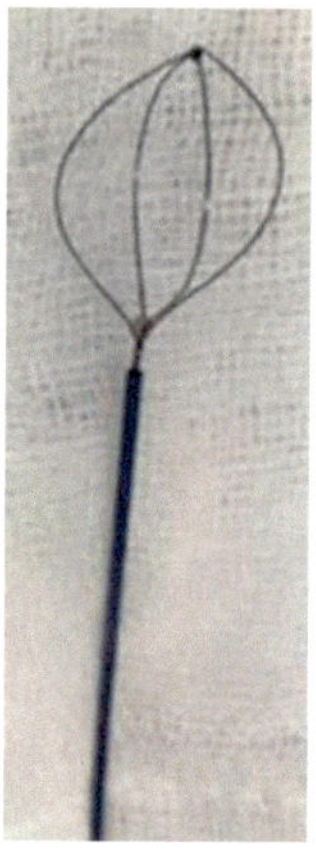

Fig. (7). Dormia basket.

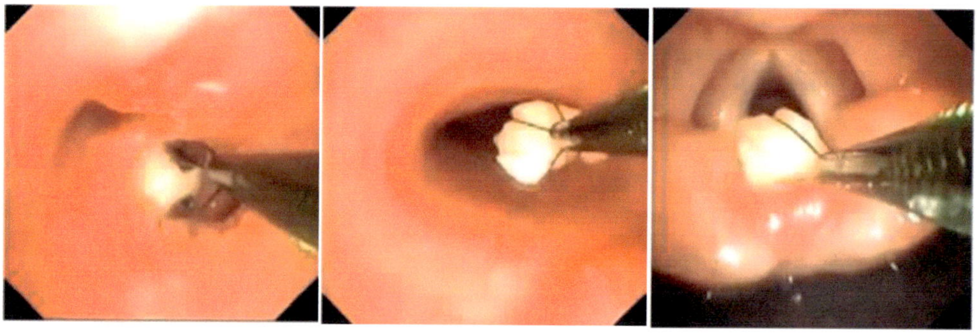

a) b) c)

Fig. (8). (a-c) Dormia basket used to capture the foreign body and remove it along the airway and vocal cords.

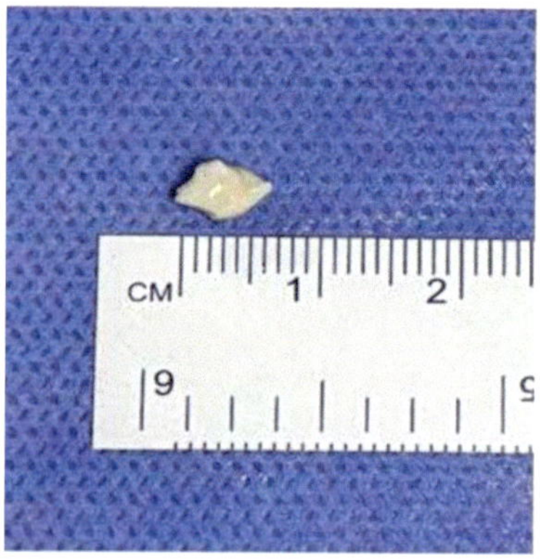

Fig. (9). Peanut retrieved from RB10.

Learning Points

- Detailed history-taking plays a very important part in the diagnosis of foreign body aspiration in children.
- Thin flexible bronchoscopes can be a replacement for rigid bronchoscopes in foreign body aspiration, especially when the foreign bodies are lodged in the distal airways.
- Fogarty balloon catheters can be useful in deep-seated foreign bodies to dislodge them into the main airways.

Video

Removal of foreign body in this 2-year-old child.

CONSENT FOR PUBLICATION

Not applicable.

CONFLICT OF INTEREST

The author declares no conflict of interest, financial or otherwise.

ACKNOWLEDGEMENT

Declared none.

REFERENCE

[1] Bounds BC. Endoscopic Retrieval Devices. Tech Gastrointest Endosc 2006; 8(1): 16-21. [http://dx.doi.org/10.1016/j.tgie.2005.12.004]

Case 2

Retrieval of Missed Foreign Bodies in Children: The Cryoextraction Method

Mohammad Ashkan Moslehi[1,*]

[1] *Pediatric Interventional Pulmonology Division, Shiraz University of Medical Sciences, Shiraz, Iran*

Keywords: Airway, Aspiration, Children, Cryoextraction, Foreign body.

Presentation

A 6-month-old male infant developed noisy breathing after a choking episode while eating. Due to repeated cyanotic cough spells and increasing difficulty in breathing, he was referred to the emergency department of Namazi hospital, Shiraz, on the same day. He was thought to have bronchiolitis or acute asthma and was given nebulized Albuterol, intravenous dexamethasone, and nebulized budesonide. One day after admission to the hospital, a little improvement was observed and he was discharged on the same day. He again continued to have noisy breathing and tachypnea. He had a history of intermittent expiratory monophasic wheezing on the right side and had been admitted twice with the impression of reactive airway disease and pneumonia, but his problem continued until his referral to our hospital after one month.

Chest Imaging

A CXR showed right sided hyperinflation and a scattered infiltration on the opposite side.

Intervention

He underwent flexible fiberoptic bronchoscopy (FFB) under slight general anesthesia using intravenous Propofol (1mg/kg) by maintaining his spontaneous breathing. The foreign body (FB) was observed in the bronchus intermedius (Fig. **1**) surrounded by thick mucosal secretion and granulation tissue; then, the left main

*__Corresponding author Mohammad Ashkan Moslehi:__ Pediatric Interventional Pulmonology Division, Shiraz University of Medical Sciences, Shiraz, Iran; E-mail: ashkanmoslehi@gmail.com

Jamalul Azizi Abdul Rahaman & Tinku Joseph (Eds.)

bronchus was checked. There was another FB that had entirely obliterated the left main bronchus (Fig. **2**).

After applying slight suctioning, diluted epinephrine was instilled to prevent bleeding. First, it was decided to remove the FB on the left side by alligator forceps as it thoroughly interrupted the airflow. Due to the friable nature of the object and after trying twice unsuccessfully, the object was removed using a 1.9mm cryoprobe (ERBE, Germany). The cryoprobe was introduced through the 2mm working channel of pediatric-sized FFB with an external diameter of 4.2mm (Olympus, Japan). Once the cryoprobe touched the FB, cryo energy was applied using the foot pedal for four seconds and then the cryoprobe was pulled out with the bronchoscope en bloc. After that, the right-side FB was also extracted *via* the same method (Fig. **3**). The whole airways were checked again with the FFB, and no additional FBs were found.

Complications

Nil.

Post-Intervention

The post-operative period was uneventful, and the patient was discharged a day after the procedure.

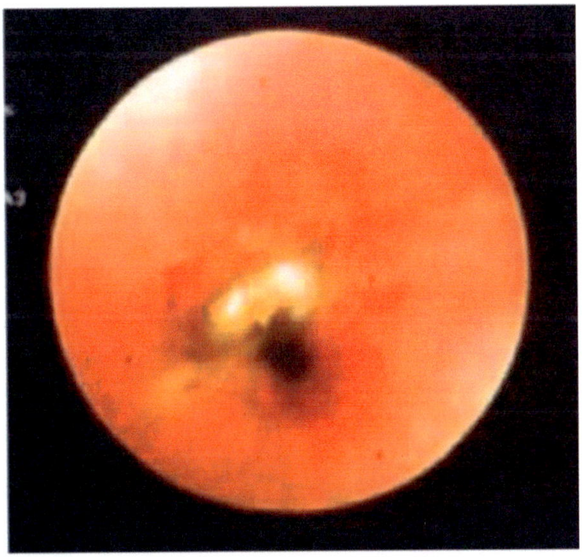

Fig. (1). Chicken cartilage in the right bronchus intermedius.

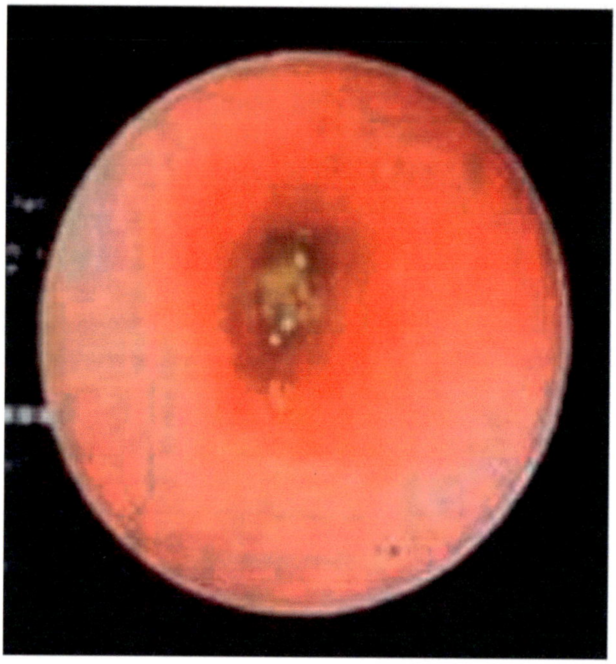

Fig. (2). Chicken cartilage in the left main bronchus.

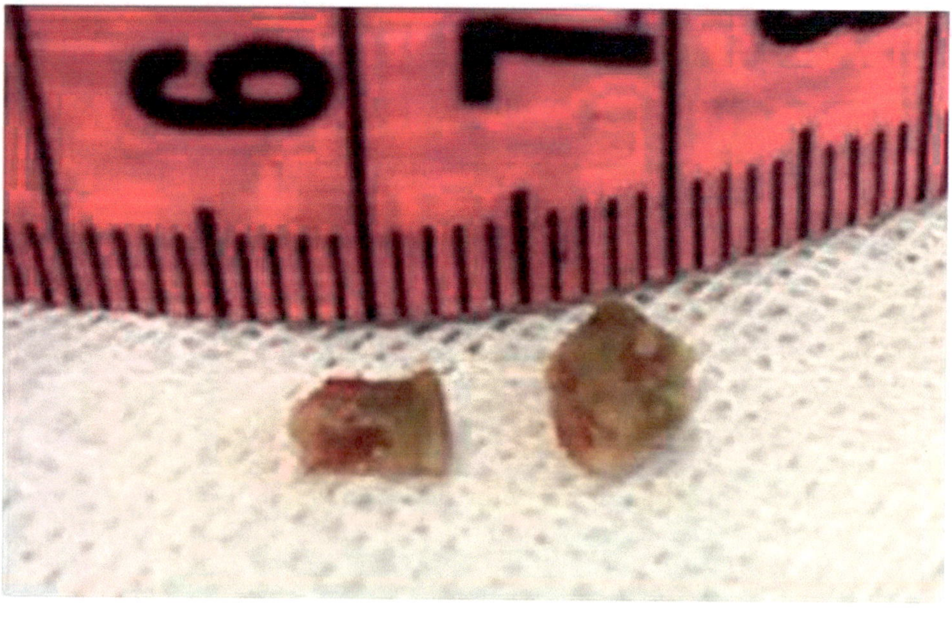

Fig. (3). Two pieces of chicken cartilages after extraction.

Learning Points

- Children can quickly inhale FB into the airways. Physical findings include cough, cyanosis, dyspnea, tachypnea, diminished breath sounds, wheezing, stridor and respiratory distress. Foreign body aspiration (FBA) is a common pediatric problem with severe complications, and delayed diagnosis can lead to serious complications. Early diagnosis and appropriate treatments may prevent many of these complications.
- FBA is a common cause of respiratory compromise in early childhood. FBA can be misdiagnosed as asthma, upper respiratory tract infection, pneumonia, bronchiolitis, or croup [1]. Delay in diagnosis is due to failure to give serious consideration to the diagnosis. FBA complications are recurrent pneumonia, atelectasis, lung abscess, bronchiectasis, pneumothorax, pneumomediastinum, bronchospasm, asphyxia, and finally, death. In one series, a delay of over three days between aspiration and removal of the FB was reported in almost 30% of children [2].
- Early diagnosis and removal of FBs using bronchoscopy is crucial to avoid such complications. In suspected cases, FFB can be used to examine more distal parts of the bronchial tree and more confidently exclude a foreign body than rigid bronchoscopy [3]. Recently, new FFB modalities, like the basket, snares, and cryoprobe have seen good results. Cryoprobe has been used to extract friable objects with high water content (*e.g.*, large mucus plugs and blood clots) [4, 5]. The success of FB extraction using a cryoprobe depends on the expertise of the bronchoscopist.
- This case highlights the importance of a thorough clinical evaluation of patients suspected of FBA. FBA is still a life-threatening event, especially among children less than four years old. FBA should be considered as a cause for unexplained sudden onset of cough, which does not respond to cough or asthma medications, especially in patients with good healthy background. FBA may not have a clear aspiration history, even in small infants. Delayed diagnosis and treatments can be associated with a high number of complications.

- Rules of FBA removal in children:
  - The bronchoscopist should always examine both sides.
  - Due to inflamed bronchial mucosa, irrigation with a mixture of diluted epinephrine and lidocaine will prevent bleeding and bronchospasm, respectively.
  - In the case of bilateral FB aspirations, the more obstructed bronchus should be approached first.

- After a successful FB removal, both sides should be re-evaluated for any remaining particles or unwanted complications.

- Although rigid bronchoscopy is still the first choice modality for FB removal in children, cryoextraction with FFB may be considered an alternative method, especially for friable objects.

CONSENT FOR PUBLICATION

Not applicable.

CONFLICT OF INTEREST

The author declares no conflict of interest, financial or otherwise.

ACKNOWLEDGEMENT

Declared none.

REFERENCES

[1] Moslehi MA. A rare case of massive foreign body aspiration mimic asthma. Respir Med Case Rep 2019; 28: 100963.
[http://dx.doi.org/10.1016/j.rmcr.2019.100963] [PMID: 31720210]

[2] Tan HKK, Brown K, McGill T, Kenna MA, Lund DP, Healy GB. Airway foreign bodies (FB): a 10-year review. Int J Pediatr Otorhinolaryngol 2000; 56(2): 91-9.
[http://dx.doi.org/10.1016/S0165-5876(00)00391-8] [PMID: 11115682]

[3] Martinot A, Closset M, Marquette CH, *et al.* Indications for flexible versus rigid bronchoscopy in children with suspected foreign-body aspiration. Am J Respir Crit Care Med 1997; 155(5): 1676-9.
[http://dx.doi.org/10.1164/ajrccm.155.5.9154875] [PMID: 9154875]

[4] Moslehi MA. Foreign Body Retrieval by Using Flexible Cryoprobe in Children. J Bronchology Interv Pulmonol 2021; 28(2): 103-6.
[http://dx.doi.org/10.1097/LBR.0000000000000698] [PMID: 32649328]

[5] Kazachkov M, Vicencio A. Foreign body removal is getting "cooler". Pediatr Pulmonol 2016; 51(9): 886-8.
[http://dx.doi.org/10.1002/ppul.23521] [PMID: 27378166]

Case 3

A Flower in the Lung

Amanil'Ula Hassan[1], **Huda Munirah Ainuddin**[1] and **Dayang Zuraini Sahadan**[1,*]

[1] *Pediatric Respiratory Unit, Serdang Hospital, Selangor, Malaysia*

Keywords: Biphasic rhonchi, Choking, Foreign body, Unilateral hyperinflation, Wheezing.

Presentation

A 1-year-7-month-old boy was referred to the Pediatric Respiratory Unit for persistent wheezing on exertion for 4 months duration which was not alleviated by bronchodilators. The child was brought to medical attention several times at a private clinic and received 3 courses of antibiotics and inhaled bronchodilators. The mother offered a history of retching and vomiting episodes prior to the initial wheezing presentation. He had no previous recurrent wheezing before, nor a personal history of atopy. At the presentation, he was active, not in respiratory distress. The lung examination revealed a hyperinflated chest bilaterally, equal breath sound, and biphasic rhonchi heard bilaterally upon exertion.

Chest Imaging

CXR showed unilateral hyperinflation and hyperlucency at the right hemithorax (Fig. **1**). There was no segmental collapse seen. CT thorax showed an intraluminal hyperdensity in the right main bronchus (Fig. **2**).

Intervention

He underwent flexible fiberoptic bronchoscopy (FFB) under slight general anesthesia *via* ETT size 5.0mm. A white spiky plastic object was visualized at the right main bronchus which was surrounded by mucus. The foreign body was successfully retrieved using a flexible forceps (Fig. **3**). No residual foreign body was noted in other subsegmental bronchi.

*__Corresponding author Dayang Zuraini Sahadan:__ Pediatric Respiratory Unit, Serdang Hospital, Selangor, Malaysia; E-mail: Zuraini.Sahadan@gmail.com

Jamalul Azizi Abdul Rahaman & Tinku Joseph (Eds.)

Complications

None.

Post-Intervention

The boy was extubated and remained well. CXR post-intervention showed an area of aeration with no focal air trapping (Fig. **4**). The clinical findings remarkably improved.

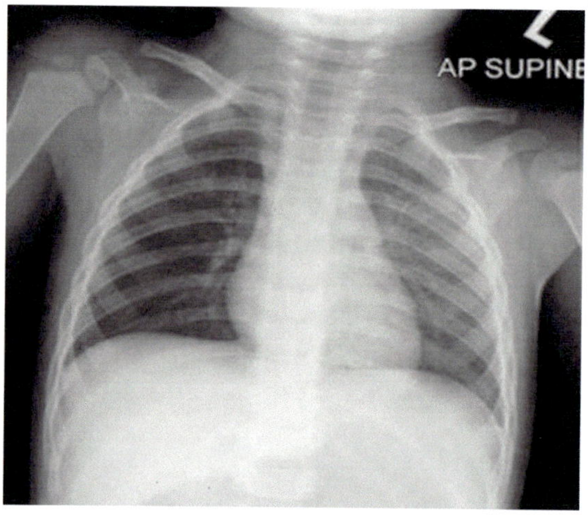

Fig. (1). CXR prior to the intervention showing unilateral hyperinflation and hyperlucency at the right hemithorax. There was no segmental collapse seen.

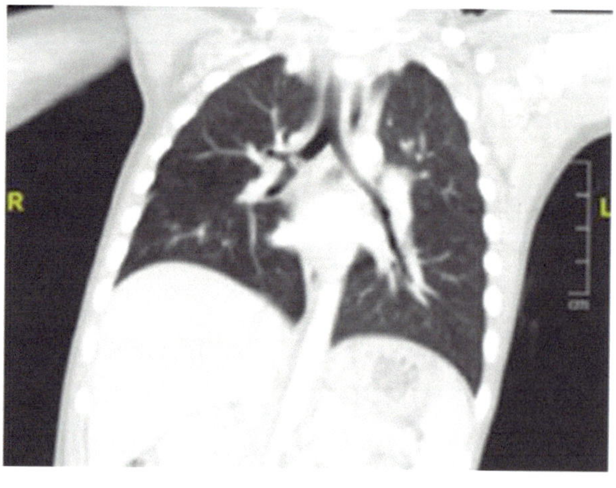

Fig. (2). CT thorax coronal view showing an intraluminal hyperdensity in the right main bronchus with patent trachea and left main bronchus lumen.

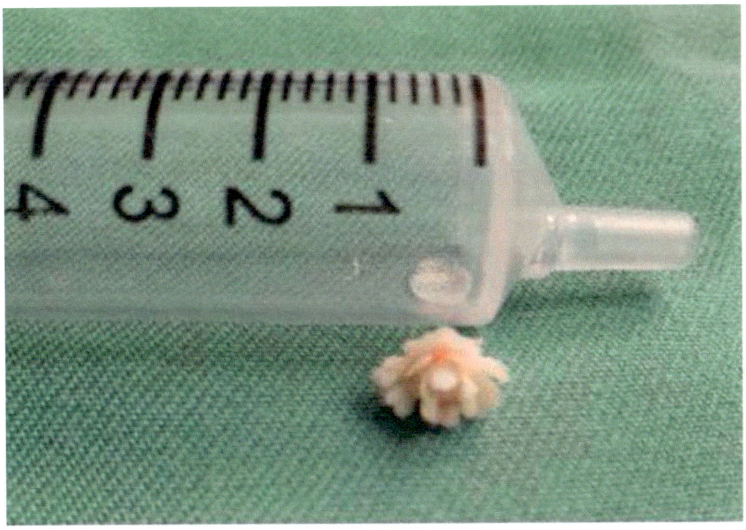

Fig. (3). The plastic flower measuring 1cm in diameter.

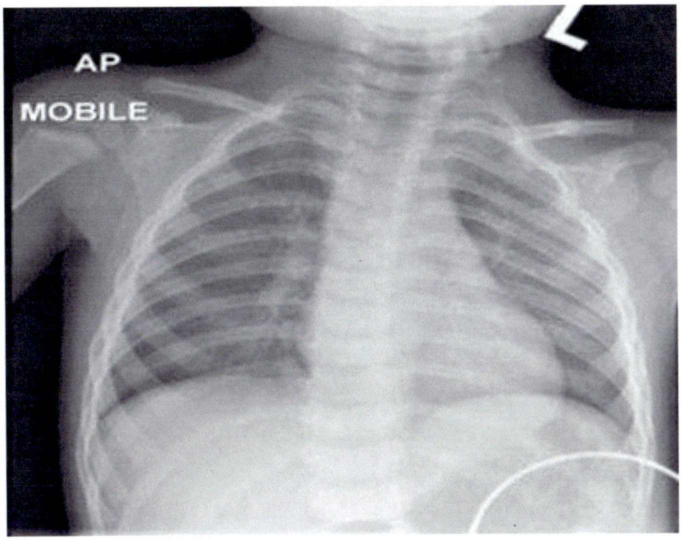

Fig. (4). CXR post-intervention showing area of aeration with no focal air trapping.

Learning Points

- Recurrent wheezing is common in children. Persistent symptoms, suspicious clinical findings and unilateral hyperinflation on chest radiograph should raise the suspicion of foreign body inhalation [1].

Video

Removal of the foreign body from the right main bronchus.

CONSENT FOR PUBLICATION

Not applicable.

CONFLICT OF INTEREST

The author declares no conflict of interest, financial or otherwise.

ACKNOWLEDGEMENT

Declared none.

REFERENCE

[1] Foltran F, Ballali S, Rodriguez H, *et al.* Inhaled foreign bodies in children: A global perspective on their epidemiological, clinical, and preventive aspects. Pediatr Pulmonol 2013; 48(4): 344-51.
[http://dx.doi.org/10.1002/ppul.22701] [PMID: 23169545]

Case 4

A Successful Foreign Body Removal with an Adverse Outcome

Amanil'Ula Hassan[1], **Huda Munirah Ainuddin**[1] and **Dayang Zuraini Sahadan**[1,*]

[1] *Pediatric Respiratory Unit, Serdang Hospital, Selangor, Malaysia*

Keywords: Flexible bronchoscopy, Foreign body inhalation, Cyanosis, Life-threatening event, Severe hypoxic event.

Presentation

A 1-year-6-month-old girl who was pre-morbidly well and thriving, was referred urgently to the Pediatric Respiratory Unit and Otorhinolaryngology Department from a nearby hospital for a life-threatening foreign body inhalation. The event happened while she was taking her lunch at the babysitter's house, when she suddenly choked. It was followed by bouts of coughing and subsequently, she turned cyanosed. She was immediately brought to a nearby hospital, with no signs of life. Initial resuscitation was given at the Emergency Department and subsequently transferred to the tertiary center for further intervention. At presentation, she was severely acidotic and required inotropic support and high-setting ventilation. There was a significantly reduced breath sound over the left side. She required stabilization in the Pediatric Intensive Care Unit before going for bronchoscopy and foreign body removal in the operation theater.

Chest Imaging

CXR revealed left upper lobe collapse (Fig. **1**).

Intervention

Flexible bronchoscopy using a bronchoscope size 3.6mm. There was a whitish foreign body noted on the left main bronchus which was identified as a piece of fish ball. It was successfully retrieved *via* suctioning through the flexible bronchoscope

*__Corresponding author Dayang Zuraini Sahadan:__ Pediatric Respiratory Unit, Serdang Hospital, Selangor, Malaysia; E-mail: Zuraini.Sahadan@gmail.com

Jamalul Azizi Abdul Rahaman & Tinku Joseph (Eds.)

(Figs. **2** and **3**). No obvious foreign body on the right side but there was oozing of blood-stained secretion from the right upper lobe.

Complications

None.

Post-Intervention

CXR post-intervention showed clearance of the left upper lobe collapse (Fig. **4**). The child required cerebral protection due to refractory seizure following the hypoxic event. Unfortunately, this had resulted in unavoidable neurological sequelae which included severe brain infarct, and she developed spastic quadriplegic cerebral palsy. Due to the prolonged ventilation, tracheostomy was done. She had multiple hospital admissions for recurrent pneumonia and eventually died at the age of 4 years and 3 months old due to severe pneumonia.

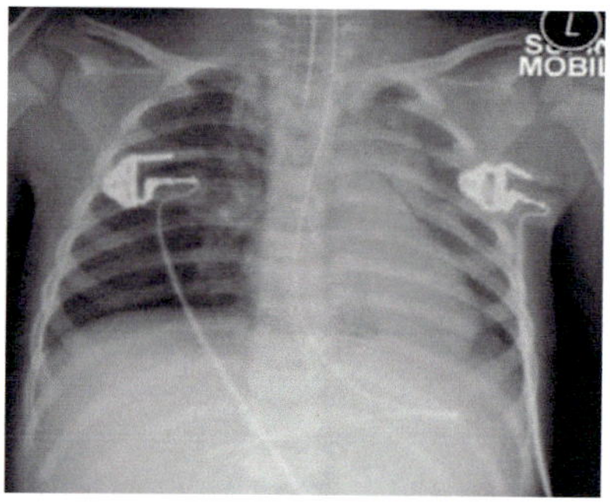

Fig. (1). CXR prior to intervention revealed left upper lobe collapse.

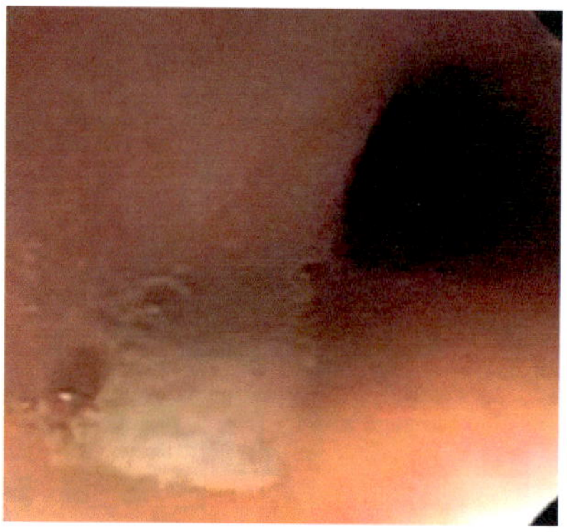

Fig. (2). A whitish object lodged and occluded the left main bronchus which was surrounded by clear secretion.

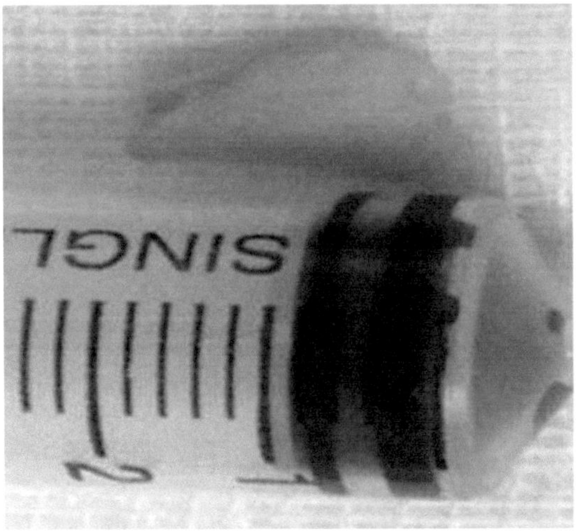

Fig. (3). A piece of fish ball, measuring 1.8cm in length identified during flexible bronchoscopy.

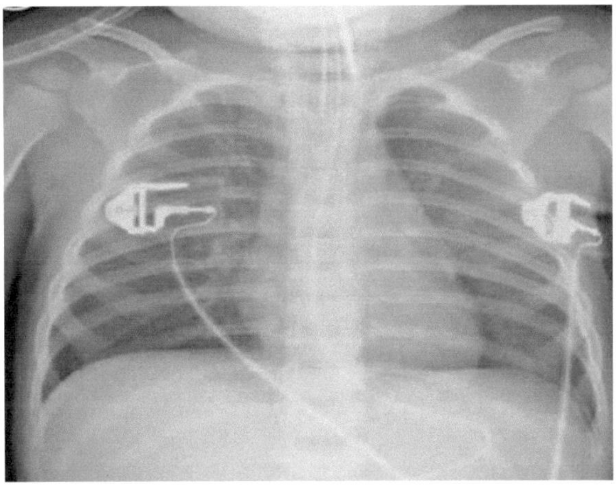

Fig. (4). CXR post intervention showed clearance of the left upper lobe collapse.

Learning Points

- Foreign body inhalation may present as an acute life-threatening event in which life-saving maneuver for removal is vital to improve the outcome [1].

Video

Removal of foreign body from the left main bronchus.

CONSENT FOR PUBLICATION

Not applicable.

CONFLICT OF INTEREST

The author declares no conflict of interest, financial or otherwise.

ACKNOWLEDGEMENT

Declared none.

REFERENCE

[1] Janahi IA, Khan S, Chandra P, *et al.* A new clinical algorithm scoring for management of suspected foreign body aspiration in children. BMC Pulm Med 2017; 17(1): 61. [http://dx.doi.org/10.1186/s12890-017-0406-6] [PMID: 28407759]

Case 5

A Plastic Cap in the Lung

Amanil'Ula Hassan[1], **Huda Munirah Ainuddin**[1] and **Dayang Zuraini Sahadan**[1,*]

[1] *Pediatric Respiratory Unit, Serdang Hospital, Selangor, Malaysia*

Keywords: Choking, Flexible bronchoscopy, Prolonged expiratory phase, Recurrent wheezing, Unilateral rhonchi.

Presentation

A 3-year-11-month-old boy who was previously well and healthy, presented with intermittent wheezing for 2 days following an episode of choking while eating a slice of honeydew. He vomited the food content after bouts of coughing. He was noted to be well and active with no signs of respiratory distress. However, the mother noted that he tended to have intermittent wheezing after playing. He had previous history of coin ingestion at the age of 2 years old, which did not require any intervention as the coin passed out during defecation. At the presentation, the boy was well, active and not tachypneic. However, there was reduced chest expansion, unilateral rhonchi, and reduced breath sound, with prolonged expiratory phase over the right chest.

Imaging

CXR showed mild perihilar haziness with no focal air trapping or collapse area (Fig. **1**).

Intervention

Flexible bronchoscopy was done using a bronchoscope size 3.6mm *via* a laryngeal mask. On approaching the main carina, a hollow oval-shaped foreign body was seen lodged at the right main bronchus. The object was removed in one attempt using a flexible forceps. It was a bright red hollow plastic cap measuring 13mm in length (Fig. **2**).

*Corresponding author Dayang Zuraini Sahadan: Pediatric Respiratory Unit, Serdang Hospital, Selangor, Malaysia; E-mail: Zuraini.Sahadan@gmail.com

Jamalul Azizi Abdul Rahaman & Tinku Joseph (Eds.)

Complications

None.

Post-Intervention

CXR was normal (Fig. **3**). The boy was well and was extubated immediately after intervention and remained well.

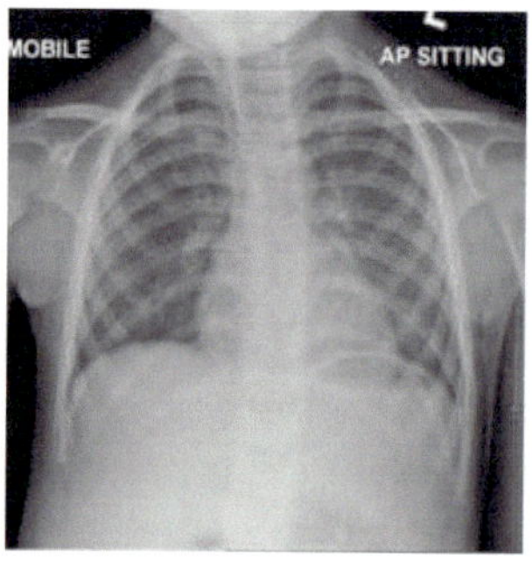

Fig. (1). CXR before intervention showed mild perihilar haziness with no focal air trapping or collapse area.

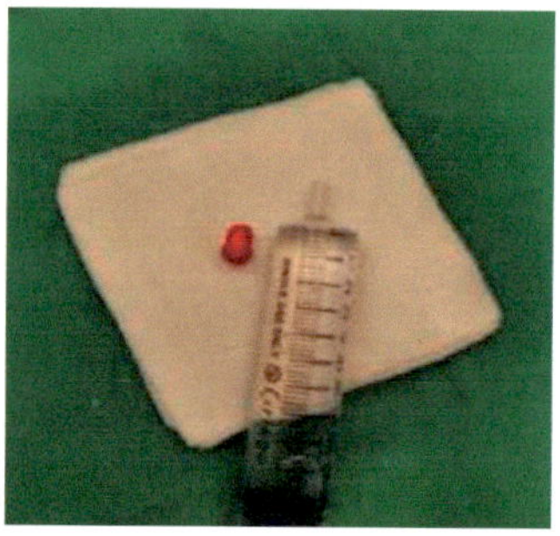

Fig. (2). A tubular hollow red plastic cap.

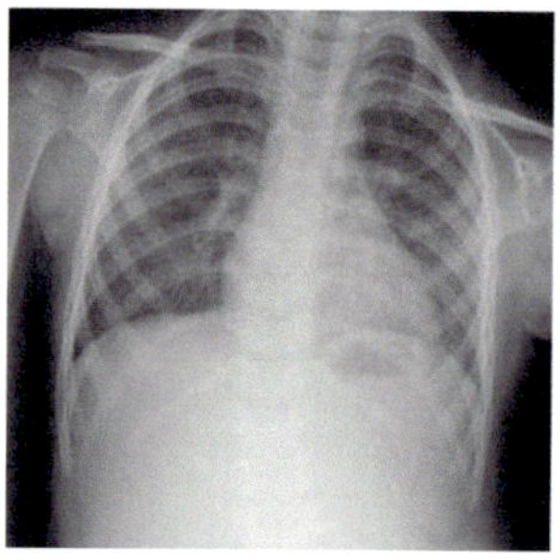

Fig. (3). CXR after the removal of the foreign body from the right main bronchus.

Learning Points

- Foreign body inhalation among toddlers is common. Recurrent wheezing with a history of choking should lead to a prompt decision for flexible bronchoscopy [1, 2]. Choking on food may present as a red herring as in this case.

Video

Removal of the foreign body from the right main bronchus.

CONSENT FOR PUBLICATION

Not applicable.

CONFLICT OF INTEREST

The author declares no conflict of interest, financial or otherwise.

ACKNOWLEDGEMENT

Declared none.

REFERENCES

[1] Janahi IA, Khan S, Chandra P, *et al.* A new clinical algorithm scoring for management of suspected foreign body aspiration in children. BMC Pulm Med 2017; 17(1): 61. [http://dx.doi.org/10.1186/s12890-017-0406-6] [PMID: 28407759]

[2] Sahadan DZ, Zainudin NM, Kassim A, *et al.* Case series of foreign body aspiration in Paediatric Institute, Hospital Kuala Lumpur. Med J Malaysia 2011; 66(5): 484-6. [PMID: 22390106]

Case 6

Transbronchial Lung Cryobiopsy in DPLD

Novel Technique of Performing Transbronchial Lung Cryobiopsy for Diagnosing Etiology of DPLD in an Infant - First Case Reported in the World

Tinku Joseph[1,*], **Sreeraj Nair**[1] and **Ajit Nambiar**[2]

[1] *Division of Interventional Pulmonology Unit, Amrita Institute of Medical Sciences, Kochi, India*

[2] *Department of Pathology, Amrita Institute of Medical Sciences, Kochi, India*

Keywords: DPLD, Ground glass opacity, Infant, Paediatric cryobiopsy, Paediatic ILD.

Presentation

11-month-old infant suffered from recurrent history of cough and breathlessness since birth. He was apparently treated for lower respiratory tract infection initially and later for viral pneumonia as well. In view of non-responsiveness to the treatment given, a CT chest was taken which was suggestive of interstitial lung disease. For further management, including a lung biopsy for histopathological confirmation, the child was referred to our hospital. Upon arrival he was tachypneic, saturation was 92% and had intermittent fever as well. He was initially admitted to the ICU and initiated on intravenous antibiotics and other necessary supportive measures. Once his general condition improved, he was shifted to the ward. Sputum and BAL sampling done prior to the present admission at another center ruled out TB, fungal and other bacterial pathologies.

Comorbidities

Nil.

Chest Imaging

CXR showed diffuse reticular shadows with bilateral lower zone alveolar opacities (Fig. **1**). CT chest revealed bilateral diffuse ground glass opacities with consolidatory patches in the lower lobes (Fig. **2**).

[*]**Corresponding author Tinku Joseph:** Division of Interventional Pulmonology Unit, Amrita Institute of Medical Sciences, Kochi, India; E-mail: tinkujoseph2010@gmail.com

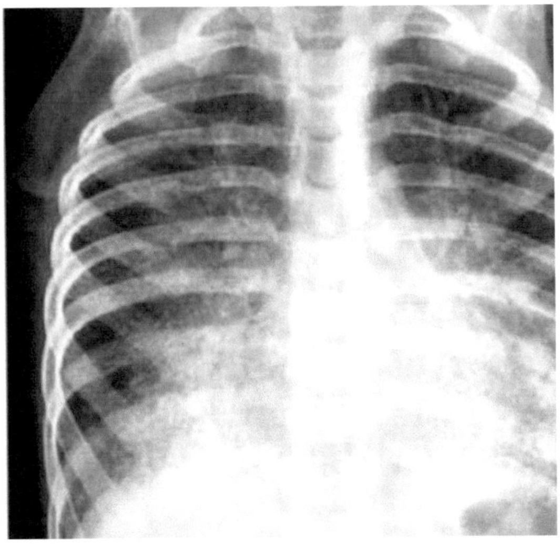

Fig. (1). CXR: Bilateral patchy alveolar opacities.

Intervention

In view of the inconclusive lab parameters and BAL reports, the case was discussed in a multidisciplinary ILD board meeting and the plan was to do lung biopsy to confirm the diagnosis. Options of VATS or cryo lung biopsy and their pros and cons were also discussed during the meeting held with the ILD MDT board members and the patient's family. Finally, the decision was made to do transbronchial lung cryobiopsy under general anaesthesia.

After obtaining written informed high-risk procedural consent, the child was intubated with a 4mm size rigid bronchoscope and airway was secured. Lung cryobiopsy was performed using a novel technique in which 1.9mm flexible cryoprobe was passed through the working channel of the rigid bronchoscope under fluoroscopic guidance into the left lower lobe basal segments. In order to obtain post-procedural haemostasis, a 2F Fogarty balloon was kept in the adjacent segment with the help of an ultrathin flexible bronchoscope (Fig. **3**). Multiple cryobiopsies were taken from the left lower lobe basal segments. Adequate haemostasis was achieved post-procedure and there was no evidence of pneumothorax on the fluoroscopic image taken immediately. The child was also extubated on the table after the procedure.

Complications

No immediate or delayed post-procedure complications.

Post-Intervention

Histopathological examination of the transbronchial lung cryobiopsy specimen showed lamellated concretions in alveolar lumina suggestive of alveolar microlithiasis (Fig. **4**). Genetic mutation analysis was sent for the SLC34A2 gene which was classified as a pathogenic variant showing exonic deletion contributing to pulmonary alveolar microlithiasis.

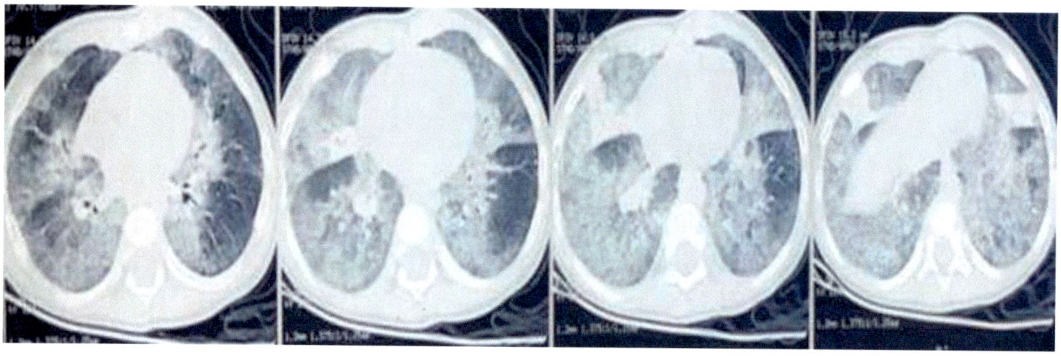

Fig. (2). CT Chest: Bilateral diffuse ground glass opacities involving the entire lung fields.

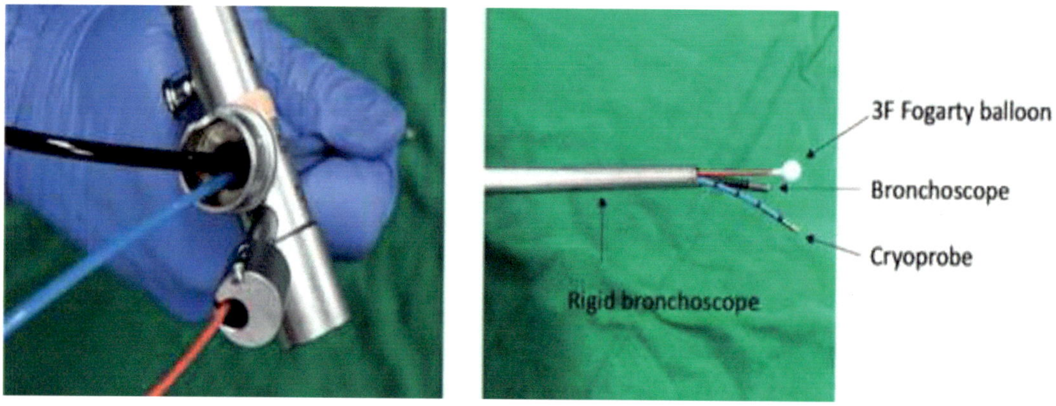

Fig. (3). Modified transbronchial lung cryobiopsy technique used in this case.

Learning Points

- Transbronchial lung cryobiopsy was introduced into clinical practice and has recently been recognized as a safe and effective tool for the diagnosis of diffuse parenchymal lung diseases. However, its role in diagnosing pediatric ILDs is not explained much in the literatures.

- Due to the non-availability of adequate tools and difficulty in its application in paediatric age group, we developed this novel technique by which we were fortunate to obtain a TBLC speci men in an 11-month-old child.
- This is the first reported case in the world of TBLC procedures in the infant age group.
- This procedure was done in 2019 and at this time, only 1.9mm and 2.4mm cryoprobes were available to perform TBLC. However, currently 1.1mm and 1.7mm cryoprobes are available, which can potentially be used for sampling lung tissue in the paediatric age group.
- More data is required to assess the safety and feasibility of the TBLC procedure and the use of various cryoprobes in the paediatric age group [1].

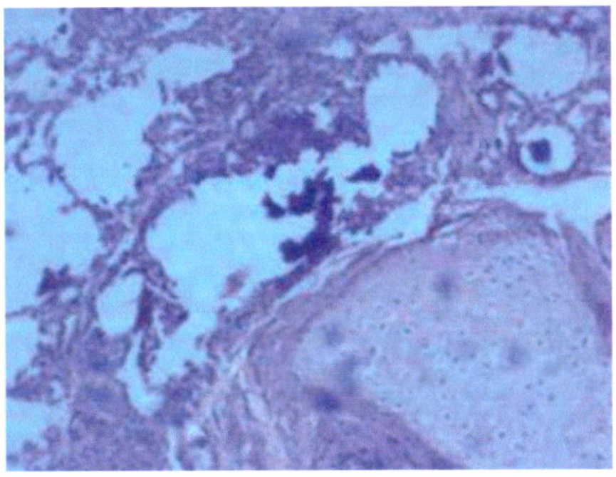

Fig. (4). Histopathology image of the transbronchial lung cryobiopsy specimen: Periodic acid–Schiff positive multiple microliths within the alveolar lumen.

CONSENT FOR PUBLICATION

Not applicable.

CONFLICT OF INTEREST

The author declares no conflict of interest, financial or otherwise.

ACKNOWLEDGEMENT

Declared none.

REFERENCE

[1] Moslehi A. Transbronchial Lung Cryobiopsy in children. Expert Rev Respir Med 2022; 16(3): 333-9.
[http://dx.doi.org/10.1080/17476348.2021.1987884] [PMID: 34602011]

Case 7

A Rare Case of "Brown Lung Induration"

Tinku Joseph[1,*], **Sreeraj Nair**[1] and **Ajit Nambiar**[2]

[1] *Division of Interventional Pulmonology Unit, Amrita Institute of Medical Sciences, Kochi, India*

[2] *Department of Pathology, Amrita Institute of Medical Sciences, Kochi, India*

Keywords: Haemoptysis, Haemosiderosis, Interstitial lung disease (ILD), Lung cryobiopsy, Rigid bronchoscope.

Presentation

A 15-year-old boy, presented with progressive breathlessness, cough and occasional haemoptysis for past 4 years. On examination, the patient was pale. Chest findings were unremarkable. Laboratory tests showed anemia and deranged liver function test. A bone marrow study showed trilineage haematopoiesis with scattered histiocytes and plasma cells and absent bone marrow Iron stores. 2D ECHO showed severe pulmonary arterial hypertension (PAH). His ANA, ANCA and RA factor were negative. Flexible bronchoscopy-guided BAL sampling and analysis from another hospital had ruled out infectious and malignant conditions.

Comorbidities

Severe PAH, anaemia.

Chest Imaging

CXR showed bilateral non-homogenous opacities in bilateral lung fields (Fig. **1**). A HRCT thorax showed diffuse ground glass opacities, inter and intra lobular septal thickening bilaterally, right upper lobe and posterobasal lobe consolidation, intra parenchymal cysts and minimal pericardial effusion (Fig. **2**).

Intervention

In view of inconclusive diagnosis, after a multi-disciplinary ILD board meeting, a decision was made to do transbronchial lung cryobiopsies (TBLC) to obtain a tissue

***Corresponding author Tinku Joseph:** Division of Interventional Pulmonology Unit, Amrita Institute of Medical Sciences, Kochi, India; E-mail: tinkujoseph2010@gmail.com diagnosis. The patient was intubated using 6.6mm size Karl storz rigid bronchoscope. The site for biopsy was localised using HRCT and real time fluoroscopy evidence. Using a 1.9mm flexible cryoprobe, multiple transbronchial lung cryobiopsies (Fig. **3**) were obtained from the right lower lobe (RB 7, RB9 segments) and right middle lobe (RB5 segment). Adequate haemostasis was achieved using a 3F Fogarty balloon and adrenaline solution.

Complications

No immediate or delayed post-procedure complications. The child was extubated on the table post-procedure.

Post-Intervention

HPE of lung biopsy specimens showed alveolar haemorrhage with alveolar septal fibrosis (ILD like) with no evidence of capillaritis or vasculitis (Fig. **4**). The case was further discussed in the ILD-MDT meeting and a final diagnosis of idiopathic pulmonary haemosiderosis was made after ruling out all possible causes leading to alveolar haemorrhage [1]. The patient was subsequently initiated on oral corticosteroids and he responded well to treatment.

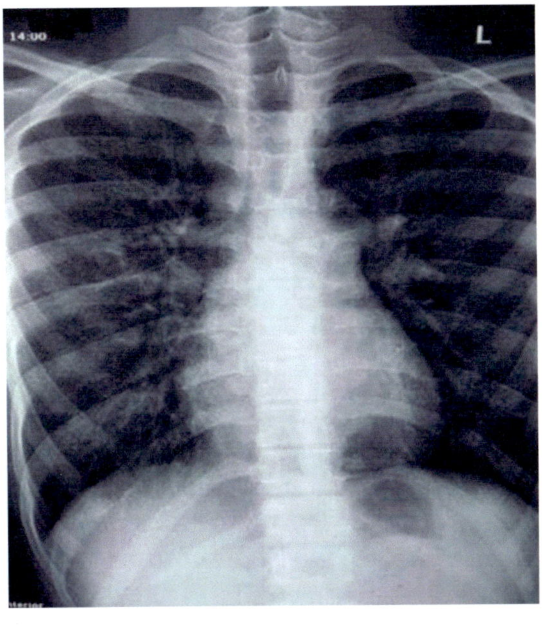

Fig. (1). CXR before intervention showed mild perihilar haziness with no focal air trapping or collapse area.

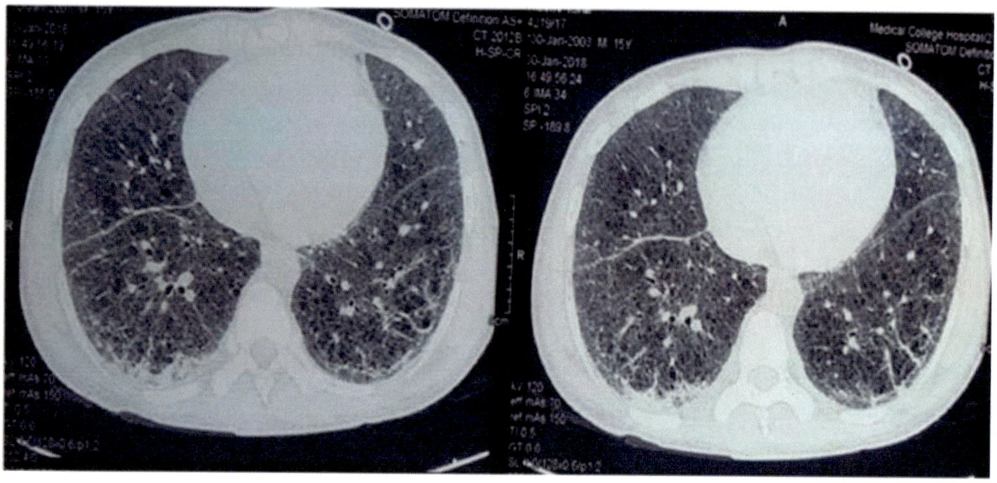

Fig. (2). Axial HRCT thorax shows diffuse ground glass opacities, inter and intra lobular septal thickening bilaterally, right upper lobe and posterobasal lobe consolidation, intra parenchymal cysts and minimal pericardial effusion.

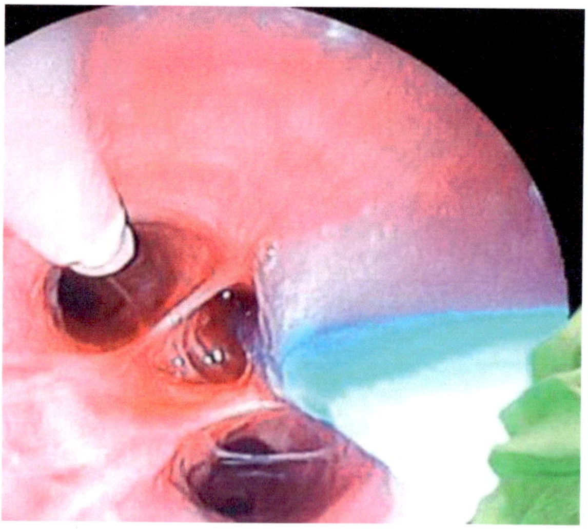

Fig. (3). Transbronchial lung Cryobiopsy (TBLC) technique.

Learning Points

- TBLC is a novel technique for sampling lung tissue for the diagnosis of Idiopathic interstitial pneumonias.

- TBLC is less invasive than surgical lung biopsy in obtaining lung biopsy, with minimal complications.
- Be wise in choosing cases for lung cryobiopsies, especially in the paediatric age group. Keep in mind the relative and absolute contraindications for this procedure.
- TBLC procedure should be done with caution among patients with severe pulmonary arterial hypertension due to the risk of a life-threatening bleed.
- All cases for TBLC procedures should be discussed in ILD-MDT meeting prior to and after the procedure.

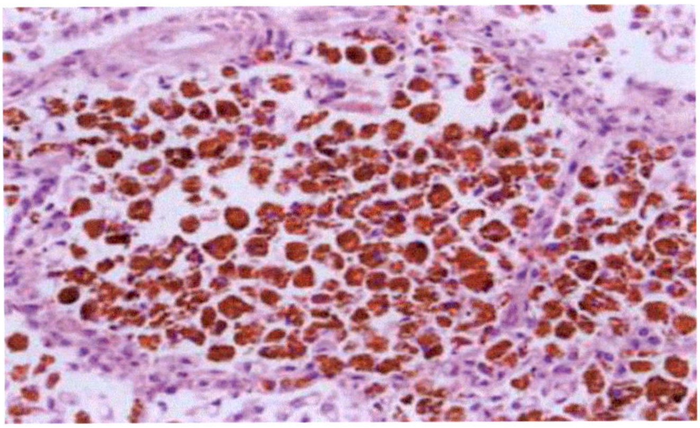

Fig. (4). Histopathology slide of TBLC specimen showed alveolar haemorrhage with alveolar septal fibrosis (ILD like) with no evidence of capillaritis or vasculitis.

CONSENT FOR PUBLICATION

Not applicable.

CONFLICT OF INTEREST

The author declares no conflict of interest, financial or otherwise.

ACKNOWLEDGEMENT

Declared none.

REFERENCE

[1] Bakalli I. Idiopathic pulmonary hemosiderosis - a diagnostic challenge. Ital J Pediatr 2014; 40: 35.
[https://doi.org/10.1186/1824-7288-40-35]

Case 8

Bronchoscopic Airway Stenosis Repair

Posterior Glottic Stenosis in a Child

Shuib Khairudin[1], **Khadijah Mohd Nor**[2], **Shantini Jaganathan**[1] and **Saraiza Abu Bakar**[1,*]

[1] *Department of Otorhinolaryngology, Serdang Hospital, Selangor, Malaysia*

[2] *Department of Otorhinolaryngology, University Putra Malaysia, Selangor, Malaysia*

Keywords: Balloon, Endoscopic, Dilatation, Posterior glottic, Stenosis, Vocal cord palsy.

Presentation

A 6-year-old boy with underlying prematurity. The child presented with persistent intermittent stridor associated with shortness of breath when having upper respiratory tract infection; otherwise, good growth and developmental milestones.

Comorbidities

Extremely preterm at 27 weeks with prolonged intubation more than 3 week's duration. Stormy neonatal period with history of multiple intubations.

Intervention

Diagnostic endoscopic direct laryngoscopy and rigid bronchoscopy were performed. Findings: Matured fibrous band over the inter-arytenoid fold (a small ligament in the posterior larynx) causing posterior glottic stenosis. The fibrous band also involved the bilateral cricoarytenoid joints (a joint connecting the cricoid cartilage and the arytenoid cartilage) causing restriction of the vocal cord mobility. The assessment of subglottic area and trachea was unremarkable. The diagnosis of posterior glottic stenosis (PGS) was confirmed (Fig. **1**).

Vocal cord spreader was used to expose the posterior glottic space. Then the fibrous band was released using sickle knife and micro-scissors (Fig. **2**), followed by balloon dilatation (Fig. **3**). The end result was good (Fig. **4**).

[*]**Corresponding author Saraiza Abu Bakar:** Department of Otorhinolaryngology, Serdang Hospital, Selangor, Malaysia; E-mail: drsaraiza@yahoo.com

Jamalul Azizi Abdul Rahaman & Tinku Joseph (Eds.)

Complications

No post-operative complications and the patient was discharged well.

Post-Intervention

Follow-up showed much improvement with occasional stridor during daytime but no stridor during sleeping.

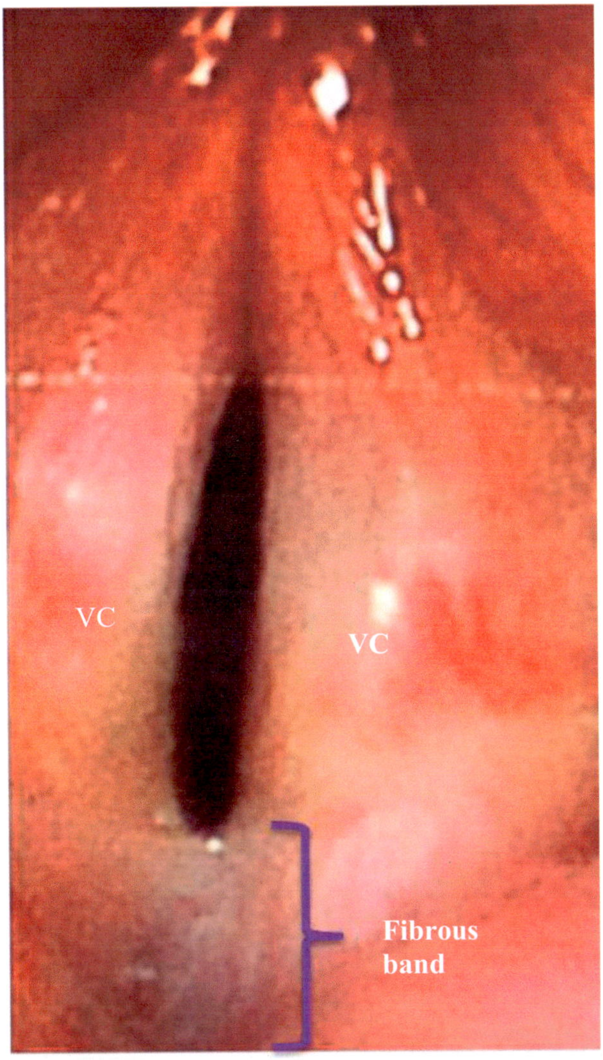

Fig. (1). Direct laryngoscopic view using vocal cord spreader to identify vocal cord (VC) and fibrous band that's causing the posterior glottic stenosis.

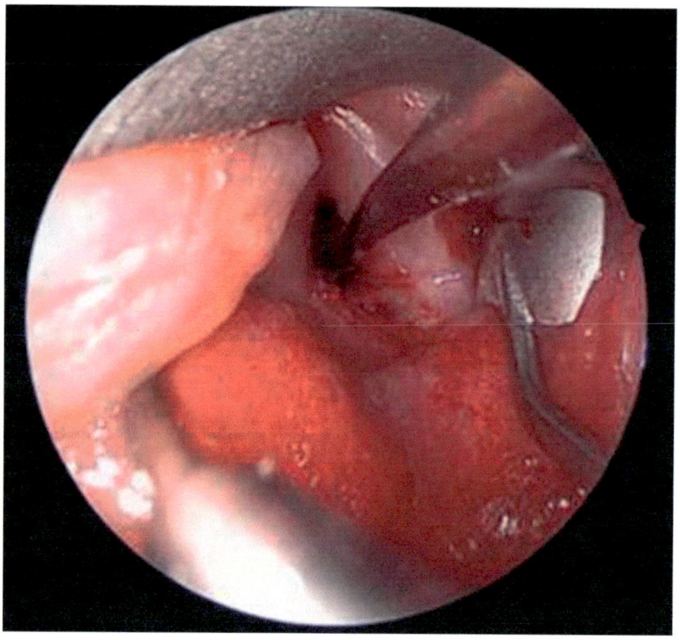

Fig. (2). Division by sickle knife.

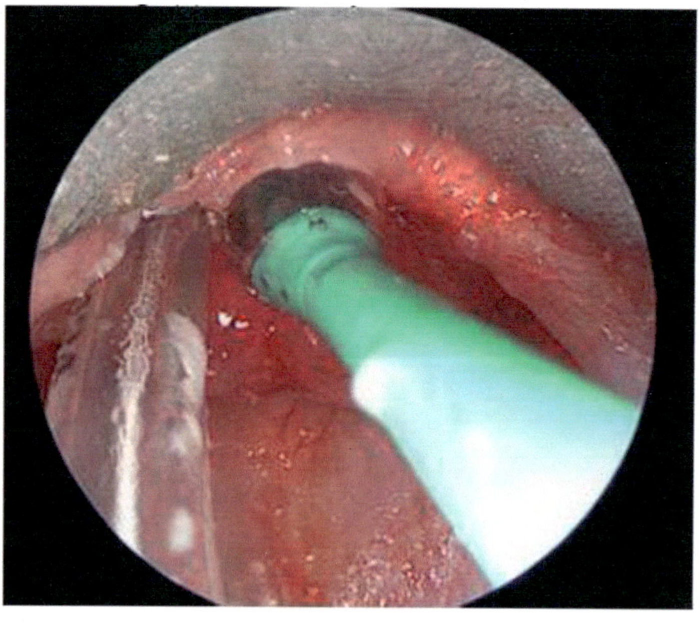

Fig. (3). Balloon dilatation.

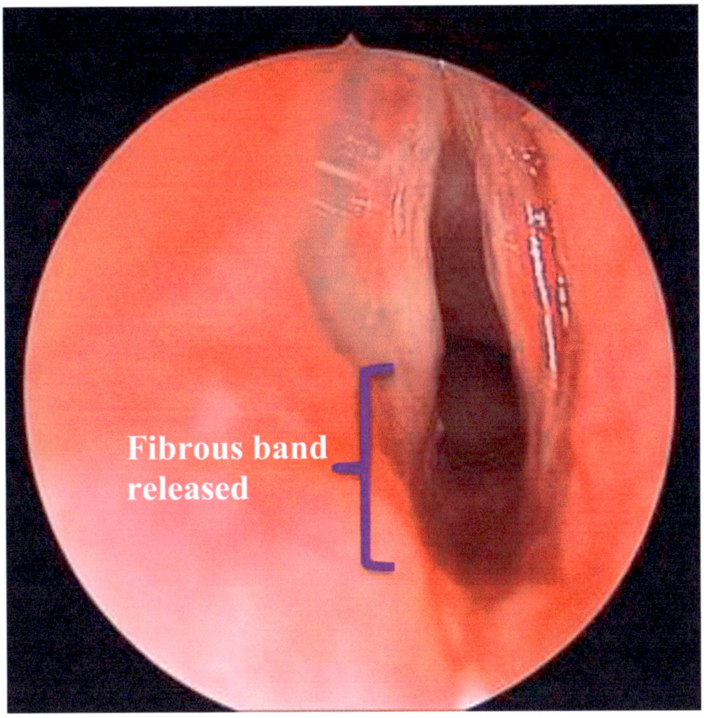

Fig. (4). Post-division by sickle knife and balloon dilatation.

Learning Points

- PGS can be classified according to a grading scale proposed by Bogdasarian and Olson:
  - Grade 1: Distinct posterior glottic scar band separate from inter arytenoid mucosa
  - Grade 2: Stenosis involving posterior inter arytenoid mucosa without cricoarytenoid ankylosis
  - Grade 3: Stenosis involving inter arytenoid mucosa with unilateral cricoarytenoid ankylosis
  - Grade 4: Stenosis involving inter arytenoid mucosa with bilateral cricoarytenoid ankylosis
- Detailed in-depth airway assessment is essential to diagnose infrequent cases of PGS and treatment *via* balloon dilation is effective [1, 2]. This is important to avoid misdiagnoses and prevent unnecessary tracheostomy in children. Treatment options for PGS are shown in Table **1**.

Table 1. Treatment options for PGS.

Treatment Options and Decision Making		
PGS 1	Endoscopic Scar Lysis	
PGS 2 or Higher	-	
Isolated	Adult	Endoscopic postcricoid mucosal advancement flap.
	Children	Posterior cricoid split with cartilage graft.
With Subglottic Stenosis	Open reconstruction with anterior and posterior grafts. If very severe, consider extended partial cricotracheal resection.	
Focal Partial Obstruction	Targeted destruction procedure. Arytenoid reduction, if subluxation present, ablate redundant mucosa.	

Videos

Direct laryngoscopy showing posterior glottic stenosis.

1

Dilatation using balloon with ETT *in situ.*

2

Post division by sickle knife and balloon dilatation.

3

CONSENT FOR PUBLICATION

Not applicable.

CONFLICT OF INTEREST

The author declares no conflict of interest, financial or otherwise.

ACKNOWLEDGEMENT

Declared none.

REFERENCES

[1] Lambercy K, Pincet L, Sandu K. Intubation Related Laryngeal Injuries in Pediatric Population. Front Pediatr 2021; 9: 594832.
[http://dx.doi.org/10.3389/fped.2021.594832] [PMID: 33643969]

[2] DeHart AN, Richter GT. Posterior glottic stenosis: management and outcomes. Curr Opin Otolaryngol Head Neck Surg 2020; 28(6): 414-24.
[http://dx.doi.org/10.1097/MOO.0000000000000671] [PMID: 33060394]

Case 9

Bronchoscopic Repair of Post Intubation Tracheal Stenosis

Tinku Joseph[1,*] and **Sathish C. Reddy**[1]

[1] *Division of Interventional Pulmonology, Amrita Institute of Medical Sciences, Kochi, India*

Keywords: Balloon dilatation, Electrocautery, Mitomycin C, Post-intubation tracheal stenosis (PITS), Subglottic stenosis.

Presentation

A 14-year-old boy with a history of road traffic accident sustained head injury and right clavicular fracture was initially admitted to a local hospital and was subsequently intubated and mechanically ventilated. After stabilization he was extubated and discharged. Later, he developed worsening breathlessness and stridor. He was evaluated with bronchoscopy at the local hospital, which showed a sub-glottic stenosis and was subsequently referred to our centre for further management.

Comorbidities

None.

Chest Imaging

CXR was normal.

Multi-detector computed tomography (MDCT) neck and chest showed circumferential thickening in the subglottic area at the level of C7 vertebral body 1.8cm below the lower border of cricoid cartilage causing 50 percent luminal narrowing (Fig. **1**). Cricoid and arytenoid cartilages appeared to be disrupted. No evidence of pneumothorax and pneumomediastinum.

Intervention

Initially under conscious sedation flexible bronchoscopy was done which showed a critical narrowing of the tracheal lumen, 3.5cm distal to the vocal cords with a pin

*Corresponding author Tinku Joseph: Division of Interventional Pulmonology, Amrita Institute of Medical Sciences, Kochi, India; E-mail: tinkujoseph2010@gmail.com

Jamalul Azizi Abdul Rahaman & Tinku Joseph (Eds.)

hole opening noted at this site (Fig. **2**). Subsequently, under general anaesthesia he was intubated with a 4F LMA tube and the stenotic web was resected using electrocautery knife followed by serial balloon dilatation using 12 and 16mm CRE balloon catheters (Figs. **3** and **4**). Post-procedure, adequate airway patency was achieved and mitomycin C was applied locally to prevent chances of re-stenosis (Fig. **5**). The tracheal lumen was completely recanalized (Figs. **6** and **7**). The patient was extubated on the table and shifted to ICU for observation. After stabilization, the patient was discharged on the next day with advice for surveillance bronchoscopy after 3 months.

Complications

No immediate post-procedure complications were noted.

Post-Intervention

Surveillance bronchoscopy was done after 3 months and it showed adequate luminal patency and the patient was advised to continue follow up at the airway clinic every 3 months until one year to rule out chances of re-stenosis.

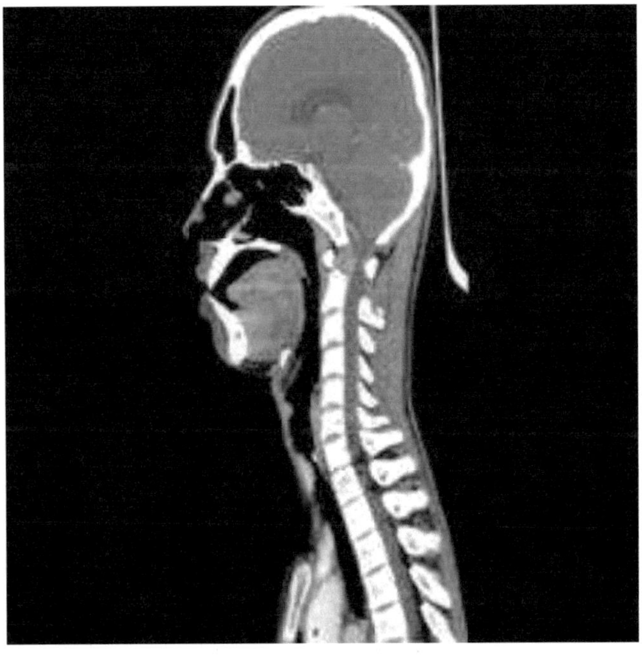

Fig. (1). MDCT neck: Stenosis noted 1.8 cm below the lower border of cricoid cartilage.

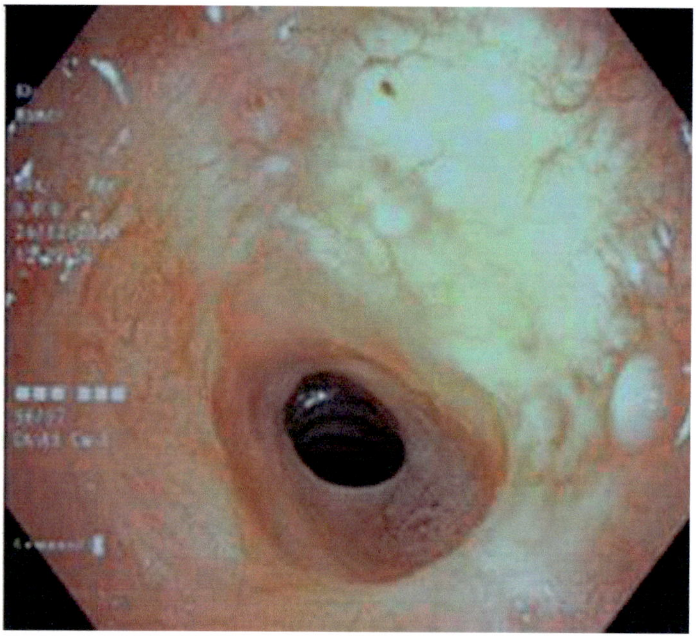

Fig. (2). Pre-Procedure: Subglottic stenosis (Pin hole opening).

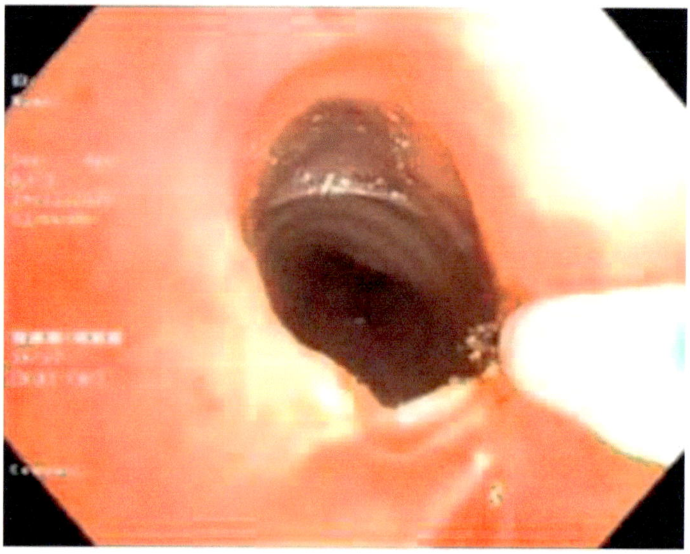

Fig. (3). Step 1: Electrocautery knife incision of stenotic segment.

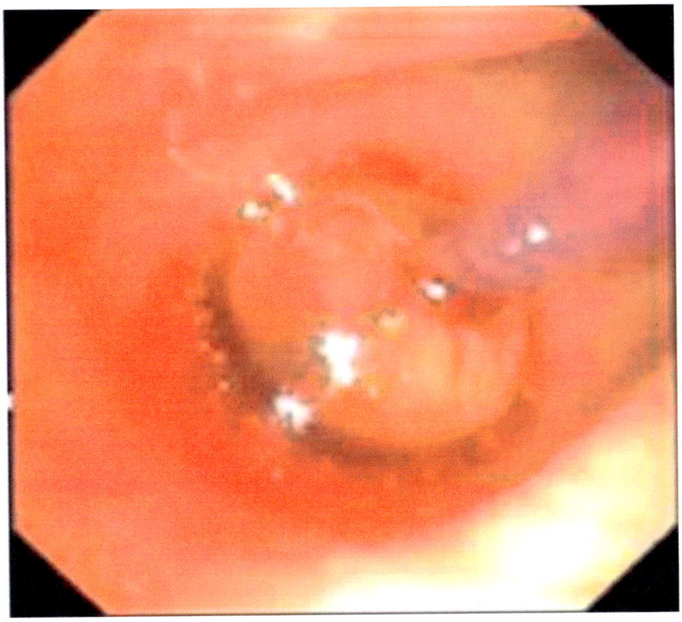

Fig. (4). Step 2: Serial CRE balloon dilatation.

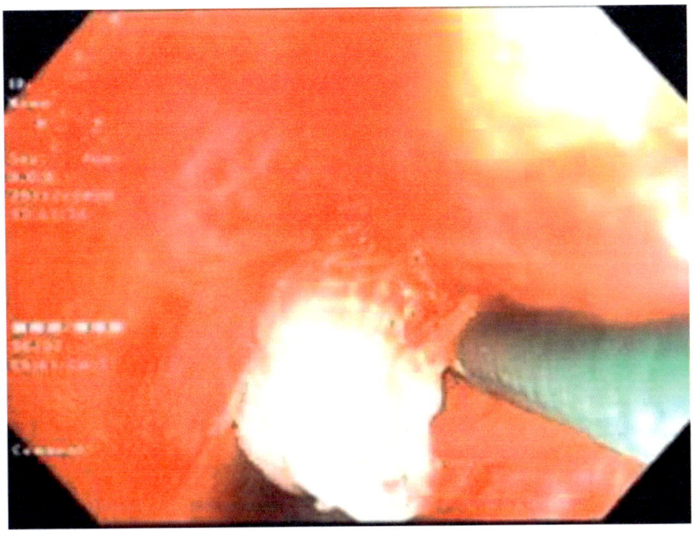

Fig. (5). Step 3: Post-procedure Mitomycin C application.

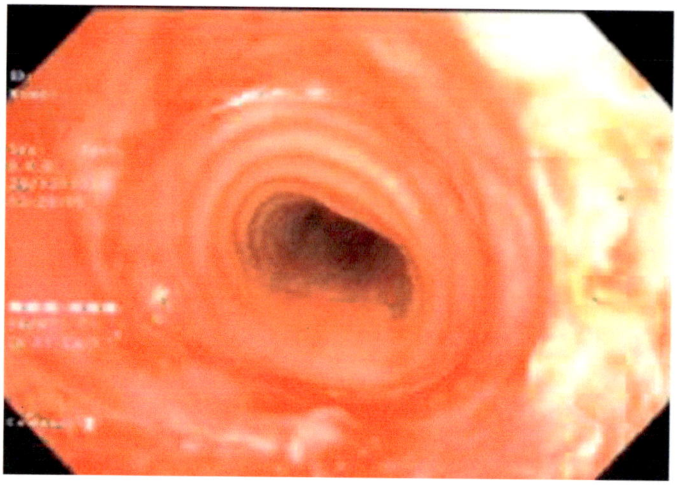

Fig. (6). Post-procedure: Completely recanalized tracheal lumen.

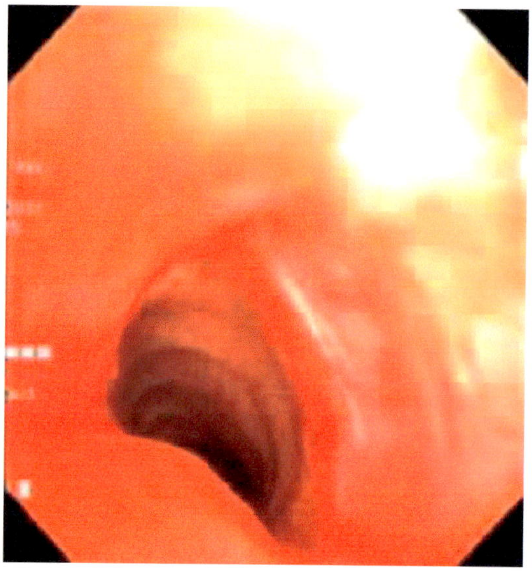

Fig. (7). Post-procedure: Completely recanalized tracheal lumen.

Learning Points

- Causes of Post-Intubation (PITS) / Post-Tracheostomy Tracheal stenosis.

  - Prolonged intubation period [1].
  - Traumatic intubation.
  - Excessive cuff pressure of endotracheal tube.

- Frequent suctioning through ET tube.
- Due to abnormal wound healing with formation of excess granulation tissue around the tracheal stoma.
- Fractured tracheal cartilage due to trauma or pressure necrosis.
- High tracheostomy site.
- History of previous intubation/tracheostomy.
- Excessive use of corticosteroids.
- Underlying disorders like autoimmune disorders, obstructive sleep apnoea, post-radiation therapy for oropharyngeal and laryngeal malignancies and gastroesophageal reflux disease.

- Types of PITS:

Type 1: Simple (web-like) stenosis

The length of stenosis is less than 1cm. No or minimal damage to tracheal cartilages.

Type 2: Complex stenosis

Longer than 1cm. Tracheal cartilages are damaged. Usually complicated with tracheomalacia.

Type 3: Pseudoglottic (A-shaped or tent-shaped) stenosis

Subtype of the complex stenosis. Occurs due to dislocation or fracture of the tracheal cartilaginous rings with localized tracheomalacia.

- Treatment Options:

Type 1: Bronchoscopic correction using electrocautery and balloon dilatation.

Type 2: Bronchoscopic correction can be attempted along with stent placement (Chances of recurrence of stenosis are high).

Type 3: Surgical correction is the treatment of choice–Tracheal resection/ reconstruction and end-to-end anastomosis.

CONSENT FOR PUBLICATION

Not applicable.

CONFLICT OF INTEREST

The author declares no conflict of interest, financial or otherwise.

ACKNOWLEDGEMENT

Declared none.

REFERENCE

[1] Caruselli M, Amici M M. Post intubation tracheal stenosis in children. Pediatr Rep 2014; 6(3): 5491.
[http://dx.doi.org/10.4081/pr.2014.5491] [PMID: 25635215]

Case 10

Neonate with Noisy Breathing and Choking Spells

Mohammad Ashkan Moslehi[1,*]

[1] *Pediatric Interventional Pulmonology Division, Shiraz University of Medical Sciences, Shiraz, Iran*

Keywords: Choking spells, Coughing, Neonate, Noisy breathing, Vascular ring malformation (VRM).

Presentation

The patient was a 20-day-old male neonate from a 25-year-old (para 3, abort 0) mother with the gestational age of 37 weeks, born *via* normal vaginal delivery. He was admitted with choking spells, respiratory distress, and persistent noisy breathing after feeding. He had been admitted and treated after delivery with the impression of aspiration pneumonia. He also had several regurgitation episodes containing vomitus after feeding and was treated as gastroesophageal reflux disease (GERD) without any improvement. There was no significant family history related to his illness. On examination, the neonate was malnourished and underweight. His weight was 2300 grams (birth weight was 2600 grams) on admission. His temperature was normal, but the respiratory rate was about 70 breaths/ minute, and he had suprasternal and subcostal retraction. He also had biphasic stridor. Although his chest expansion was symmetrical, he had fine crackles in the basal part of both lungs on auscultation. Other systems were unremarkable on physical examination. Laboratory investigations were normal.

The patient was referred to our center with an impression of tracheoesophageal fistula (TEF).

Comorbidities

Nil.

Chest Imaging

CXR showed diffuse infiltrations in the lung fields (Fig. **1**).

*Corresponding author **Mohammad Ashkan Moslehi:** Pediatric Interventional Pulmonology Division, Shiraz University of Medical Sciences, Shiraz, Iran; E-mail: ashkanmoslehi@gmail.com

Jamalul Azizi Abdul Rahaman & Tinku Joseph (Eds.)

Intervention

Fiberoptic endoscopic evaluation of swallowing (FEES) was normal. Bronchoscopy revealed grade two laryngomalacia, arytenoiditis, and thick milky secretions. Vocal cords were normal and had symmetrical movements. After suctioning, there was no aberrant orifice in favor of TEF. The trachea had slight malacia and protrusion in the middle third due to external pulsatile pressure. In view of the persistent stridor and bronchoscopy findings, a neck and chest CT scan with contrast was obtained. The epiglottis, vallecula, supraglottic, pyriform sinuses, aryepiglottic folds, larynx, and ventricles were normal on CT scan. There was no pathological enhancement after administration of IV contrast in the neck region. However, there was evidence of bilateral alveolar infiltration in favour of aspiration pneumonia.

After IV contrast, the right-sided aorta with the aberrant left subclavian artery (SCA) and a dilated esophagus was seen (Fig. **2**).

Barium swallow with cine-esophagram revealed irregular and abnormal peristalsis, occasional skipping of peristaltic waves, and inhibition of normal cardio-esophageal relaxation to the passage of the barium bolus (Fig. **3**). Moreover, there were no external pressure effects on the entire length of the esophagus.

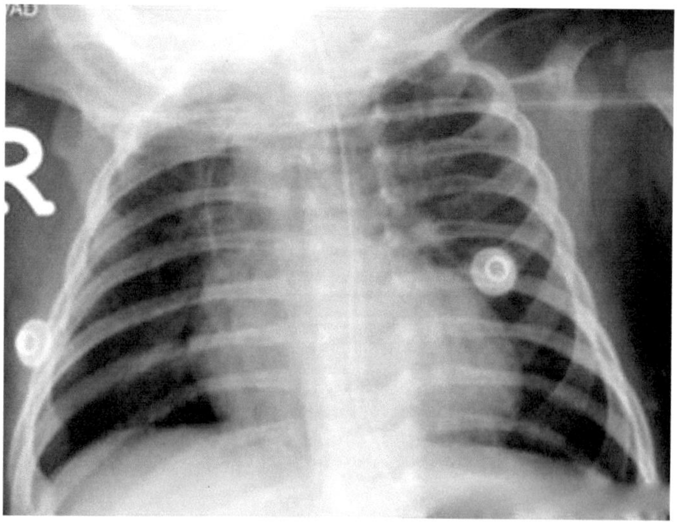

Fig. (1). CXR: Diffuse infiltrations in both lung fields.

Vascular ring malformation (VRM) was diagnosed and he was referred for surgery. A schematic picture of VRM is shown in Fig. (**4**).

Post-Intervention

The post-operative period was uneventful, and the patient became asymptomatic. His general condition and weight improved through conservative treatment, including accurate energy consumption calculation after surgery.

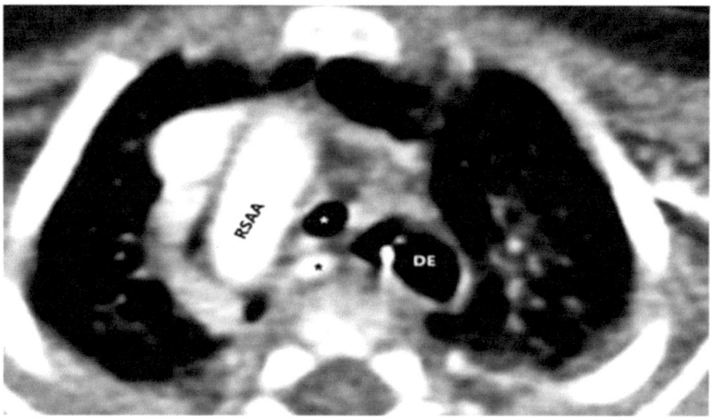

Fig. (2). CT scan: Right-sided aortic arch (RSAA) with the aberrant left subclavian artery (Black asterisk), a dilated esophagus (DE) and trachea (White asterisk) (Blurred vision is due to low dose radiation protocol for neonates and respiratory motion artifacts).

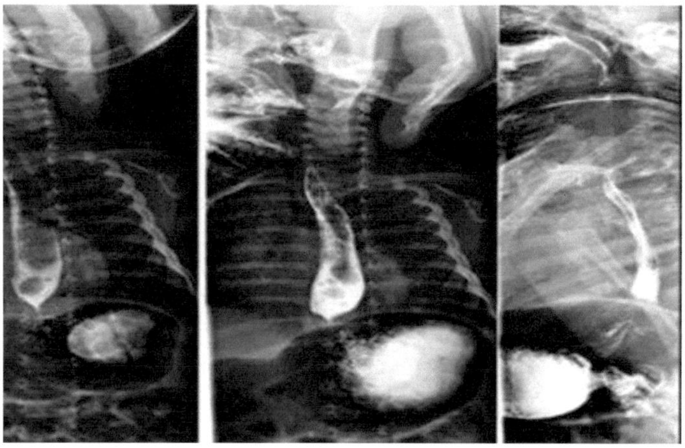

Fig. (3). Barium swallow with cine-esophagogram: Irregular and abnormal peristalsis, occasional skipping of peristaltic waves, and inhibition of normal cardioesophageal relaxation to the passage of the barium bolus.

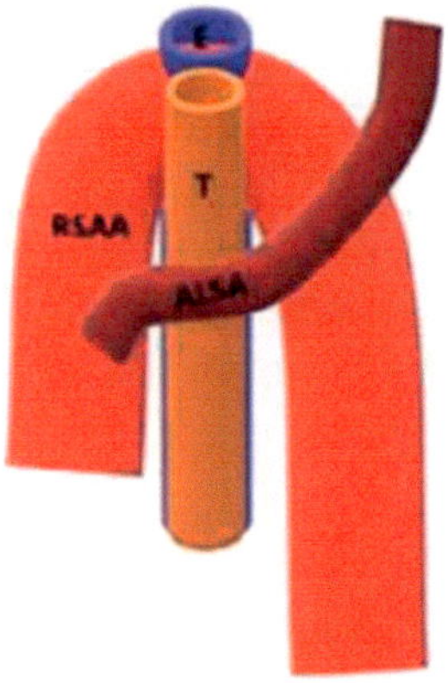

Fig. (4). Schematic picture of VRM (Right-sided aortic arch (RSAA) with the aberrant left subclavian artery (ALSA), esophagus (E) and trachea (T).

Learning Points

- The term vascular ring malformation (VRM) refers to the obstruction of the trachea and esophagus by an unusual combination of derivatives of the aortic arch system, which forms a complete or incomplete ring around them, representing approximately 1% of congenital cardiovascular abnormalities. On the other side, esophageal achalasia is defined as an inability of the coordinated rest mechanism of the lower esophageal sphincter (LES) muscle after a peristaltic contraction of the esophageal body, inspired *via* deglutition. The etiology is unknown, and it is not a common disorder during childhood.
- Esophageal achalasia is a rare disease with an unknown origin that affects about 1:100000 of the population. Just 4% to 5% of these cases are described in children and less than 1% in infants. However, the number of reported cases in the neonatal period is limited [1]. Achalasia involves failure of the LES in conjunction with reduced motility in the esophagus itself. Symptoms of achalasia in infants vary from recurrent milk regurgitation to aspiration pneumonia. The usual symptomatology includes dysphagia, regurgitation, pulmonary infection, and weight loss. Retardation of growth and development and the severity of pulmonary symptoms have been much more profound in this age group. The vomiting of uncurdled milk is a characteristic symptom of achalasia. The disease is often misdiagnosed as overfeeding, GERD, increased intracranial pressure and neurological insults, sucking and swallowing discoordination, and other anatomical problems (like cleft palate, esophageal stenosis, and TEF), which all are causing delays in the specific treatment.

- Esophageal achalasia is a failure of the coordinated muscle relaxation mechanism of the LES following a peristaltic contraction of the esophagus stimulated by a deglutition. Plain radiograph features include the absence of the fundus air bubble and a mediastinal air-fluid level. In most infants, a barium swallow with a cine-oesophagogram will reliably provide the diagnosis. Features include the dilated esophagus, decreased peristalsis with a smooth narrowing of the distal esophagus, and esophagogastric junction described as the "bird-beak" sign. Although motility studies are desirable for definitive diagnosis, manometry is per formed very infrequently in children due to technical difficulty. Management should reduce the patient's symptoms, improve eso-phageal emptying, and prevent mega-esophagus. Achalasia can be treated with botulinum toxin injections, pneumatic dilatation, or esophagotomy, but among these, the most effective treatments are pneumatic dilation and surgical myotomy. A modified Heller's oesophagocardiomyotomy with fundoplication by open or laparoscopic surgery considered the gold standard of management. Although some authors suggest that balloon dilatation in children with cardiac achalasia is the treatment of choice or even as the only possible treatment [2].
- On the other hand, the patient had coughing, biphasic stridor, and fine bilateral crackles in conjunction with his choking spells and vomiting. In this situation, the aerodigestive system should be investigated carefully. The aerodigestive system consists of the upper and lower airways and the esophagus. Accordingly, FEES and bronchoscopy are another two crucial and non-invasive investigations even in neonates [3]. FEES study revealed normal findings. Bronchoscopy showed laryngomalacia, normal vocal cord function, and mild tracheomalacia. No abnormal orifice to suggest TEF, only a pulsatile non-obstructing bulging inward the middle third of the trachea due to external pressure was observed, which was in favor of VRM. The whole tracheobronchial tree was patent with a normal airflow. VRMs are unusual congenital anomalies that occur early in the aortic arch development, and great vessels occur very early in embryologic development. Abnormal or incomplete regression of embryonic branchial arches correlates with 22q11 deletion. A right aortic arch and associated aberrant left SCA can be associated with a left ligamentum arteriosum (LA) that forms a complete VRM and leads to airway compression. This form is a complete type of VRM, and the defect is in the involution of the left fourth branchial arch and remnant of the right. In this anomaly, the right arch is first branching out the left carotid artery, which moves to the anterior aspect of the trachea. It then gives off the right carotid, followed by the right SCA, and, lastly, the left SCA, which courses in a retroesophageal position and gives rise to the LA from its base. The LA

connects the left SCA. Both the trachea and esophagus are anteriorly surrounded by the ascending aorta, the aortic arch on the right, the descending aorta posteriorly, and the LA and left pulmonary artery on the left.

- Bronchoscopy should be done in neonates with persistent or recurrent noisy breathing.
- Bronchoscopy should start from both oral and nasal routes. Checking airway dynamics and anatomy, including nares, nasopharynx, oropharynx, epiglottis, VCs, glottis, subglottis, and the whole length of the tracheobronchial tree is mandatory.
- In most cases, the symptoms of VRM are mild, and the condition can go undiagnosed until a child becomes older or even in adulthood.
- The symptoms that may be present in children with VRM consist of noisy or labored breathing, especially with eating, difficulty in eating and swallowing, regurgitation of milk or other food, persistent cough, and acid reflux.
- Diagnosis of VRM may require some or all of the following tests: CXR, bronchoscopy, cardiac MRI, Chest CT, echocardiography and barium swallow.
- Surgical division of VRM is indicated in all symptomatic patients. Surgery should not be delayed, especially in patients with symptoms of airway compression, to prevent serious complications such as sudden death or significant damage to the trachea or bronchi.
- Achalasia and VRM can be seen as simultaneous events and should be kept in mind in the differential diagnosis of intractable regurgitation and noisy breathing in infants with recurrent or persistent stridor, choking, or cyanotic spells, regurgitations, and aspiration pneumonia. An early diagnosis would result in prompt surgical relief.

CONSENT FOR PUBLICATION

Not applicable.

CONFLICT OF INTEREST

The author declares no conflict of interest, financial or otherwise.

ACKNOWLEDGEMENT

Declared none.

REFERENCES

[1] Shettihalli N, Venugopalan V, Ives NK, Lakhoo K. Achalasia cardia in a premature infant. BMJ Case Rep 2010; 2010(nov04 1): bcr0520103014. [http://dx.doi.org/10.1136/bcr.05.2010.3014] [PMID: 22791855]

[2] Hamza A, Awad H, Hussein O. Cardiac achalasia in children. Dilatation or surgery? Eur J Pediatr Surg 1999; 9(5): 299-302. [http://dx.doi.org/10.1055/s-2008-1072268] [PMID: 10584188]

[3] Moslehi MA, Fallahi F. Fiberoptic Bronchoscopy as a Diagnostic Tool in Neonatal Intensive Care Unit: A Single Center Experience. Iranian Journal of Neonatology 2021; 12(1): 70-7.

Case 11

Congenital Tracheal Stenosis and Successful Slide Tracheoplasty

Amanil'Ula Hassan[1,*], Dayang Zuraini Sahadan[1], Saraiza Abu Bakar[1], Ani Suraya Abd Ghani[1], Koh Gee Tiong[1], Hamdan Leman[1] and **Zakaria Zahari[2]**

[1] *Serdang Hospital, Selangor, Malaysia*

[2] *Tunku Azizah Hospital, Kuala Lumpur, Malaysia*

Keywords: Congenital long segment tracheal stenosis, Cyanosis, Continuous positive airway pressure (CPAP), Recurrent stridor, Slide tracheoplasty.

Presentation

A 7-month-old girl was referred to the Pediatric Cardio-thoracic center for further intervention of congenital long segment tracheal stenosis and ventricular septal defect (VSD). She was born term, with an uneventful postnatal period. She presented with recurrent wet cough and stridor since she was 2 months old which required multiple hospital admissions. At 4 months old, she was diagnosed with peri-membranous VSD when she showed signs of heart failure and anti-failure medications were commenced. However, she continued to show signs of respiratory distress and started to develop cyanotic episodes during crying. Apart from that, she had frequent episodes of choking and coughing post feeding.

Chest Imaging

CXR showed bilateral hyperinflation with pulmonary congestion. Bilateral bronchi were not well aerated (Fig. **1**).

Intervention

Slide tracheoplasty (Fig. **2**) and VSD repair were done in the same sitting. Flexible bronchoscopy was done prior to the procedure using bronchoscope size 2.8mm. There was a long segment stenosis from distal third tracheal ring to the main carina (Figs. **3** and **4**). Right main bronchus was normal in caliber.

*Corresponding author Amanil'Ula Hassan: Serdang Hospital, Selangor, Malaysia; E-mail: amani_hassan83@yahoo.com

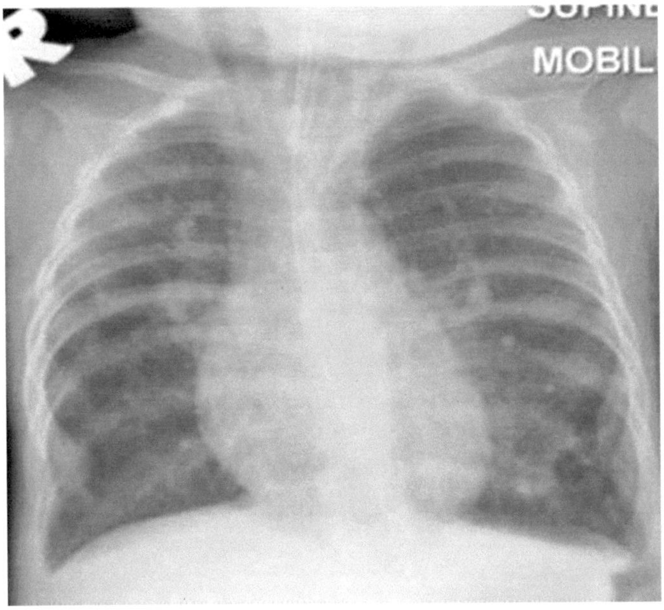

Fig. (1). CXR prior to surgical intervention showing bilateral hyperinflation with pulmonary congestion. Bilateral bronchi are not well aerated. The endotracheal tube tip is at the level of T3 with feeding tube just entering the stomach. There is no cardiomegaly.

Complications

The girl was kept intubated for a week post-procedure as she contracted nosocomial pneumonia and localised left lower zone pneumothorax (Fig. **5**).

Post-Intervention

She required home continuous positive airway pressure (cPAP) for 6 months. She remained well with good weight gain and no longer had recurrent cough or cyanosis or respiratory infections after the cPAP support was discontinued. Currently she is doing very well, on regular review every 6 monthly by the local paediatric respiratory physician.

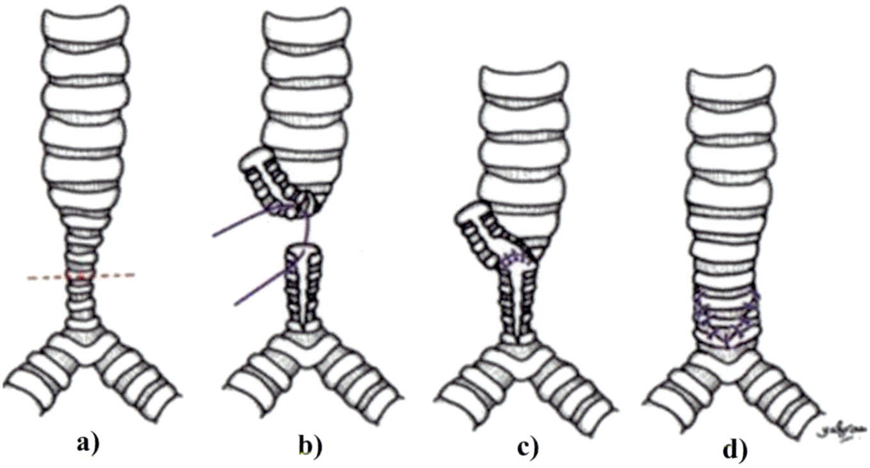

Fig. (2). Slide tracheoplasty illustration. **(a)** The stenosis was identified at the distal trachea, just above the main carina. Transection was made at the middle portion of the stenotic segment. **(b)** Vertical slits were made posteriorly for the proximal end and anteriorly for the distal end of the trachea. **(c)** The prepared trache al ends were approximated and brought together for an end-to-end anastomosis. **(d)** Complete anastomosis. (Image illustrations are courtesy of Dr. Mohd Yusran Othman, Paediatric Surgeon, Tunku Azizah Hospital, Kuala Lumpur, Malaysia).

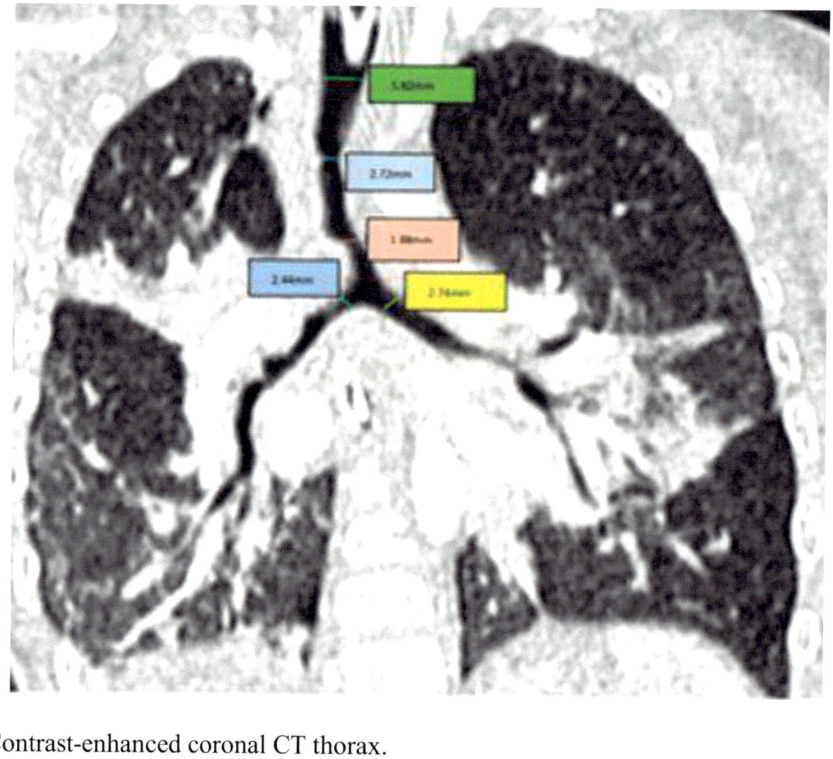

Fig. (3). Contrast-enhanced coronal CT thorax.

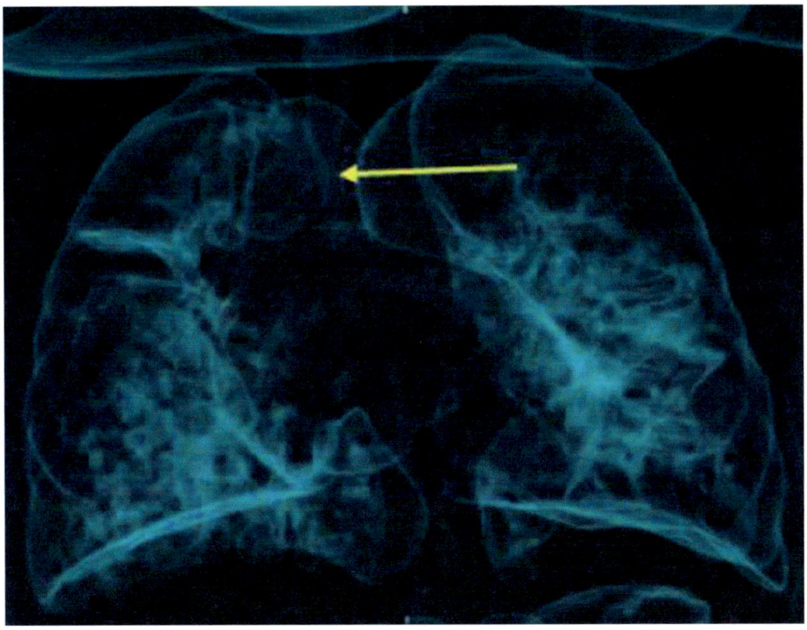

Fig. (4). CT reconstruction showing airway narrowing (yellow arrow) at distal tracheal level (at the T1/T2 level) till the main carina, narrowest at T3 level measuring only 1.88mm in diameter. The length of the stenosis is 2.4cmw (Images are courtesy of Dr. Hasyma Abu Hassan, Paediatric Radiologist, Universiti Putra Malaysia).

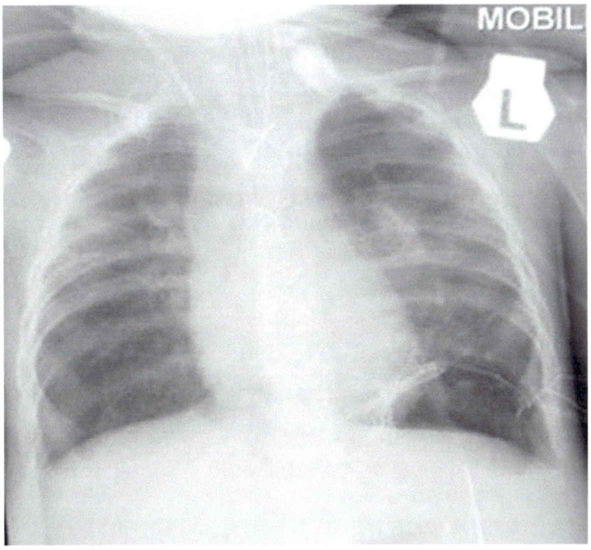

Fig. (5). CXR post VSD repair and slide tracheoplasty showing consolidation over bilateral upper zone with loculated pneumothorax at the left lower zone.

Learning Points

- Congenital tracheal stenosis is frequently associated with an underlying cardiovascular anomaly.
- The patient has no vascular compression on the airway and hence this makes the prognosis good post-tracheoplasty [1].

Video

Flexible bronchoscopy demonstrating long segment tracheal stenosis prior to slide tracheoplasty.

CONSENT FOR PUBLICATION

Not applicable.

CONFLICT OF INTEREST

The author declares no conflict of interest, financial or otherwise.

ACKNOWLEDGEMENT

Declared none

REFERENCE

[1] Yokoi A. Congenital tracheal stenosis: what should we look at for successful tracheoplasty? Transl Pediatr 2018; 7(3): 229-32.
[http://dx.doi.org/10.21037/tp.2018.07.01] [PMID: 30159250]

Case 12

Recurrent Tracheal Stenosis and Tracheomalacia

Amanil'Ula Hassan[1,*], **Dayang Zuraini Sahadan**[1], **Saraiza Abu Bakar**[1], **Ani Suraya Abd Ghani**[1], **Koh Gee Tiong**[1] and **Hamdan Leman**[1]

[1] *Serdang Hospital, Selangor, Malaysia*

Keywords: Biphasic stridor, Balloon dilatation, Bilevel positive airway pressure (BIPAP), Left pulmonary artery (LPA) sling, Slide tracheoplasty.

Presentation

A 5-month-old-boy who was an ex-premature 34 week, diagnosed to have left pulmonary artery (LPA) sling with tracheomalacia at 4 months of age. The diagnosis was confirmed by the CT Pulmonary Angiography (CTPA). He had an initial uneventful neonatal period and never required intubation. He was noted to have biphasic stridor with chest recession at 1 month old which improved with continuous positive airway pressure (cPAP) support. He was transferred to the Pediatric Cardio-thoracic Centre initially for further intervention for his cardiac lesion. Flexible bronchoscopy done prior to LPA reimplantation -Tracheal rings normal shaped, narrowing at the lower third of the trachea, unable to advance the 2.8 bronchoscope, there was sign of external compression whereby pulsation could be seen.

He underwent LPA reimplantation at 5 months old. Pre-implantation CXR revealed prominent right heart border due to the presence of LPA sling (Fig. **1**). Post-implantation showed normal cardiac border (Fig. **2**). However, he had a stormy post-operative period whereby it was complicated with chylothorax, left diaphragm paralysis and deep sternal wound infection with mediastinitis that required prolonged ventilation and hospital stay. There were 3 episodes of acute life-threatening events during his stay in intensive care unit due to airway obstruction. Therefore, a flexible bronchoscopy was done that showed a short segment tracheal stenosis at the lower third of the trachea with complete tracheal ring (short segment) about 0.5cm from main carina. The boy was subsequently subjected to slide tracheoplasty (Fig. **3**) 4 weeks after the initial cardiac surgery. Post-procedure, he remained well on cPAP and was transferred back to the referring hospital in northern Peninsular Malaysia.

*__Corresponding author Amanil'Ula Hassan:__ Serdang Hospital, Selangor, Malaysia; E-mail: amani_hassan83@yahoo.com

Jamalul Azizi Abdul Rahaman & Tinku Joseph (Eds.)

However, 2 months later, he had recurrent tracheal stenosis when he presented with worsening respiratory distress and significant biphasic stridor. Contrast-enhanced CT Thorax showed a short segment distal tracheal stenosis and hence he was transferred back to our center for further management.

Chest Imaging

CT thorax showed a stenotic segment at the distal third of the trachea with narrowest segment measuring 1.51mm in diameter (Figs. **4** and **5**).

Intervention

Direct laryngoscopy, tracheoscopy, and balloon dilatation of trachea for recurrent tracheal stenosis. Tracheal stenosis seen 3.9cm from the vocal cords, circumferential, immature segment, Cotton Myers Grade II, thickness is 0.6cm.

Complications

None post-balloon dilatation.

Post-Intervention

The boy required home BiPAP and gradually improved after the intervention. He was admitted twice for mild pneumonia later which required short hospital stay. He is currently well, on regular follow up and thriving.

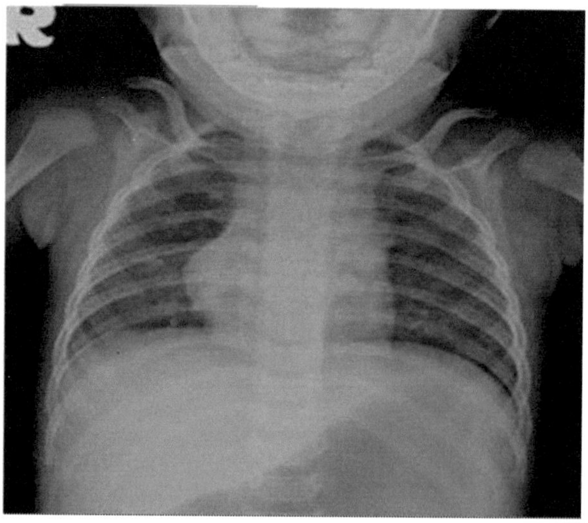

Fig. (1). CXR pre-LPA reimplantation.

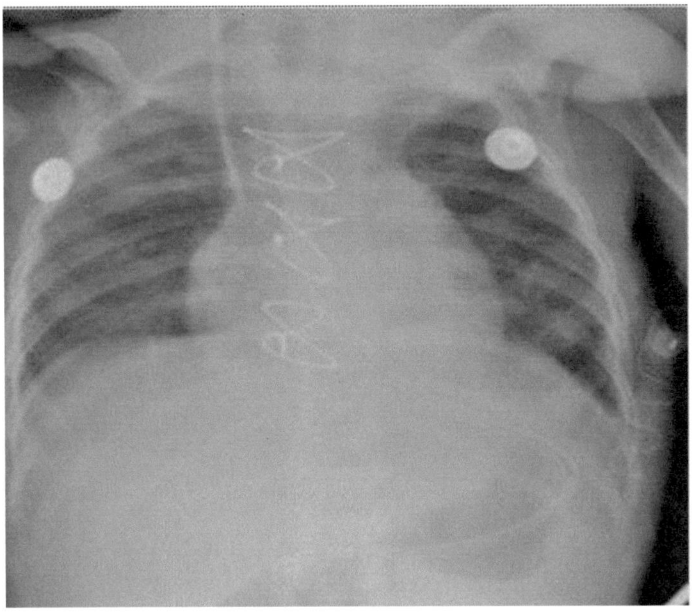

Fig. (2). CXR post-LPA reimplantation.

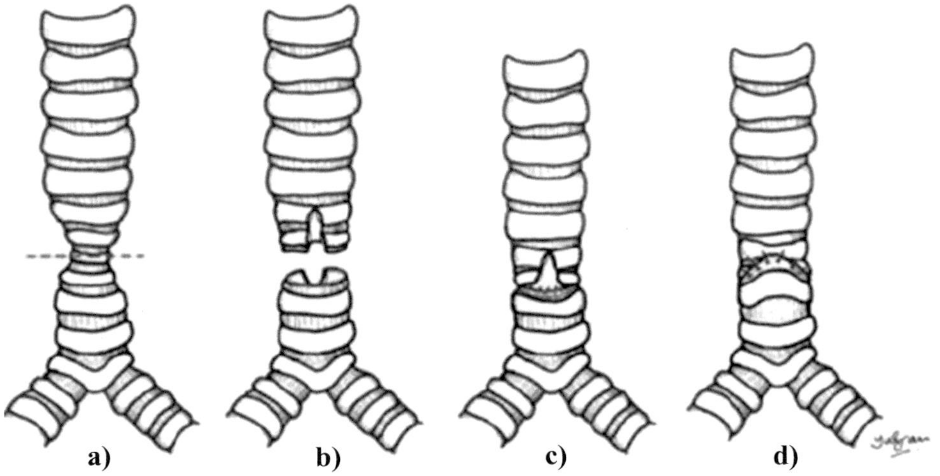

Fig. (3). Slide tracheoplasty illustration. **(a)** The trachea was transected in the middle portion of stenosis and lumen examined. **(b)** Vertical slits were made anteriorly for the proximal end and posteriorly for the distal end of the trachea. The slit ends were spatulated over the edges. **(c)** The prepared tracheal ends were approximated and brought together for an end-to-end anastomosis. **(d)** Complete anastomosis (Image illustrations are courtesy of Dr. Mohd Yusran Othman, Paediatric Surgeon, Tunku Azizah Hospital, Kuala Lumpur, Malaysia).

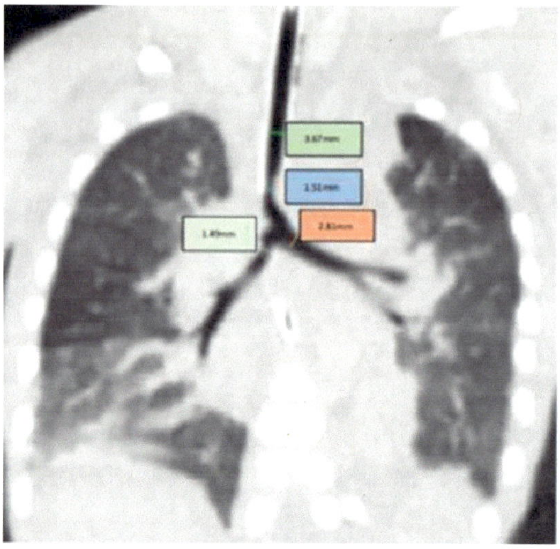

Fig. (4). Coronal CT thorax view.

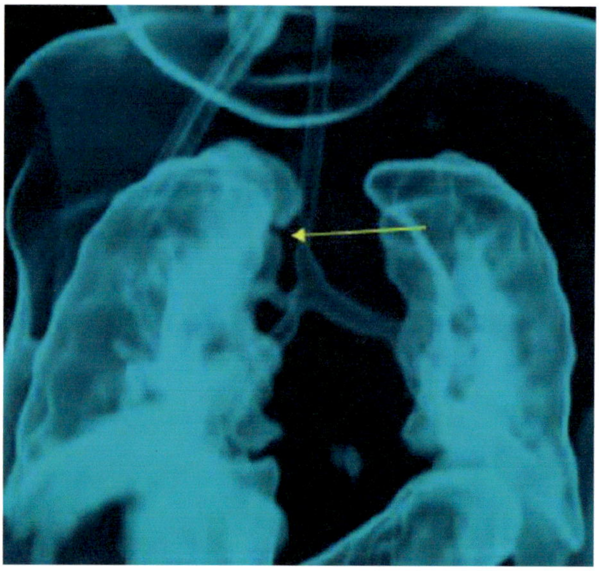

Fig. (5). CT reconstruction done 4 weeks after initial cardiac surgery. There is a stenotic segment at the distal third of the trachea (yellow arrow) with narrowest segment measured 1.51mm in diameter (Images are courtesy of Dr. Hasyma Abu Hassan, Paediatric Radiologist, Universiti Putra Malaysia).

Learning Points

- Tracheal restenosis is a recognized complication post-slide tracheoplasty. This may require airway intervention either balloon dilatation or airway stenting [1].

Videos

(1) Stenosis at the lower third of the trachea, (2) improvement of the stenosis post-tracheoplasty and (3) balloon dilatation to treat the recurrent tracheal stenosis.

1

2

3

CONSENT FOR PUBLICATION

Not applicable.

CONFLICT OF INTEREST

The author declares no conflict of interest, financial or otherwise.

ACKNOWLEDGEMENT

Declared none.

REFERENCE

[1] Hofferberth SC, Watters K, Rahbar R, Fynn-Thompson F. Management of congenital tracheal stenosis. Pediatrics 2015; 136(3): e660-9. [http://dx.doi.org/10.1542/peds.2014-3931] [PMID: 26304826]

Case 13

Tracheobronchomalacia

An Infant with Laryngomalacia

Mohammad Ashkan Moslehi[1,*]

[1] *Pediatric Interventional Pulmonology Division, Shiraz University of Medical Sciences, Shiraz, Iran*

Keywords: Airway malacia, Barking cough, Flexible bronchoscopy, Neonate, Stridor.

Presentation

An 11-month-old boy was admitted to the emergency unit of our hospital because of inspiratory stridor, barking cough, and desaturations while feeding for four days. On admission, the infant's temperature was 37.9 °C. The heart and respiratory rate was 100 beats/minute and 75 breaths/minute, respectively. Oxygen saturation levels were unstable (between 75 to 90%) while the patient was breathing room air (21 % oxygen). He had respiratory distress with subcostal, suprasternal notch retractions. Upon physical examination, inspiratory stridor was noted, and on auscultation, both lungs had noticeable fine rales and rhonchi especially in the lower zones. He had been delivered by uneventful vaginal delivery at a gestation age of 38 weeks with a normal weight (3500 grams). His APGAR scores were eight, nine, ten at 1, 5, and 10 minute, respectively. On the seventh day of life, the patient presented with noisy breathing that gradually worsened until the tenth month of life. Since then, he had had several bouts of cyanosis with coughing spells while feeding and was admitted three times with the impression of aspiration pneumonia. Due to this history, a barium swallow study was performed that revealed severe gastroesophageal reflux (GERD). Echocardiography showed normal findings. After stabilization by administration of nebulized epinephrine, intravenous dexamethasone, and pantoprazole, the infant was transferred to our unit for further assessment.

Intervention

The patient underwent flexible fiberoptic bronchoscopy using a thin (2.8mm) flexible bronchoscope (Olympus Company, Japan) *via* the nasal route when he was on spontaneous breathing. For maintaining spontaneous breathing through to severe elongation of the epiglottis and arytenoids with a redundancy of the

*Corresponding author **Mohammad Ashkan Moslehi:** Pediatric Interventional Pulmonology Division, Shiraz University of Medical Sciences, Shiraz, Iran; E-mail: ashkanmoslehi@gmail.com aryepiglottic folds and the arytenoid mucosa. Moreover, there was a foreshortening conscious sedation and lessening the secretions during the procedure, small doses of propofol and atropine were used, respectively. Bronchoscopy revealed moderate of the bilateral aryepiglottic folds (Fig. **1**). After that, the patient underwent a supraglottoplasty procedure which consisted of the bilateral opening of the tightened bilateral aryepiglottic folds and retrieving redundancy of the arytenoid mucosa through the rigid laryngoscope (Fig. **2**).

Complications

None.

Post-Intervention

The postoperative period was uneventful, and the patient became asymptomatic after the intervention and remained asymptomatic in follow-ups after the management.

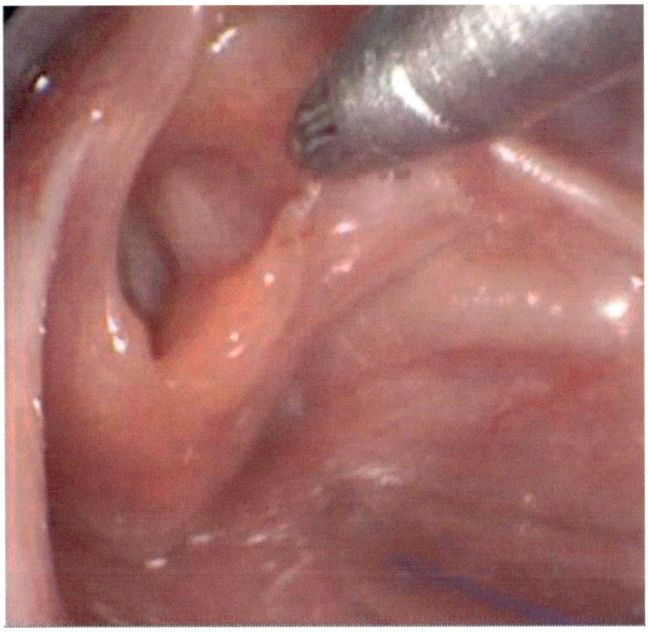

Fig. (1). Bilateral opening of the tightened bilateral aryepiglottic folds.

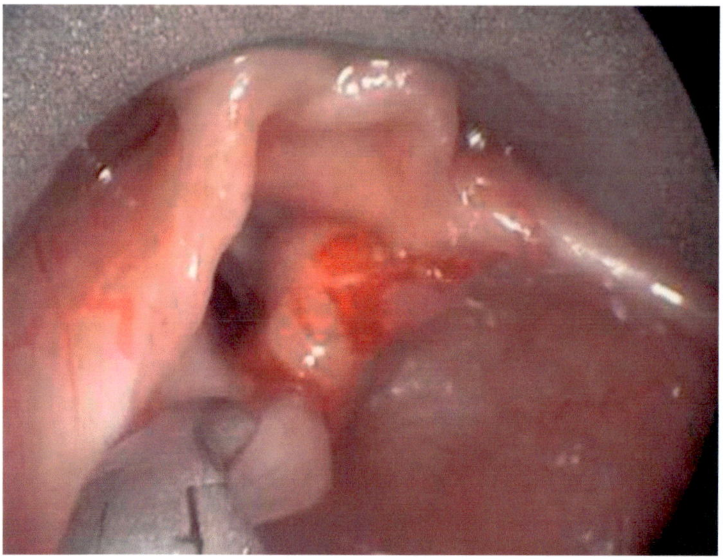

Fig. (2). Retrieving redundancy of the arytenoid mucosa.

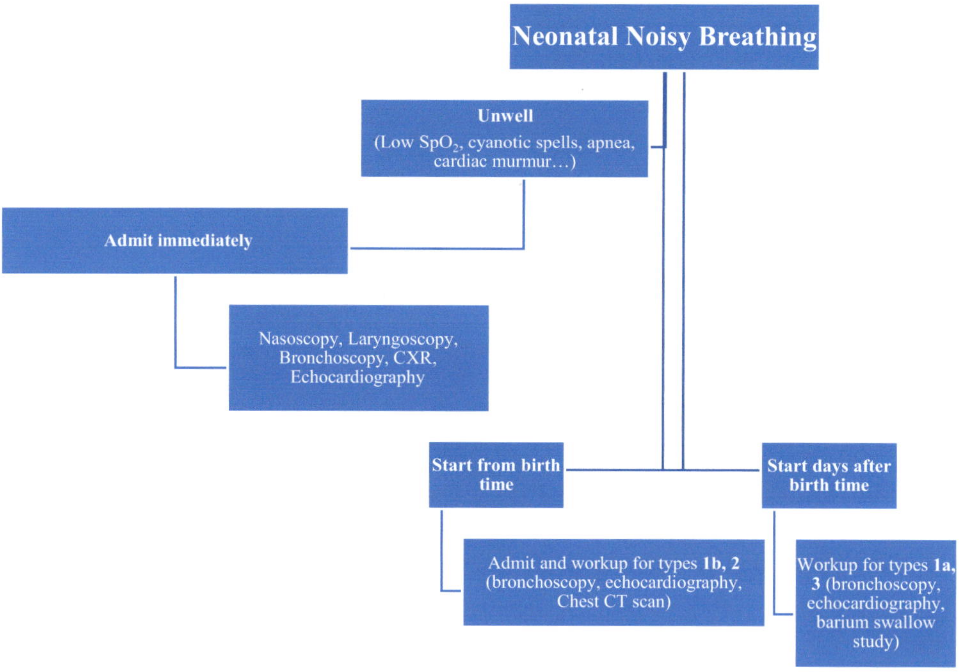

Fig. (3). Algorithmic approach to neonates with noisy breathing.

Learning Points

- Laryngomalacia is a common problem primarily seen in early infancy. Regularly it is present in the first to second week after delivery with progressive noisy breathing. Laryngo/Tracheomalacia is defined as excessive collapsibility of the laryngeal/tracheal structures due to misappropriate cartilage integrity or laxity.
- Airway malacia occurs when the changes in dynamic thoracic pressures make dynamic narrowing or collapse due to defective cartilaginous support and can occur in different levels of airways, including hypopharynx, larynx, trachea, and bronchus.
- Concomitant malacia lesions range from 24% for laryngotra-cheobroncho-malacia to 47% for tracheobronchomalacia and were found in association with other disorders such as congenital heart disorders (13.7%), tracheoesophageal fistula (9.6%), and various syndromes (8%) [1, 2].
- Disease progression is benign in the first two years of life in most affected newborns, with self-healing symptoms without further operative interventions.
- There are three types of airway malacia:

  - Type 1a: Congenital due to simple abnormal development (simple malacia).

  - Type 1b: Congenital due to complex abnormal development (esophageal atresia with or without fistula).

  - Type 2: acquired due to extrinsic compression (vascular rings, cardiomegaly due to congenital heart disease, cystic hygromas, or space occupying lesions).

  - Type 3: acquired as a result of irritation/inflammation (intubation, GERD).

- The clinical manifestation of these dynamic narrowings is noisy breathing and can contribute to coughing, cyanotic spells, feeding intolerance, respiratory discomfort, retractions, sleep apnea, and sleep disturbance. Based on our experiences and for a better approach to neonates with noisy breathing, we suggest the above algorithm (Fig. **3**).
- Laryngomalacia is the commonest cause of noisy breathing in neonates and infants.
- Laryngomalacia is common in male neonates.
- Laryngomalacia is considered severe if the ratio of the length of the arytenoepiglottis to the epiglottis is less than 0.380.
- In concomitant respiratory infection, the symptoms may consist of brassy or barking cough, cyanotic spells, low-pitched expiratory monophasic wheezing, and stridor.

- The vast majority of infants will improve over time without any intervention.
- Medical treatments for laryngomalacia consist of empirical use of anti-reflux drugs, modification in feeding techniques, and appropriate anti-reflux repositioning.
- Surgical treatments for laryngomalacia include supraglottoplasty epiglottoplasty, and tracheostomy.

CONSENT FOR PUBLICATION

Not applicable.

CONFLICT OF INTEREST

The author declares no conflict of interest, financial or otherwise.

ACKNOWLEDGEMENT

Declared none.

REFERENCES

[1] Moslehi MA. Pharyngomalacia in neonates: the missed issue. Front Pediatr 2020; 8: 555564. [http://dx.doi.org/10.3389/fped.2020.555564]

[2] Masters IB, Chang AB, Patterson L, *et al.* Series of laryngomalacia, tracheomalacia, and bronchomalacia disorders and their associations with other conditions in children. Pediatr Pulmonol 2002; 34(3): 189-95. [http://dx.doi.org/10.1002/ppul.10156] [PMID: 12203847]

Case 14

Post-Adenovirus Bronchiolitis Obliterans with Tracheobronchomalacia in a Young Child

Kah Peng Eg[1,*] and **Anna Marie Nathan**[1]

[1] *Division of Paediatric Respiratory & Sleep Medicine, Department of Paediatrics, University of Malaya Medical Centre, Kuala Lumpur, Malaysia*

Keywords: Adenovirus, Bronchiolitis obliterans, Child, Persistent wheeze, Tracheobronchomalacia.

Presentation

A 16-month-old boy presented with persistent wheeze following an adenovirus pneumonia. He required recurrent hospitalisations and did not respond to inhaled corticosteroids or bronchodilators. On examination, he had audible wheeze, mild tachypnoea with chest retractions. Chest auscultation revealed decreased breath sounds with prolonged expiratory phase and generalized monophonic wheeze.

Comorbidities

A previously well term baby until he was hospitalised at 14 months of age for adenovirus pneumonia requiring high flow nasal cannula oxygen support. He was discharged after 10 days with respiratory sequelae.

Chest Imaging

Chest HRCT three months after pneumonia showed patchy ground glass opacities in both lung fields giving a mosaic attenuation pattern suggestive of bronchiolitis obliterans (Fig. **1**).

Intervention

A fibreoptic flexible bronchoscopy showed severe tracheobronchomalacia, excessive protrusion of the pars membranacea into the tracheal lumen during expiration, occluding the main bronchi particularly the right main stem. The occlusion resolved when continuous positive airway pressure (cPAP) was applied (Fig. **2**). The child was subsequently discharged with nasal cPAP with a PEEP (positive end-expiratory pressure) of 8cm H_2O.

[*] **Corresponding author Kah Peng Eg:** Division of Paediatric Respiratory & Sleep Medicine, Department of Paediatrics, University of Malaya Medical Centre, Kuala Lumpur, Malaysia; E-mail: kah.peng@um.edu.my

Complications

None.

Post-Intervention

The wheeze resolved with cPAP. There was no hospitalisation throughout the subsequent year.

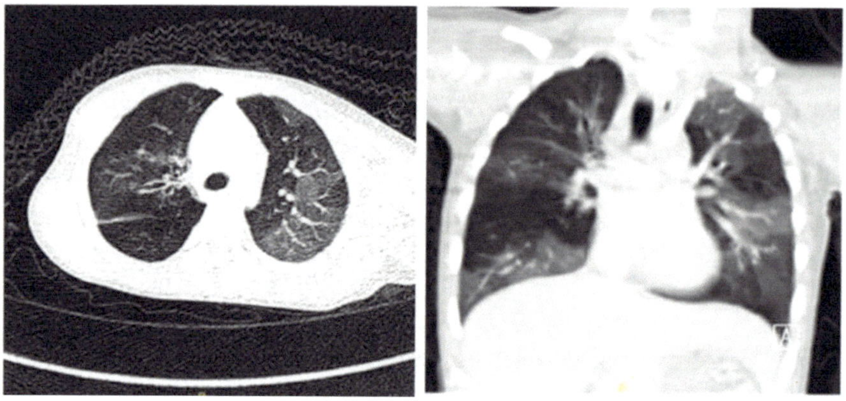

Fig. (1). Axial and coronal Chest HRCT showing patchy ground glass opacities with mosaic attenuation pattern of both lung fields.

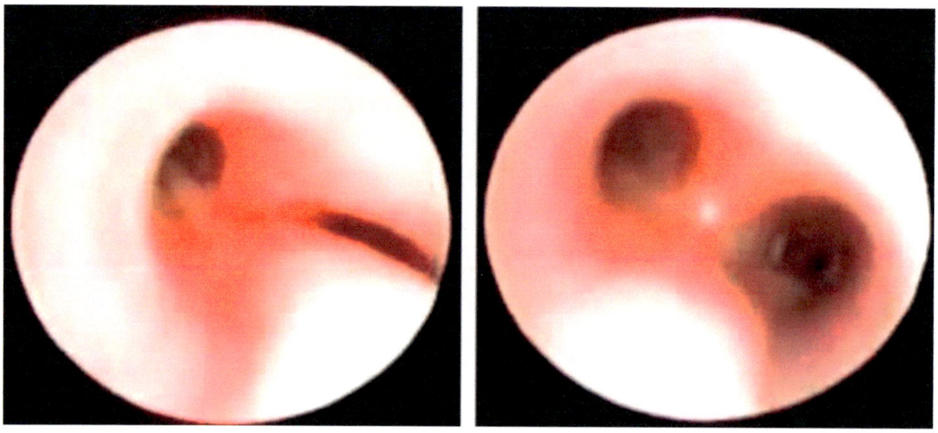

Fig. (2). Bronchoscopic view of the lower trachea and main carina. (Left) Malacic airway on spontaneous breathing during expiration. (Right) Malacia resolved when cPAP was applied.

Learning Points

- Tracheomalacia/bronchomalacia should always be considered in the differential diagnosis of infants and pre-school children with atypical wheeze [1].
- It is difficult to determine whether the malacia is primary (congenital) or secondary.
- Treatment is likely to be individualized and respiratory support with cPAP is an option.

Video

Flexible bronchoscopy in a child with tracheobronchomalacia.

CONSENT FOR PUBLICATION

Not applicable.

CONFLICT OF INTEREST

The author declares no conflict of interest, financial or otherwise.

ACKNOWLEDGEMENT

Declared none.

REFERENCE

[1] Wallis C, Alexopoulou E, Antón-Pacheco JL, *et al.* ERS statement on tracheomalacia and bronchomalacia in children. Eur Respir J 2019; 54(3): 1900382. [http://dx.doi.org/10.1183/13993003.00382-2019] [PMID: 31320455]

Case 15

Left Bronchomalacia Secondary to Vascular Compression

Dayang Zuraini Sahadan[1,*]

[1] *Paediatric Respiratory Unit, Serdang Hospital, Selangor, Malaysia*

Keywords: Bronchomalacia, Continuous positive airway pressure (CPAP), Persistent lung collapse, Partial anomalous pulmonary venous drainage (PAPVD), Vascular ring.

Presentation

An 8-month-old girl was referred for persistent left lung collapse for 2 months. She initially presented with cough and worsening respiratory distress in a district hospital. She had a persistent left lung collapse despite treatment with intravenous antibiotics and chest physiotherapy.

Comorbidities

She was noted to have a murmur at day four of life. Echocardiography revealed that she had partial anomalous pulmonary venous drainage (PAPVD) with a large patent ductus arteriosus (PDA) and atrial septal defect.

Chest Imaging

Her initial CXR showed near total collapse of the left lung with left main bronchus obstruction (Fig. **1**). CT pulmonary angiography showed partial anomalous pulmonary venous drainage with dilated and patent ductus arteriosus. There was obliteration at the left main bronchus causing left lung collapse. The left main bronchus was sandwiched between the descending thoracic aorta and right main pulmonary artery (Fig. **2**).

Flexible bronchoscopy revealed the main carina was pulled to the left and the left main bronchus was compressed by an external structure likely a vascular entity as pulsation could be seen at the main carina and left main bronchus.

[*]**Corresponding author Dayang Zuraini Sahadan:** Paediatric Respiratory Unit, Serdang Hospital, Selangor, Malaysia; E-mail: Zuraini.Sahadan@gmail.com

Intervention

Repair of PAPVD. Anastomosis of left upper pulmonary vein to left atrial appendage and the PDA was ligated.

Complications

None.

Post-Intervention

CXR Post-PAPVD repair showed resolution of left lung collapse (Fig. **3**). Flexible bronchoscopy 3 weeks post-surgery showed left bronchomalacia which was distensible with positive end expiratory pressure. She was discharged well with home cPAP (Continuous Positive Airway Pressure). Clinically and radiologically, the left lung expanded with PAPVD repair and cPAP therapy. She was thriving well with no recurrent chest infection. Her cPAP was ceased at the age of 3 years old.

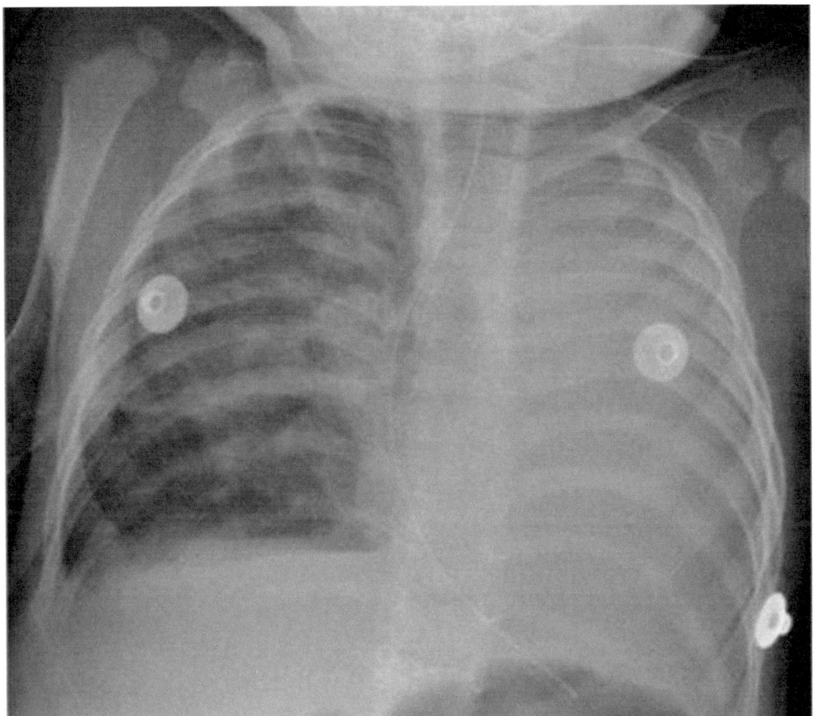

Fig. (1). CXR showed left lung collapse.

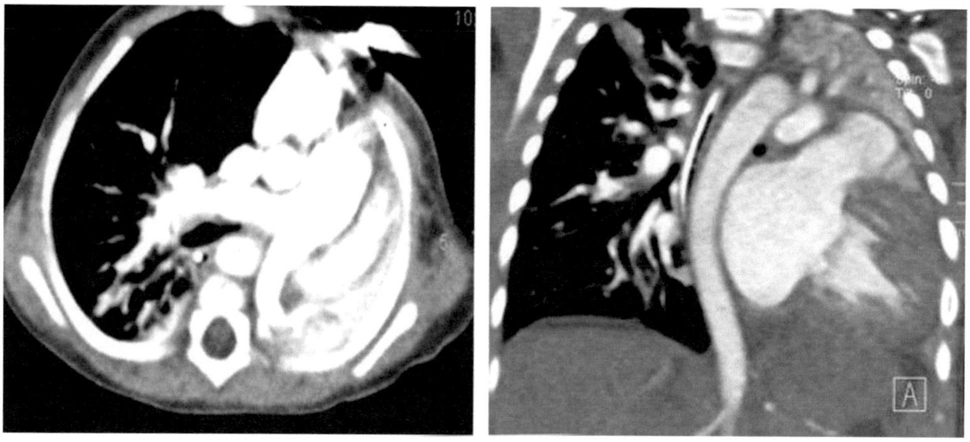

Fig. (2). CT pulmonary angiography: Partial anomalous pulmonary venous drainage with dilated and patent ductus arteriosus. There was obliteration at the left main bronchus causing left lung collapse. The left main bronchus is sandwiched between the descending thoracic aorta and right main pulmonary artery.

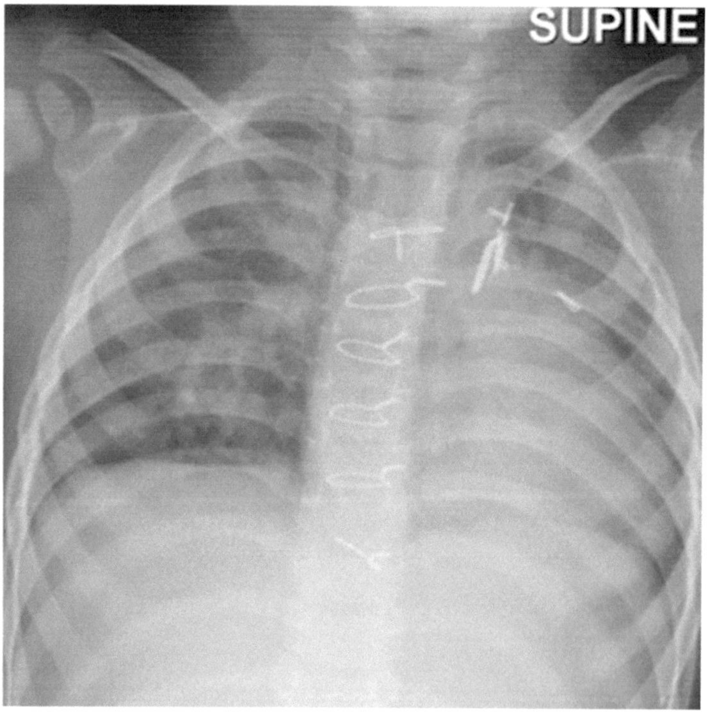

Fig. (3). CXR Post-PAPVD repair showed resolution of left lung collapse.

Learning Points

- Bronchomalacia is commonly associated with abnormal vessel/vascular ring. It should be suspected in those patients with persistent lung collapse or hyperinflation and having underlying congenital cardiovascular anomaly. cPAP can be used as a modality of treatment for bronchomalacia to buy time till the patient outgrows the malacic segment [1, 2].

Videos

(1) External compression of left main bronchus with presence of pulsation. (2) Post PAPVD repair showing remaining left bronchomalacia distensible with PEEP.

1

2

CONSENT FOR PUBLICATION

Not applicable.

CONFLICT OF INTEREST

The author declares no conflict of interest, financial or otherwise.

ACKNOWLEDGEMENT

Declared none.

REFERENCES

[1] Kamran and Jennings. Tracheobronchomalacia in Pediatrics: Evaluation, Management, Treatment. Front Pediatr 2019; 7: 512.
[http://dx.doi.org/10.3389/fped.2019.00512]

[2] Wallis C, Alexopoulou E, Antón-Pacheco JL, *et al.* ERS statement on tracheomalacia and bronchomalacia in children. Eur Respir J 2019; 54(3): 1900382.
[http://dx.doi.org/10.1183/13993003.00382-2019]

Case 16

Central Airway Obstruction

Central Airway Obstruction due to a Rare Tracheal Tumour

Tinku Joseph[1,*] and **Sathish C. Reddy**[1]

[1] *Division of Interventional Pulmonology, Amrita Institute of Medical Sciences, Kochi, India*

Keywords: Cryoprobe, Central airway tumour, Emergency debulking, Electrocautery, Paediatric rigid bronchoscope, Tracheal schwannoma.

Presentation

9-year-old child with history of breathlessness, cough and episodic wheezing was managed as a case of bronchial asthma at multiple hospitals for the past one year. Gradually her condition started to deteriorate and was admitted at a tertiary care hospital for stridor. Soon she was initiated on mechanical ventilatory support in view of worsening type 1 respiratory failure.

Comorbidities

Hyperthyroidism.

Chest Imaging

Initial CXR done at the time of hospital admission was normal. CT chest and neck was done once the patient was ventilated, which showed a soft tissue density lesion with heterogeneous area (1.2x1.2x1.2cm), with poorly defined posterior margin projecting into the tracheal lumen, at a distance of 0.96 cm above the main carina (Fig. **1**). CXR done 24 hours after ventilation showed near total collapse of the left lung (Fig. **2**).

Intervention

Flexible bronchoscopy done immediately after intubating the child showed a large growth at the lower tracheal level arising from the lateral wall (0.5cm) above the main carina causing critical airway narrowing (95% of the tracheal lumen and left main bronchus was occluded) (Fig. **3**). Tracheal tumour resection and

*__Corresponding author Tinku Joseph:__ Division of Interventional Pulmonology, Amrita Institute of Medical Sciences, Kochi, India; E-mail: tinkujoseph2010@gmail.com

Jamalul Azizi Abdul Rahaman & Tinku Joseph (Eds.)

reconstruction surgery were suggested initially and due to the high risk of morbidity/mortality associated with the procedure, patient's relatives deferred it. Subsequently the patient was shifted to our hospital for rigid bronchoscopy guided debulking of the lesion. In view of progressive hypoxemia on ventilator support, she was shifted to the operation theatre for an emergency debulking procedure. The child was intubated with a 6.5mm rigid bronchoscope initially. Airway was secured and VV ECMO was kept as a backup during the pro cedure. The lesion was initially ablated using 1.9mm size cryoprobe (30-40 seconds) at multiple sites of the lesion to reduce the chances of a potential major bleed during debulking procedure. 3F Fogarty balloon was also placed adjacent to the lesion to attain haemostasis after debulking. The entire lesion was grasped initially using a snare electrocautery and was debulked subsequently (Fig. **4**). The debulked tissue (Fig. **5**) was removed immediately using flexible cryoprobe (Cryoadhesion technique). The base of the lesion was ablated using blunt probe electrocautery and cryoprobe. Adequate haemostasis was achieved post-procedure. The entire tracheal lumen was recanalized (Fig. **6**). Impacted mucus in the left main bronchus, which caused collapse of the left lung was cleared. The child was weaned off the ventilator after 2 hours and was shifted out of ICU within 24 hours.

Complications

No immediate/delayed post-procedure complications.

Post-Intervention

CXR post-debulking showed the left lung completely expanded (Fig. **7**). Histopathological examination of the debulked tissue was suggestive of primary tracheal schwannoma. Whole body PET CT scan done after a few days of the procedure ruled out any active pathology at the debulked site and other locations.

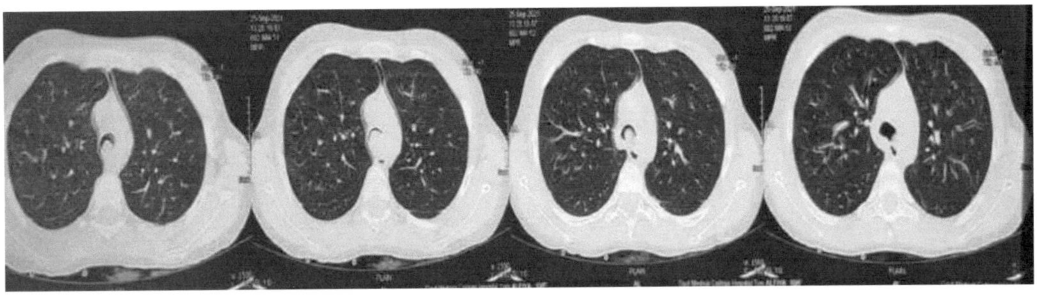

Fig. (1). CT Chest showing a large endotracheal lesion causing near total occlusion of the lumen.

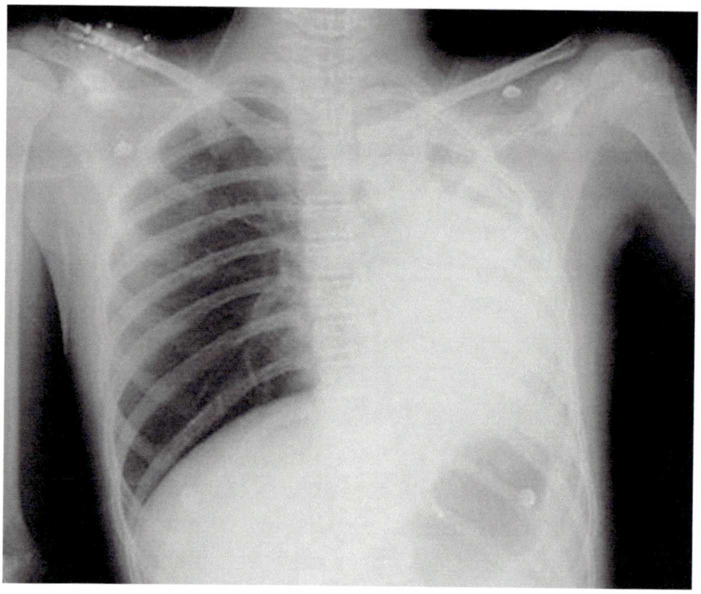

Fig. (2). CXR pre-debulking: Near total collapse of the left lung.

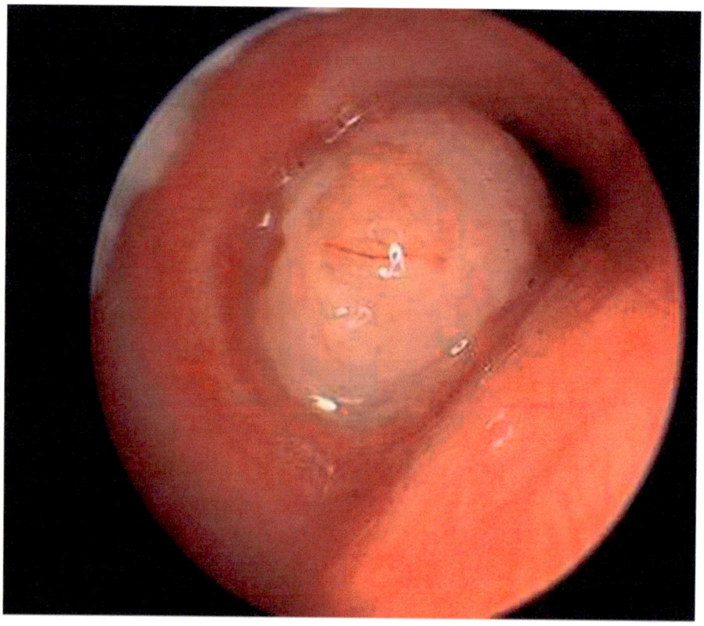

Fig. (3). Bronchoscopic image: Large growth arising from the left lateral wall of lower trachea causing near total occlusion of the tracheal lumen and entire left main bronchus.

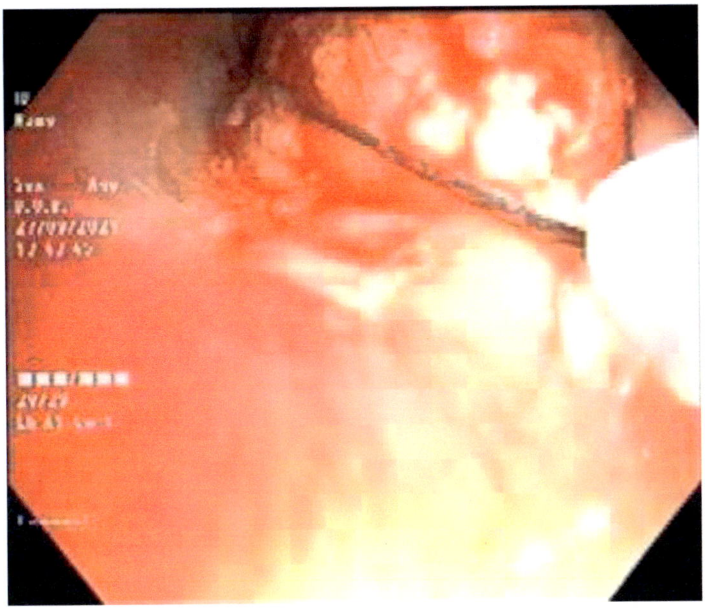

Fig. (4). Bronchoscopic Image: Debulking of the tracheal growth using snare electrocautery.

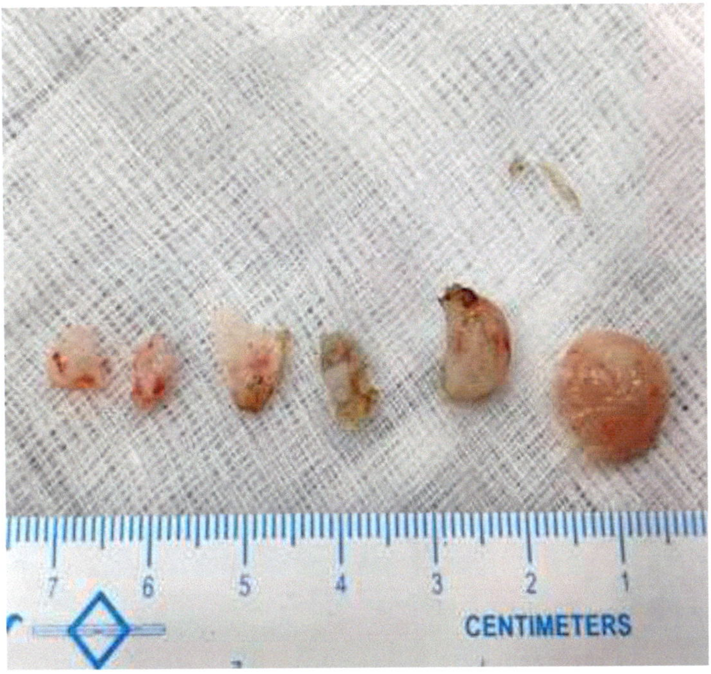

Fig. (5). Debulked tissue.

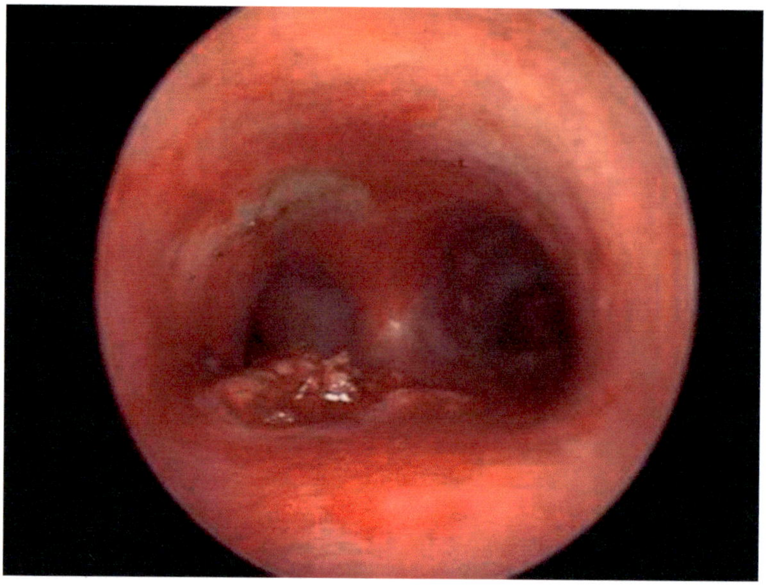

Fig. (6). Bronchoscopic Image: Completely recanalized tracheal lumen after debulking procedure.

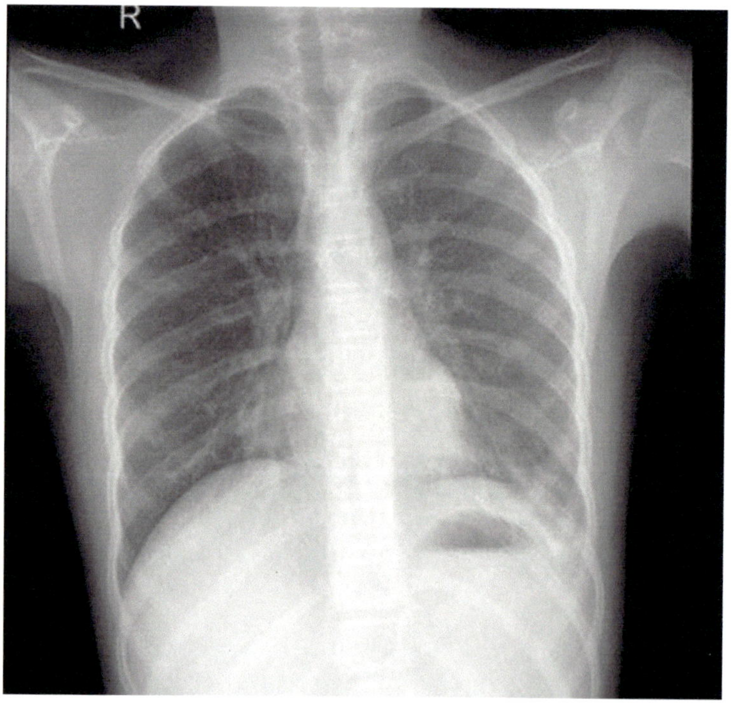

Fig. (7). CXR post-debulking: Left lung completely expanded.

Learning Points

- Not all cough and wheezes in children are asthma.
- Think about the possible alternate pathologies when your patient is not responding to treatment.
- Suspect a central airway obstruction when your patient develops stridor.
- Early bronchoscopic evaluation helps to clinch the diagnosis in such instances.
- Debulking of central airway tumours in paediatric age group should be done only by an experienced interventional pulmonologist, with adequate backup facilities such as the availability of a paediatric thoracic surgeon, critical care support, perfusionist and a dedicated ECMO team to manage all potential complications associated with the procedure.
- Primary tracheal schwannomas are rare and comprise only 1% of all neoplasms [1]. Less than 50 cases have been reported in the world to date. Most often these are benign lesions. Bronchoscopic surveillance is mandatory for a few years to rule out recurrence.

CONSENT FOR PUBLICATION

Not applicable.

CONFLICT OF INTEREST

The author declares no conflict of interest, financial or otherwise.

ACKNOWLEDGEMENT

Declared none.

NOTE

As the QR codes may expire in the future, you are recommended to download all the videos in this book for future viewing.

REFERENCE

[1] Isaac BTJ, Christopher DJ. Tracheal schwannoma: Completely resected with therapeutic bronchoscopic techniques. Lung India 2015; 32(3): 271-3.

SUBJECT INDEX

A

B

C

D

E

F

G

H

I

L

M

N

O

P

S

T

U

V

Z

Made in the USA
Las Vegas, NV
04 November 2026

57436786R00333